Perspectives in Performing Arts Medicine Practice

Sang-Hie Lee • Merry Lynn Morris
Santo V. Nicosia
Editors

Perspectives in Performing Arts Medicine Practice

A Multidisciplinary Approach

Springer

Editors
Sang-Hie Lee
University of South Florida
Tampa, FL
USA

Merry Lynn Morris
University of South Florida
Tampa, FL
USA

Santo V. Nicosia
University of South Florida
Tampa, FL
USA

ISBN 978-3-030-37479-2 ISBN 978-3-030-37480-8 (eBook)
https://doi.org/10.1007/978-3-030-37480-8

This Springer imprint is published by the registered company Springer Nature Switzerland AG
The registered company address is: Gewerbestrasse 11, 6330 Cham, Switzerland

Foreword

It was a beautiful day when the newly formed Council for the Visual and Performing Arts at the Texas Medical Center got off to its spectacular start. Our first event was a performance by the Houston Symphony. By chance, I sat next to the personnel manager at the post-concert lunch. He bemoaned the fact that although we were sitting in one of the largest medical centers in the country, orchestra musicians went to Chicago or Cleveland if they had instrument-related medical problems. That was the spark that got me going.

I dove into the then-sparse literature and quickly found the names of Alice Brandfonbrener in Chicago and Richard Lederman in Cleveland. Since I, too, am a neurologist, I had many contacts with Dr. Lederman. After a year of study, attending the first (for me) of many of the conferences in Aspen, Colorado, and with some trepidation, I hung out the proverbial shingle after enlisting the support of a talented hand surgeon and physical therapist. Musicians came, I got smarter as I gained experience, and, to my relief, most of my patients got better.

Interest in the field has grown steadily since the 1977 publication of *Music and the Brain: Studies of the Neurology of Music* edited by Critchley and Henson and the initiation of the Aspen meetings by Alice Brandfonbrener. Many of the early publications were whimsical letters to the editor that described an unusual phenomenon. Others, somewhat predictably, were the results of surveys. To the astonishment of many, instrument-related medical problems were more common than expected. More efforts are needed to bridge the gap between the arts and health sciences.

Perspectives in Performing Arts Medicine Practice: A Multidisciplinary Approach addresses the health of performing artists as a collaborative effort by artists, educators, and healthcare professionals. In the first chapter, Richard Lederman describes the growth of the field. Now, an affected performer needn't travel long distances to find help. There are several prerequisites to successful treatment: an empathic provider, recognition that problems that might be an annoyance to a typical person can end the career of a performer, maintenance of an open mind, and, above all, listening to the patient. When I taught neurology residents, I emphasized what is known as "multiple working hypotheses," an analytical strategy supported in an 1897 paper in *The Journal of Geology* by T.C. Chamberlin that "avoids the dangers of parental affection for a favorite theory." Each element of the history and physical examination should give rise to multiple hypotheses. A diagnosis should then be based on an evidence-based decision.

Some of the topics are relatively straightforward and within the scope of many practitioners, such as treatment of performance anxiety and avoiding complications of undernutrition in dancers. Others are more exploratory, such as defining a role for traditional Chinese medicine in the health of musicians.

Science has helped us understand the pathophysiology of some of the most vexing problems, such as the focal dystonias. Electrophysiological techniques such as event-related potential studies of deep brain structures recorded and analyzed with software dependent on scalp electrodes and neuroimaging, particularly functional magnetic resonance imaging, have shown what happens in the nervous system with increasing clarity. Unfortunately, the development and the treatment of this disorder still remain elusive for all but a few individuals.

Science has yet to come to the rescue of those hoping to understand some of the most common problems I encountered when I was an active practitioner. Chief among these perhaps are the repetitive strain injuries such as carpal tunnel syndrome, tendonitis, and bursitis. Molecular medicine and gene editing with CRISPR are nowhere to be found. These appear to be the prerequisites needed to gain grant support from the National Institutes of Health and others who fund research.

The gains in interest and expertise in the medical problems of performers of all types along with conferences and publications such as the present volume are causes for optimism. Chapters cover the spectrum of the field. These include musculoskeletal problems, an important focus on mental health issues, and the development of exercise programs designed to prevent injuries. Others stress the importance of multimodal approaches and collaborative efforts among those with varied fields of expertise. Inclusiveness is an important contemporary watchword in organizations. Chapters that probe culturally oriented topics in dance and medical practice fulfill that mandate. The strength and diversity of topics in this volume are indicators of progress.

Over a century ago, Louis Pasteur is reported to have said that "Chance favors the prepared mind." Success and inspiration are the result of attention to evidence, hard work, and careful thought. Go to it!

Oberlin, OH, USA Alan H. Lockwood, MD, FAAN, FANA

Preface

This compilation of work brings a novel addition to the field of Performing Arts Medicine. The chapters are written by selected invited participants of 2014, 2015, and 2018 Performing Arts Medicine Conferences at the University of South Florida. Artists, educators, and health professionals offer their research and practice-based perspectives within a broad landscape of arts and medicine intersections. *The Editors*, comprised of Sang-Hie Lee, Merry Lynn Morris, and Santo V. Nicosia, shaped and coordinated the book with creative collaboration.

The book has four parts. Part One has five chapters each contributing a unique perspective to the overview of performing arts medicine. Chapter 1 depicts a lived history of performing arts medicine by one of the founders of the International Performing Arts Medicine Association, Dr. Richard Lederman. Chapter 2, authored by Dr. Daniel Hall-Flavin, elucidates the themes of empathy and presence across theatrical practice and medical practice. In Chap. 3, Dr. William Dawson conveys a conscripted account of a lifelong dual role as an orthopedic surgeon and performing musician. Chapter 4 is an analysis of the current health issues of performing artists observed by Drs. Brandi Niemeier and Dawn Larsen. Part One ends with an essay exploring the intersections of arts and medicine through the lenses of significant painters' works by Dr. Santo V. Nicosia

Part Two contains seven research chapters, each making an original contribution to the field. In Chap. 6, Dr. Adadeyo Ajidahun and colleagues present an innovative exercise program for violin players to prevent injuries based on surveying the literature and exploring the biomechanics involved in violin playing. Dr. Evgeny Chugunov launches a probing strategy applying Bernstein's theory of motor control to piano playing and teaching in Chap. 7. Efficient and healthy breathing for vocalists is addressed through an integrated mind-body program in Chap. 8 by Emily Lopez and coauthors. In Chap. 9, Dr. Kyaien O. Conner and collaborators trace evidence-based benefits of cultural dance practice. In Chap. 10, Dr. Merry Lynn Morris and coauthors apply in-depth analysis to attend to one of the more common and anatomically difficult positions utilized in ballet training, the fifth position. Dr. Sang-Hie Lee and colleagues examine a pianist affected by focal dystonia, implement a rehabilitation strategy, and conclude with a design of a computerized integrative system for future testing in Chap. 11. Lastly, Pablo Arencibia meticulously examines the differences between digital and acoustic pianos in hopes of divulging the bodily implications for pianists who may be using both types of pianos.

In Part Three, diverse, rich, and contemporary practices in performing arts medicine are introduced with vivid details. Chapter 13 by Dr. Dusty Marie Narducci contains an extensive analysis of instrumental musicians' musculoskeletal and associated conditions. Another dimension of musicians' health is explored in Chap. 14 by Dr. Julia Clearman, who investigates the factors contributing to music performance anxiety (MPA) and emphasizes the need for pedagogical intervention. The following chapter, authored by Elizabeth Johnson, delves into the cultivation of movement proficiency through an application of the Dart Procedures and the Alexander Technique. In the next chapter, Dr. Tom Welsh examines movement proficiency from another perspective, illustrating the value of an individualized approach to dance training through specific research examples. In Chap. 17, Drs. Virginia Wilmerding and Donna H. Krasnow cite their previous work, *Motor Learning and Control for Dance: Principles and Practices for Performers and Teachers*, to promote a motor learning model for dance training. In Chap. 18, Jennie Morton directs attention to musical theater performers who must be proficient in multiple performing arts disciplines and offers effective and healthful training approaches. Dr. Lauri Wright and Casey Colin address in Chap. 19 the role of nutrition in ballet training, an important and often neglected subject in performing arts medicine. Closing Part Three, Dr. Carina Joly explains the rationale behind an exercise regimen specifically designed to improve musicians' body awareness and overall posture and to target typical strength imbalances in key muscle groups.

Chapters in Part Four describe the implementation and evaluation of educational programs in performing arts medicine. In Chap. 21, Dr. David Kaplan and Stephanie Mayer-Sattin report on a moving-mindfulness intervention program integrating the teachings of traditional Chinese medicine into an instrumental music enhancement curriculum. Chapter 22 by Juanita Patterson-Price details an approach to identify dance fundamental movement skills (DFMS) and the creation of assessment metrics to evaluate progress in these DFMS. In Chap. 23, Dr. Emily Wright and Miranda Layman introduce an institutional initiative addressing the complexity of mental health issues in dance students and explore the benefits of including mental health wellness practices within dance educational curricula. Regina Campbell describes a highly charged new initiative at Boston University Tanglewood Institute to help music students "stay well to play well" in Chap. 24. The book concludes with Chap. 25 by Dr. Jeffrey Russell who describes a successful model of comprehensive healthcare for performing art students and delineates the roles of arts and health professionals in such a context. The case is made here that incorporating essential principles of current healthcare delivery will enhance educational programs in performing arts medicine.

Finally, we thank the contributing authors for their good work and patience throughout the editing process. We gratefully recognize the editorial review panel, Dr. Ruth Bahr, Dr. Candace Burns, Dr. Stephanie Carey, and Dr. Dustin Hardwick, for their guidance.

Tampa, FL, USA
August 9, 2019

Sang-Hie Lee
Merry Lynn Morris
Santo V. Nicosia

Contents

Part IV Program Implementation

Contributors

Adedayo Tunde Ajidahun, PhD Department of Physiotherapy, Faculty of Health Sciences, University of the Witwatersrand, Johannesburg, South Africa

Pablo Arencibia, MM University of South Florida, Tampa, FL, USA

Ruth Bahr, PhD Office of Graduate Studies & Department of Communication Sciences and Disorders, Tampa, FL, USA

Regina Campbell, PT, CPAM Performing Arts Physical Therapy, PC, Winchester, MA, USA

Stephanie L. Carey, PhD Department of Mechanical Engineering, Center for Assistive, Rehabilitation, & Robotics Technologies (CARRT), University of South Florida, Tampa, FL, USA

Evgeny Chugunov, PhD, DMus Department of Music, Lakehead University, Thunder Bay, ON, Canada

Julia A. Clearman, MA Wheaton College Graduate School, Wheaton, IL, USA

Casey Colin, MS, RDN Department of Nutrition & Dietetics, University of North Florida, Jacksonville, FL, USA

Kyaien O. Conner, PhD, LSW, MPH Department of Mental Health Law and Policy, College of Behavioral and Community Sciences, The Florida Mental Health Institute, University of South Florida, Tampa, FL, USA

William J. Dawson, MD Department of Orthopaedic Surgery, Feinberg School of Medicine, Northwestern University, Northbrook, IL, USA

Performing Arts Medicine Association, Northbrook, IL, USA

Niche Faulkner, MS Department of Dance, College of Arts and Architecture, University of North Carolina- Charlotte, Charlotte, NC, USA

Ashleigh Fults, BS Department of Mechanical Engineering, Center for Assistive, Rehabilitation & Robotics Technologies (CARRT), University of South Florida, Tampa, FL, USA

Daniel K. Hall-Flavin, MD, MSc Mayo Clinic Delores Lavins Center for the Humanities in Medicine, Mayo Clinic, Rochester, MN, USA

Dustin Hardwick, DPT, PhD School of Physical Therapy & Rehabilitation Sciences, Morsani College of Medicine, University of South Florida, Tampa, FL, USA

Elizabeth Johnson, MFA School of Theatre and Dance, Nadine McGuire Theatre and Dance Pavilion, University of Florida, Gainesville, FL, USA

Carina Joly, DMA, CAS Music Department, Universidade Federal de São João del-Rei, São João del-Rei, MG, Brazil

David B. Kaplan, MD Wudang Wellness, Rockville, MD, USA

Edgewood Surgical Hospital, Transfer, PA, USA

Eun Sook Kim, PhD Department of Measurement and Evaluation, College of Education, USF, Tampa, FL, USA

Donna H. Krasnow, PhD York University, Toronto, ON, Canada

Dawn Larsen, PhD Minnesota State University-Mankato, Mankato, MN, USA

Miranda Layman, MS, ATC Belhaven University, Jackson, MS, USA

Matthew Lazinski, PT, DPT, OCS School of Physical Therapy and Rehabilitation sciences, USF, Tampa, FL, USA

Richard J. Lederman, MD Center for General Neurology, Neurological Institute, Cleveland Clinic, Cleveland, OH, USA

Sang-Hie Lee, PhD, EdD, MM School of Music, College of the Arts, University of South Florida, Tampa, FL, USA

Emily Lopez, MM School of Music, University of South Florida, Tampa, FL, USA

University of Florida, College of Pharmacy, Department of Medicinal Chemistry, Gainesville, FL, USA

Stephanie L. Mayer-Sattin, BA, MA Instrumental Music Department, Bullis School, Potomac, MD, USA

Wudang Wellness, Rockville, MD, USA

Kaitlin Morgan, BFA Florida State University, Tallahassee, FL, USA

Merry Lynn Morris, MFA, PhD School of Theatre and Dance, University of South Florida, Tampa, FL, USA

Jennie Morton, BSc, MS, MSc The Colburn School, Los Angeles, California, USA

Brittany Mott, MS Department of Mechanical Engineering, Center for Assistive, Rehabilitation & Robotics Technologies (CARRT), University of South Florida, Tampa, FL, USA

Witness Mudzi, PhD Department of Physiotherapy, Faculty of Health Sciences, University of the Witwatersrand, Johannesburg, South Africa

Ryan Murtagh, MD, MBA Department of Neurology, Morsani College of Medicine, University of South Florida, Tampa, FL, USA

Hellen Myezwa, PhD Department of Physiotherapy, Faculty of Health Sciences, University of the Witwatersrand, Johannesburg, South Africa

Dusty Marie Narducci, MD, CAQSM Morsani College of Medicine, University of South Florida, Tampa, FL, USA

Santo V. Nicosia, MD, MS Department of Pathology and Cell Biology, University of South Florida Morsani College of Medicine, Tampa, FL, USA

Brandi S. Niemeier, PhD University of Wisconsin-Whitewater, Whitewater, WI, USA

Paula Nunez School of Theatre and Dance, University of South Florida, Tampa, FL, USA

Juanita Patterson-Price, MSc Department of Mental Health Law and Policy, College of Behavioral and Community Sciences, University of South Florida, Tampa, FL, USA

Jeffrey A. Russell, PhD, AT, FIADMS Clinic for Science and Health in Artistic Performance, Division of Athletic Training, School of Applied Health Sciences and Wellness, College of Health Sciences and Professions, Ohio University, Athens, OH, USA

Juan Sanchez-Ramos, MD, PhD Department of Neurology, Morsani College of Medicine, University of South Florida, Tampa, FL, USA

Andee Scott, MFA School of Theatre and Dance, University of South Florida, Tampa, FL, USA

Tuan Vu, MD Department of Neurology, Morsani College of Medicine, University of South Florida, Tampa, FL, USA

Tom Welsh, PhD Florida State University, Tallahassee, FL, USA

Gabriel Williams, MFA Florida State University, Tallahassee, FL, USA

Virginia Wilmerding, PhD University of New Mexico, Albuquerque, NM, USA

Wendy-Ann Wood, PhD Department of Physiotherapy, Faculty of Health Sciences, University of the Witwatersrand, Johannesburg, South Africa

Lauri Wright, PhD, RDN Department of Nutrition & Dietetics, University of North Florida, Jacksonville, FL, USA

Emily Wright, MFA, PhD Independent Scholar, Charlottesville, VA, USA

Part I
Overview

Chapter 1
Overview of Performing Arts Medicine

Richard J. Lederman

Background

Participants in the various performing arts have, of course, always suffered from medical problems and have always required the attention of healthcare practitioners. However, it has only been in the last 40 years that this need has been widely recognized as deserving of specialized attention. Too often in the past, performers, particularly instrumentalists, who sought advice from physicians or other providers for pain and other symptoms impairing function, were advised to simply stop playing. Several explanations may account for this problematic advice. First, very little information was available in the medical literature regarding the specific problems afflicting musicians; thus, physicians may have been simply unaware of these unique issues. Additionally, there was, at times, a perception, perhaps unrecognized or unacknowledged, that "playing" could more easily be stopped or reduced than "working," because a performing artist's work may have been incorrectly viewed as supplementary to other types of work or in the category of a hobby. Furthermore, healthcare providers may, at times, have underestimated the impact of a small impairment of fine motor control that might have seemed *minor* in some other occupation or avocation but is *debilitating* for an instrumentalist. It might have been difficult for non-musician healthcare providers to recognize that advanced students or young professionals have already invested 10–20 years and thousands of hours in training and simply cannot be advised to stop playing or do something else for a living. Musicians have been notably reluctant to divulge that they were having difficulty playing, whatever the reason and at whatever level of accomplishment, for fear of being labeled as unable to work or less desirable to hire.

This chapter will provide an overview of the development of the field of performing arts medicine and introduce the origin of Performing Arts Medicine

R. J. Lederman (✉)
Center for General Neurology, Neurological Institute, Cleveland Clinic, Cleveland, OH, USA

S.-H. Lee et al. (eds.), *Perspectives in Performing Arts Medicine Practice*,
https://doi.org/10.1007/978-3-030-37480-8_1

Association (PAMA) in the 1980s. Harmon [1] has provided a more comprehensive and detailed review, which should be consulted by the interested reader.

Developmental Steps in the Field of Performing Arts Medicine

Bernardino Ramazzini, considered the father of occupational medicine, did not ignore the health problems of performers. In his classic monograph, *De Morbis Artificum Diatriba* (Diseases of Workers) of 1700/1713, he described the following [2]:

> *In the same class of the infirm are flutists and those who play the pipes; all in short who play wind instruments with cheeks puffed out; for from violent exertion of the breath necessary for blowing trumpets and flutes they incur not only the maladies above-mentioned but far more serious ones,* e.g. *ruptures of the vessels of the chest and sudden discharges of blood from the mouth. In his Observations, Diemerbroeck gives a pitiable case of a flutist who, when certain others were playing the trumpet, was so ambitious to play louder than they that he ruptured a large vein in the lung, had a violent hemorrhage, and died within two hours.*

Over the subsequent two centuries, occasional reference was made to a variety of medical problems encountered in performers, mostly musicians. In his monumental textbook, translated into English as *A Manual of the Nervous Diseases of Man* in 1853 [3], Moritz Heinrich Romberg referred to a case reported by Stromeyer [4] of a pianist whose thumb involuntarily flexed into his palm as he played. Probably representing focal dystonia, the disorder was allegedly cured by performing a tenotomy, a treatment not likely to be endorsed by today's medical community. G. Vivian Poore, a London physician, collected a series of 21 pianists (19 of them women) with what he called "piano failure," involving the left more often than the right hand [5]. From his description, these likely represented a variety of disorders, mechanical and neurological, some of which were helped with treatment. Also in London, Sir William Gowers, probably the most revered figure in neurology at the time, included occupational cramps (writer's cramp was almost epidemic at the time among "scribes") in pianists, violinists, harpists, and drummers in his widely used textbook of 1888 [6].

In what appears to have been the first book devoted to health problems among performers, Kurt Singer, MD, himself a professional musician (founder and conductor of the Berlin Doctors' Choir and general director of Stadtische Oper,1927–1932) as well a neurologist, published in 1926, *Die Berufskrankheiten der Musiker* (subsequently translated into English in 1932 as *Diseases of the Musical Profession*), chronicles a host of ailments among musicians [7]. Heavily weighted toward psychological issues (and I suspect significantly influenced by Freudian thinking), the book nonetheless represents a landmark in the field of performing arts medicine. Tragically, he was terminated from his post at the Opera in 1932 because he was Jewish. He subsequently founded the Jüdischer Kulturbund in Berlin in 1933. This organization and branches following his example in Frankfurt, Cologne, Hamburg, and other cities sponsored concerts and theatrical performances, enabling at least temporary employment for some of the many hundreds, if not thousands, of Jewish musicians and other performing artists who were dismissed from orchestras and theaters throughout Germany. In 1938, he came to the USA to visit his sister and lectured at Harvard. He returned to Europe, committed to continuing his work in Berlin but was persuaded not to continue on to Germany and remained in Rotterdam until he was deported from occupied Holland in 1943 to the concentration camp, Terezin, where he died in 1944 at age 58.

Another landmark publication in the field was a remarkable "case report" [8] of the composer, Maurice Ravel, by the eminent French neurologist Th. Alajouanine, who had extensively studied and attempted to treat Ravel's disabling illness. Ravel had lost his ability to both play and compose, but had relative preservation of his recognition and comprehension of music. The precise diagnosis has been extensively debated in the neurologic literature, but it clearly represented some form of neurodegenerative disorder. Just as clearly, it was not going to be helped by the ill-conceived neurosurgical procedure that precipitated his demise in 1937.

The publication in 1977 of a book edited by two prominent British neurologists, Macdonald Critchley and R.A. Henson, entitled Music and the Brain, [9] based on a symposium held in Vienna in 1972, may, as stated by Lockwood in a 1989 article in the New England Journal of Medicine [10], "mark the beginning of performing-arts medicine as a discipline." This came at a time when a number of brief case reports were appearing in the medical literature describing generally mild but often annoying problems experienced by instrumental musicians, collectively referred to as "musical medicine" [11]. Also in the late 1970s and early 1980s, musicians were speaking out about more disabling problems. Most notably, two internationally renowned pianists, Gary Graffman and Leon Fleisher, who had both attained the very highest level in their professional careers, spoke out about their debilitating injuries (focal limb dystonia) and their frustration in dealing with medical professionals. Graffman was particularly critical of the level of expertise in the medical profession, their inability to recognize his affliction, and the lack of understanding of the nature of his problem and the impact it had on his ability to play [12]. This is but one example of the lack of information available at the time. Once the correct diagnosis was made and after considerable efforts at rehabilitative therapy, Graffman largely abandoned his illustrious career as a concert pianist and moved on as an administrator and sometime left-handed pianist. Fleisher after countless hours of multiple forms of treatment and 40 years of lapse has managed a remarkably successful "comeback" playing a somewhat limited but still extraordinary four-handed repertoire. This was also a time when the news media were beginning to pay attention to such phenomena as performance anxiety among artists in multiple performing disciplines and its potentially destructive effects on their careers.

Two events in this country in 1983, in the opinion of the author, set the stage for the emergence of a new phenomenon that has come to be known as performing arts medicine. The first was the publication of an article in the Journal of the American Medical Association by Hochberg and colleagues [13] reviewing their experience in treating musicians (including both Graffman and Fleisher) with hand problems at the Massachusetts General Hospital, which was the first to establish a "musicians' clinic."

This article served to provide some legitimacy and scientific credibility to a developing area of medical practice. The other event in 1983 was the planning and actual implementation, singlehandedly by Alice G. Brandfonbrener, MD (in my view against all odds), of the first symposium on Medical Problems of Musicians held in Aspen, Colorado, co-sponsored by the Music Associates of Aspen and the Aspen Music Festival, with the support of the Aspen Valley Hospital. This meeting, which has evolved into arguably the premier gathering place internationally for scholars of performing arts medicine, has kindled the enthusiasm and interest of many hundreds, if not thousands, of practitioners in this field, myself included. The above is not meant to diminish or demean other pioneering efforts in the development of performing arts medicine in this country and in many other parts of the world. Within a year after the Aspen conference, two important meetings for music and medicine were held in the USA, one on the Biology of Music Making in Denver, CO, organized by Franz L. Roehmann and Frank R. Wilson, resulting in the publication of its proceedings [14] and another by the American String Teachers Association in Chicago, the first by a musicians' organization as far as I know [15]. Far too many to list have followed since then.

Music Medicine

By this time in Germany, Christoph Wagner, MD, had for many years been carrying out his elegant studies of hand function and anatomy in musicians [16]. This eventually led to the establishment of a center for study and ultimately treatment of performance-related disorders in Hannover, Germany, currently under the dynamic leadership of Eckart Altenmüller, MD.

Also, in the early 1980s, Hunter Fry, a plastic hand surgeon in Australia, was beginning his extensive surveys of "overuse" in instrumental musicians [17] and establishing what, at that time, seemed an unexpectedly high frequency of pain and playing-related problems among the members of symphony orchestras, adding further incentive to the need to establish a specialty that was beginning to set its sights on meeting that challenge. This high prevalence of pain and injury had been suggested by other early epidemiologic studies [18] and was confirmed and extended by a large-scale survey of the 48 orchestras comprising the International Conference of Symphony and Opera Musicians (ICSOM). The survey was conducted in the mid-1980s and initially published in the ICSOM newsletter, *Senza Sordino*, in 1987. It was reprinted in the then recently founded specialty journal Medical Problems of Performing Artists in 1988 [19].

Additionally, in the mid-to-late 1980s, clinics and healthcare facilities began springing up throughout North America and Europe as well as Australia and Asia to provide the required specialized care for musicians. In the UK, Dr. Ian James, a pioneer in studying and treating performance anxiety in musicians, established a musician's clinic at the Royal Free Hospital, London, in 1984. He also founded the British Performing Arts Medicine Trust, which later evolved into the British Association for Performing Arts Medicine (BAPAM).

Dance and Vocal Medicine

By this time, there were a few ongoing and established programs involved in healthcare for performing artists in other disciplines. Dance medicine had evolved primarily under the leadership of a small group of highly specialized orthopedists and physical therapists, many of whom had become interested in the injuries specific to dancers after being involved in the management of sports-related injuries. Scientific investigation of factors contributing to hip, knee, and ankle injuries and the therapeutic approaches to these problems began appearing in increasing numbers during the 1970s and 1980s. A formal organization, the International Association of Dance Medicine and Science (IADMS), was established in 1987, and the Journal of Dance Medicine & Science was first published in 1997. IADMS grew from initial membership of 48 to over 900, testimony to the popularity of the various forms of dance and the level of interest in the health of performers.

Problems associated with vocal dysfunction have attracted scientific attention for many centuries but, again, it is only relatively recently that a cadre of laryngologists began systematically studying vocal disorders. The Voice Foundation, founded in 1969 by Wilbur James Gould, MD, for the purpose of fostering the scientific study and communication among those investigating and treating problems of the vocal apparatus, has provided the major focus of this effort, currently under the leadership of Dr. Robert T Sataloff, a prominent laryngologist as well as a singer and choral director. The Journal of Voice first appeared in 1987, only a year after the initial issue of Medical Problems of Performing Artists.

The Concept of Performing Art Medicine

Where and when did the term "performing arts medicine" first enter the lexicon? It is, of course, likely that this terminology had been utilized many times in the past and was, as mentioned previously, a part of the name of the British organization founded by Ian James. Discussions regarding the need to establish a clear scope in the burgeoning field of healthcare for performers first began at informal get-togethers at the Aspen meetings as early as 1984. There were two rather divergent approaches to the subject. One, championed particularly by Dr. Richard Lippin, a Philadelphia-based physician and the organization which he had founded in the early 1980s, the International Arts Medicine Association, favored a broad approach to the field [20]. They preferred to emphasize the importance of including all forms of arts in the proposed specialty, including not only performers but also those involved in the visual arts and literature, for instance. Thus, as their organization's title might suggest, they supported the term "arts medicine." At the other end of the spectrum, there were those who primarily were involved in the healthcare of instrumentalists and, like many of our European colleagues, liked the idea of using the term "music medicine," which had already appeared in the news media in its coverage of some of the early efforts. It was also appealing to those whose main interest was in research in performing arts medicine including how the brain processes music and how music might affect the anatomy and physiology of the brain. The closely related term "musical medicine" had been used in describing a variety of maladies affecting instrumentalists and submitted as brief case reports or letters to medical journals. Some in the group who were primarily clinicians seeing "injured" performers as patients preferred the inclusion of performers in instrumental music, singing (our ENT colleagues often referred to "vocal instrumentalists"), and dance but did not feel a strong clinical connection (albeit a highly sympathetic intellectual connection) to the visual and literary arts. Hence, the group eventually settled on promoting use of the term *performing arts medicine* for this "new" specialty.

Along with adopting a name for the type of practice, physicians who were primarily engaged in this part-time subspecialty, the members in the group, also began, as early as 1984, discussing the need for some type of organizational structure with several goals: (1) to promote quality care for performers, (2) to expand and perpetuate the meeting at which topics of mutual interest would be presented and discussed, (3) to support and conduct programs for education and research in this developing field, (4) to establish some form of communication and coordination among the clinical centers already in place and those being planned, and (5) to foster dialogue and cooperation among performing arts organizations, educational institutions in the performing arts, and healthcare associations and schools. By 1986, the organization was blessed with a vehicle for facilitating communication and education, the journal Medical Problems of Performing Artists (MPPA), which had been incubating for a couple of years before its appearance in March of 1986. Over the following 2 years, there were spirited discussions regarding a name for the proposed organization (including, but not limited to, Association of Clinical Care for Performing Artists and Association of Performing Arts Medicine Clinics). By 1988, the Performing Arts Medicine Association (PAMA) had been established and had a mission statement and bylaws, a set of officers and a board of directors, an official journal (MPPA), at least one annual meeting planned (in Aspen, Colorado), and an annual dues structure of $100 for physician members. By the following year, PAMA was officially incorporated as a non-profit organization with a Federal Employer Tax ID number and 16 members, with another 10 preparing to apply. The association's account balance in 1989 was $2570.00.

The Last 30 Years

To say that a lot has happened over the last 30 years would obviously be an understatement and something no one participating in those early meetings would have predicted or believed possible. Literature in the field of performing arts medicine has increased exponentially. Whereas finding studies regarding medical problems producing impairment in musicians and particularly relating playing an instrument to specific ailments was extremely difficult in the late 1970s and early 1980s, case studies and reviews began to appear in the late 1980s, not only in the journal MPPA but in many general and specialty publications. PAMA began to keep track of relevant literature in a bibliography which has, at the present time, reached some 15,000 citations! MPPA has roughly doubled in size from 142 pages published in 1986 to close to 290 pages in 2018. A number of books began to appear on this subject, notably, *The Musician's Hand: A Clinical Guide* by Winspur and Wynn Parry, pioneer clinicians from the UK [21], *Medical Problems of the Instrumentalist Musician* by Tubiana and Amadio [22], and the first *Textbook of Performing Arts Medicine* by Sataloff, Brandfonbrener, and Lederman in 1991 [23]. Performing arts, music, and its connection with medicine, especially related to brain function, became a subject of increasing interest and research. Perhaps no individual was more responsible for highlighting this relationship than the late Oliver Sacks, MD, a neurologist and prolific writer who provided fascinating insights into the brain's function and dysfunction as it relates to the arts, culminating in his Musicophilia in 2007 [24]. How music and the arts can influence brain development and function has also been the subject of increased scrutiny and investigation. There is now abundant evidence that the brains of musicians can differ significantly from those of non-musicians as the result of musical training and playing an instrument [25].

As the field of performing arts medicine became recognized, performing artists began seeking the expertise of practitioners with knowledge in this area, leading to the establishment of specialized clinics and groups throughout the USA and worldwide. Unfortunately, many of these subsequently folded or simply disappeared, often for lack of support from parent institutions and inability to sustain the necessary energy and financial resources to keep them going. Educating healthcare practitioners in dealing with problems of performing artists has been an ongoing concern of PAMA and other professional organizations. The meeting held in Aspen each summer, and more recently in other venues, and now having evolved into an annual international symposium, has served this function admirably, and the excitement generated among attendees at this meeting and workshops is palpable by the closing day. A number of regional meetings and courses have supplemented the annual event, now expanded to include not only lectures, workshops, and open communications but a pre-symposium certification course dedicated to educational objectives. Attendance at these symposia has more than doubled since the early meetings.

PAMA itself has grown dramatically from the original 16 members to the current 342, representing 19 countries. Most encouraging is the inclusion of 87 students and resident trainees and 67 representatives from the performing arts community. Membership was initially limited to medical professionals, trainees, and students, purposefully and after sometimes heated debate among the founders. The reasoning, viewed as possibly elitist by some, was that the concept of such an organization was sufficiently unusual that it was necessary to establish its scientific legitimacy and peer respect in the medical community before opening membership to performing artists and therapists of all types. This was finally accomplished in 1993, 4 years after its establishment. While PAMA remains truly international, similar organizations have been established in other countries, including the UK, France, Germany, Holland, and Australia.

Performing arts medicine has achieved a substantial degree of name recognition. There are still many in the performing arts community and, indeed, many healthcare professionals who remain unaware that such services exist or, if aware, how to access knowledgeable healthcare practitioners. There is work to be done to increase the knowledge base of performing arts medicine through clinical and basic research, disseminate that information to healthcare professionals who can incorporate it into their practices, expand the number and availability of knowledgeable practitioners, and educate the entire performing arts community that their particular and, at times, special needs can and should be adequately met. We are not there yet.

References

1. Harmon SE. The evolution of performing arts medicine. In: Sataloff RT, Brandfonbrener AG, Lederman RJ, editors. Performing arts medicine. 3rd ed. Narbarth: Science & Medicine, Inc; 2010. p. 1–23.
2. Ramazzini B. Diseases of workers (*De Morbis Artificum Diatriba,* 1713). Translated by Wilmer Cave Wright. New York: Hafner; 1964. p. 335.
3. Romberg MH. A manual of the nervous diseases of man, vol. 1. Translated and edited by Edward H Sieveking. London: Sydenham Society; 1853. p. 322–324.
4. Stromeyer L. Ueber den Schreibekrampf (*spasmus habitualis musculi flexoris pollicis longi) und dessen Heilung durch die Tenotomie*. Medicinisches Correspondenz-Blatt bayerischer Aerzte. 1840;8:113–23.
5. Poore GV. Clinical lecture on certain conditions of the hand and arm which interfere with the performance of professional acts, especially piano-playing. Br Med J. 1887;1:441–4.
6. Gowers WR. A manual of diseases of the nervous system, vol. II. 2nd ed. (1893). Darien: Hafner; 1970. p. 710–730.
7. Singer K. Diseases of the musical profession: a systematic presentation of their causes, symptoms and methods of treatment. Translated by Wladimir Lakond. New York: Greenberg; 1932.
8. Alajouanine T. Aphasia and artistic realization. Brain. 1948;71:229–41.
9. Critchley M, Henson RA, editors. Music and the brain: studies in the neurology of music. London: Heinemann; 1977.
10. Lockwood AH. Medical problems in musicians. N Engl J Med. 1989;320:221–7.
11. Dawson JB. Musical medicine [letter]. N Engl J Med. 1975;292:322.
12. Graffman G. Doctor, can you lend an ear? Med Probl Perform Art. 1986;1:3–6.
13. Hochberg FH, Leffert RD, Heller MD, Merriman L. Hand difficulties among musicians. JAMA. 1983;249:1869–72.
14. Roehmann FL, Wilson FR, editors. The biology of music making: proceedings of the 1984 Denver conference. St. Louis: MMB Music; 1988.
15. Mischakoff A, editor. *Sforzando*! Music medicine for string players. Bloomington: American String Teachers Association; 1985.
16. Wagner C. Success and failure in musical performance: biomechanics of the hand. In: Roehmann FL, Wilson FR, editors. The biology of music making: proceedings of the 1984 Denver conference. St Louis: MMB Music Inc.; 1988. p. 154–79.
17. Fry HJH. Incidence of overuse syndrome in the symphony orchestra. Med Probl Perform Art. 1986;1:51–5.
18. Caldron PH, Calabrese LH, Clough JD, Lederman RJ, Williams C, Leatherman J. A survey of musculoskeletal problems encountered in high-level musicians. Med Probl Perform Art. 1986;1:136–9.

19. Fishbein M, Middlestadt SE, Ottati V, Straus S, Ellis A. Medical problems among ICSOM musicians: overview of a national survey. Med Probl Perform Art. 1988;3:1–8.
20. Lippin RA. Arts medicine: a call for a new medical specialty. Phila Med. 1985;81:14–5.
21. Winspur I, Christopher B, Parry W, editors. The musician's hand: a clinical guide. London: Martin Dunitz Ltd. Distributed in the United States by Blackwell Science, Inc; 1998.
22. Tubiana R, Amadio PC, editors. Medical problems of the instrumentalist musician. London: Martin Dunitz; 2000. ISBN 1-85317-612-5.99.50.
23. Sataloff RT, Brandfonbrener AG, Lederman RJ, editors. Textbook of performing arts medicine. New York: Raven Press; 1991.
24. Sacks O. Musicophilia: tales of music and the brain. New York: Alfred A Knopf; 2007.
25. Jäncke L. The motor representation in pianists and string players. In: Altenmüller E, Wiesendanger M, Kesselring J, editors. Music, motor control and the brain. Oxford: Oxford University Press; 2007. p. 153–72.

Chapter 2
This Wide and Universal Stage: How Empathy and Presence Inform the Contribution of Theatrical Practice to the Physician's Art

Daniel K. Hall-Flavin

'Begotten by one,
I should know better. "Healing,"
Papa would tell me,
"is not a science,
but the intuitive art
of wooing Nature…"
…
"Every sickness
is a musical problem."
So said Novalis,
"and every cure
A musical solution":
you knew that also.'
W. H. Auden, *The Art of Healing* [1, p. 22–47]

Introduction

The British poet Wystan Hugh Auden, born into a medical family, throughout his career demonstrated an abiding interest in the interface between poetry and medicine. He composed *The Art of Healing* in memory of his own physician, Dr. David Protech. His words conjure images of the vulnerability, creativity, focus, capacity for true listening, and strength that characterize presence.

Presence occupies the time and space between medical caregivers and their patients. It is perhaps the most critical interpersonal process that exists in the medical encounter. In June 2017, the noted Harvard anthropologist and psychiatrist

D. K. Hall-Flavin (✉)
Mayo Clinic Delores Lavins Center for the Humanities in Medicine, Mayo Clinic, Rochester, MN, USA
e-mail: flavin.daniel@mayo.edu

S.-H. Lee et al. (eds.), *Perspectives in Performing Arts Medicine Practice*,
https://doi.org/10.1007/978-3-030-37480-8_2

Arthur Kleinman announced his retirement after 50 years of scholarship and practice in *The Lancet*, in a deceptively simply entitled essay *Presence* [2]. Kleinman describes presence as, '...the intensity of interacting with another human being that animates both being there for, and with, that person. It is…active…built out of listening intensely…ordinary yet with the potential to be exhilarating…, a moral act' [p. 2466]. With a nod to the American psychologist and philosopher William James, he notes: 'I personally believe it is the clinician's repeated experience of presence that sustains clinical work over the long and difficult journey of a career in medicine' [p. 2467]. Kleinman's words are important because of his unique and extended experience as master physician, healer, and humanist reflecting upon what he considers to be the most important lesson of his career. Framed within the realities of a digital age, the importance of a careful curation of presence helps us to navigate relationships within a world faced with the promise of a more humane globalization and the threat of jingoism and authenticity in crisis. Indeed, the casual use of the word 'presence' has now made its way into competitive marketing in the field of medicine.

I will use the term 'presence' in an interpersonal sense that can be as applicable in the health-care encounter as well as in the experience of performance. It is characterized by existential, spatial, temporal, linguistic, and ethical demands between an authentic self-awareness and alterity. It is embodied and occurs in dimensions of engagement. It is predicated on a critically assessed concept of empathy, on alterity, and on capacity for engagement in a broader sense.

The space of presence is evocative of the British paediatrician and psychoanalyst Donald Woods Winnicott's concept of the 'transitional space', which he defined as '…that space of experiencing between the inner and outer worlds, and contributed by both self and other in which primary creativity or illusion exists and can develop' [3, pp. 1795–1796]. In adulthood, this space is transformed into an intermediate arc of experience…throughout life it is retained in an intense experiencing that is arts and religion and to imaginative living, and to creative scientific work [4]. In this sense it is porous and allows personal interaction between two or more individuals in which a sense of time is temporarily suspended.

The philosopher Michael Brannigan describes levels of engagement with the alterity of the other in active presence [5]. Calling upon the work of Emmanuel Levinas and working from a Buddhist spiritual perspective, Brannigan, like Kleinman, emphasizes the importance of 'active listening' as a moral responsibility in which 'presence to the other induces presence from the other' [pp. 25–47].

Entry into the interpersonal space of presence requires empathy, altruism, and capacity, much as the combination on a padlock. The latter refers to physical factors such as the level of fatigue and physical capability, an emotional readiness to engage alterity, and the ability to house and manipulate both the knowledge and skills of one's profession. Of these three, the concept of empathy has been a focus of attention in the Humanities literature for a number of reasons, not the least of which has been concern regarding its conceptual validity and reliability. Yet, it is a critical cornerstone for other elements of the clinical encounter to build upon, most notably altruism and capacity. It has been conflated with sympathy, altruism, compassion, emotional contagion, and personal distress [6–8].[1,2]

Empathy fundamentally requires imagination in our interactions with others in our daily lives and represents a cognitive journey of discovery that animates our lives and has promoted our survival. The essayist Leslie Jamison notes that 'empathy is always perched precariously between gift and invasion' [9, p. 5]. There is significant overlap between the experience of presence in medicine and its expression in the arts, as Auden reminds us.

Medicine contains a substantial theatrical element, with representational scenery, roles (doctors, nurses, patients), costumes (white coats, indiscrete patient gowns), performance (lectures, bedside rounds, Morbidity and Mortality conferences), and simulation of mentoring models. There is rehearsal, repetition, and interruption. It requires imagination and is a journey of discovery, one journey made with patients, with colleagues, with mentors, and between patients. Medicine is at its core an examination of embodiment and its contents and discontents. Performance through embodiment promotes healing through being present to the other.

It is the purpose of this chapter to explore how empathy informs presence within the space between self and other and thereby how theatrical practice may be used within the field of medicine to promote more compassionate and resiliency in providers of the healing art.

The Nature of Empathy

Empathy is untidy and complex, and there is a moral force that emanates from empathy [10, 11]. In the practice of medicine, its primary purpose is to help open a space within which a person, whose life's trajectory has been turned to disadvantage by any number of physiologic, social, and/or psychological factors, may, with the help of care providers, build an illness narrative that gives meaning to their experience and sinew to the 'new normal' of altered human agency. Empathy functions as a 'proactive search engine'; it has been an essential component in our evolution as a species, with both nurturing and destructive capabilities [12–14].

There has been progress in our understanding of empathy and how it may impact work in both medicine and the theatre. This has been associated with increased research interest by social and developmental psychologists during the last two decades of the twentieth century, advances in research methodologies including

[1] Amy Coplan and Peter Goldie (2011) said that Altruism is a pro-social behaviour performed for the sake of benefitting the other person. Compassion may be thought of as a sympathetic state in which there is a strong motivation for the authentic observer to help the other, p.xxiv.

[2] Klimecki and others (2013) using fMRI concluded that brain plasticity changes were associated with 'compassion training' in reversing negative emotion associated with 'empathy training' after a negative visual exposure. Neither variable was described, however, and empathy was confused with emotional contagion.

imaging studies in cognitive neuroscience, complex changes in social communications, in how time itself is perceived, political changes, and an expanding void in the depth of personal connectivity in social communication. In addition, a landmark 2013 study by Kidd and Castano demonstrated in a series of five experiments that reading literary fiction can improve at least temporarily the capacity of the reader to identify and understand others' subjective affective and cognitive mental states compared with reading non-fiction [15]. As neuroscience has not yet outdistanced theory, there remains a continued interest in the phenomenological understanding of empathy within Theory of Mind studies.

At the same time, the use of the term 'empathy' has become encumbered. This is due to a variety of factors including lack of scholarly rigor in definition, its widespread intuitive appeal, its appropriation in the discourse of 'disciplines within silos', and severe limitations on how diverse research measurements and methodologies may be compared. In his recent book *Against Empathy*, the Yale University psychologist Paul Bloom criticizes the concept of 'affective empathy', privileges reason over empathy in defence of the concept of 'rational compassion', and argues that the concept of empathy is 'parochial, narrow-minded, and innumerate', leading to many examples of empathy misapplied, at times with peril [16]. Empathy is still of a young age, and a closer look reveals that it has never been without controversy or criticism about its use or overuse. In 1935, the pioneer of lay psychoanalysis Theodor Reik stated, 'The concept of empathy in psychological discussion has come to mean so much that it is beginning to mean nothing' [17, pp. 356–357]. More recently, the American psychoanalyst Warren Poland most eloquently and succinctly described the potential danger of reaching for more facile explanations in science, when he referred to the overuse of the concept of empathy specifically, '…introduced as a valuable contribution that is expanded before its time…used to close off questioning…as a shibboleth of parochial allegiance…in the face of unending uncertainty, compromising discipline in a search for final answers' [18, pp. 87–88]. It has also been criticized as a political means to appropriating 'others' and in reinforcing support to political and social power [19, 20].

These cautions are credible and deserving of our full attention. Yet empathy is critical to human agency, our status as social and moral agents, and in the study of philosophy and the human evolutionary sciences, including cognitive, social, and developmental psychology, and behavioural economics [6]. It requires more circumspection in its precise characterization and, in particular, its curation, if it is to be of value.

There are many definitions of empathy. For purposes of this discussion, a phenomenological definition authored by the philosopher Amy Copland and refined by more recent multidisciplinary studies within the arts and sciences seems to be more directly applicable in medicine and in theatrical practice [21]:

> Empathy is a complex imaginative process in which an observer simulates another person's situated psychological states while maintaining clear-self other differentiation. To say that empathy is 'complex' is to say that it is simultaneously a cognitive and affective process. To say that empathy is 'imaginative' is to say that it involves the representation of a target's states that are activated by, but not directly accessible through, the observer's

> perception. And to say that empathy is a 'simulation' is to say that the observer replicates or reconstructs the target's experiences, while maintaining a clear sense of self-other differentiation [pp. 5–6].

Empathy and the Theatre

In a sense we are all refugees in search of a better place. Theatre offers us a delimited space and time of creativity and imagination demarcated from that of our daily cognitive routine. It is a place to see and be seen, a place to contemplate our sense of vulnerability as a key to empathy, and ultimately presence. Whether within the staged poetic drama of Tennessee Williams, an evening with the Tyrone family in Eugene O'Neill's autobiographical play *Long Day's Journey into Night*, contemplating the meaning of justice and mercy in the plight of Shylock in Shakespeare's *The Merchant of Venice*, or being an eyewitness to one of the most moving moments of empathy and presence that theatre can offer, the freezing gaze between *The Tempest's* Prospero and Caliban at the end of *The Tempest*, the ineluctable but commanding cognitive experience of presence is felt by the engaged spectator.

Theatre, good theatre, invites, not always comfortably, and perhaps at its best uncomfortably, reconsideration of alterity and ourselves. It 'happens' according to the Shakespearean director Peter Brooks, when actors and audience occupy the same space [20]. It also happens in the 'proto-performance', a term coined by the father of Performance Studies, Richard Schechner, which includes workshops, rehearsals, the review of the director's notes, the response of the critics, post-performance dialogue with the audience, and archiving an experience that is singular, in the moment, and not to be repeated [22]. It happens at intermissions with audience members interacting with others and after the experience. It happens inexplicably and almost imperceptibly between audience members while watching a particularly poignant moment in a production that is in resonance with our common humanity. The director Bryan Doerries notes '…I often know how an audience is reacting to a performance by the way people are breathing. Sometimes during powerful moments, when actors are able to convey the truth of an experience, audience members begin breathing together, inhaling and exhaling as one…the quality of the silence deepens' [23, p. 437].

I had an opportunity to witness this myself in the closing moments of the London West End production of Jez Butterworth's *The Ferryman* [24]. The audience silence was profound, I and my fellow spectators were breathing in unison, and we all were leaning forward in our seats in anticipation of a finale of tragic proportion that made it clear that redemption and freedom can carry a very high price. The British woman of letters and super-naturalist fiction, Vernon Lee, aka Violet Paget, proposed at the turn of the last century that an individual can empathize with a work of art when the object stimulates memories which may lead to *unconscious* bodily changes in posture or breathing [25].

The American theatre scholar Lindsay Cummings has proposed that empathy is dialogical in nature and requires that we be open to change if our theatrical experience is to have meaning [20]. The communications scholar Julia Wood comments that, '…dialogue is emergent (rather than stagnant), fluid (rather than static), performative (rather than representational), and never fully finished (rather than completed)' [26, p. xvii].

For Cummings, dialogic empathy is embodied; it is cognitive, affective, and sensorial [20]. The key question is not whether we empathize, but why do we empathize and what does the process of doing this afford us? As empathy is moved from destination to journey, it may create ambiguity and anxiety and a challenge to respond to what we may not fully recognize as therein lies our ethical obligation [27].

To help achieve this, the theatrical techniques of interruption, repetition, and rehearsal are used. For the actor, repetition and rehearsal are central in creating a character that is to be presented to the spectator. As a spectator, lingering on the concept of the interruption, the cognitive dissonance between the observed and the expected is worth understanding more. It is what moves us forward according to Zahavi, Brecht, cognitive and social psychologists, and others [28]. What does Cummings mean by interruption and the gap that follows?

An interruption may occur when the behaviour or verbal presentation of a character on stage is not of the sort we might expect; there is an interruption in the flow of our empathic imagination that may or may not be settled at the time, later, or ever. Lingering in the gaps of time, imagination, and emotion requires attention, active listening, and an ability to tolerate contradiction and critical analysis. From the actor's perspective in the gap, there is a fear of exposure and vulnerability that comes from contact with alterity.

Within this gap there is a thinking space in which prior assumptions of both actor and spectator can be examined. Here there is a charisma marked by contradicting thoughts and feelings, such as strength and vulnerability, innocence and experience, and singularity and typicality, which nurtures empathy through the process of validation and of being seen. Making the other feel seen adds to a sense of affective resonance which adds to a sense of authenticity and personhood which help to create the conditions for change [29]. This grants the spectator the permission to consider change to our embodied relationship to past experience and bias and be sensitive to the need for equity in any meaningful dialogue.

Theatre, perhaps more than any other art form other than dance, relies on our visceral connection to the body to make meaning [30]. Its potential contribution as an art form to medicine lies in its 'uniquely compelling emotional quality, making it difficult to avoid or intellectualize the struggles and suffering portrayed'. Within the cognitive sciences, which link language, linguistics, cognition, and embodiment, we are reminded by Amy Cook that theatre has the capacity to change minds and touch bodies at the deepest level [31]. Cook argues that the 'interplay between cognitive science and performance theory' provides important information of what Louis Montrose has called the 'cognitive and therapeutic instrument' of drama and performance [31, 32].

The theatre is a complex multidimensional space in which there are important interpersonal relationships between audience participants and actor, between audience participants themselves, between actor and actor, and between director and actor, set in a context of place and time that is represented in embodied time. Within performance there are gaps, or episodes of cognitive difference, that are crucial in the development of new knowledge and attitudes [33]. The cognitive basis for understanding the nature of empathy as an embodied phenomenon has gained epistemic traction within the past decade with the assistance of more advanced imaging techniques in the neurosciences.

Failure, Finitude, and Presence

> Sweet are the uses of adversity; Which, like the toad, ugly and venomous, Wears yet a precious jewel in his head and this our life exempt from public haunt Finds tongues in trees, books in the running brooks, Sermons in stones and good in every thing. I would not change it.
>
> *Duke Senior*
> *As You Like It, Act II, Sc* [34]

It is ironic that the status of Medicine as a healing art is threatened by a crisis in the health and professional sustainability of its own providers. Physician burnout, characterized by emotional exhaustion, depersonalization, and a sense of reduced fulfilment and accomplishment, is at an all-time high, and physician and patient health and quality of care are put at risk [35]. Physicians have traditionally been trained to be kind but withhold emotion, and expectations are high; traditionally physicians have been selected by victories. Isolation, long work hours, sleep deprivation, increasing stringent institutional requirements on time limits with patients, the lack of mentoring, an increasing lack of autonomy, and a failure of institutional culture to support physicians are all factors involved with this physician health crisis, which includes suicide [36–38].

Ultimately, it is the inability to successfully negotiate ambiguity and the fear of being defined by failure if we fail, a feeling of shame in ultimately being unable to attain unattainable expectations, and a perceived or real lack of permission to discuss vulnerability that places physicians at risk. Death is the traditional metaphorical enemy that physicians battle daily; it will ultimately overcome any therapeutic weapon that can be aimed on a patient's behalf in its direction. It is difficult if not impossible to establish empathy and enter the space of presence fully without considering our own potential for failure, suffering, and, ultimately, our own finitude. The perimeter set up by these factors establishes the space of our existential anxiety.

In her book, *This Republic of Suffering: Death and the Civil War*, the Lincoln Professor of History and Immediate Past-President of Harvard University Drew Gilpin Faust begins the preface to her book with five words: 'Mortality defines the human condition' [39]. So does suffering, and in particular suffering alone. But by taking on these issues, as existentially challenging as they may be, we engage in an ongoing, iterative, and powerful process of making and remaking meaning as we make and remake meaning at the theatre, a meaning which we come to know is uniquely our own. A physician cannot truly achieve the presence and the authenticity that patients seek without a visceral willingness to take on this most human of vulnerabilities that binds us together. To paraphrase Brannigan, our openness invites the trust and the openness of the other.

The social scientist Walter Benjamin wrote: 'Death is the sanction of everything the story-teller can tell. He has borrowed his authority from death' [40, p. 94]. To extend the argument put forth by Doerries [23], theatre can be a very effective tool of helping the physician in this journey. It is in many ways the most familiar art form that he or she may know, a safe space for permission to embrace our vulnerabilities and in so doing nurture the potential for creativity.

Theatre in Healing the Healer and the Patient

There is a growing literature testifying to the effectiveness of theatre arts in medical school curricula, with various definitions of effectiveness. The use of specific theatre techniques is reported to be an effective tool in curricula development [41–44]. These include standardized patient encounters which emphasize reflection upon the actual experience of the individual being observed. The use of particular theatrical genres, such as *Commedia dell'arte*, emphasizes a focus on deliberate movement and embodiment in the use of space, voice, and eye contact. Other techniques include staged theatrical readings, improvisation, specific theatrical training exercises and storytelling, the use of opera, specific plays (e.g. *Wit*), and film [45]. Theatre has been used to help provide insight and nurture empathy in conditions such as post-traumatic stress disorder, traumatic brain injury, autistic spectrum disorder, and Parkinson's disease [46–48].

The space between self and other that is part of the daily medical interaction is recreated in the space between self and other in the theatre. It is a place of holding and containing, a place of permission, and a model of a space of creativity, space, and problem-solving in place of one of waiting, confusion, isolation, fear, ambiguity, and shame that can characterize the medical encounter. Recalling the contextual aspects of Cummings' dialogic empathy, the caregiver is given permission for interruption, for lingering in the gaps of cognitive dissonance, to attend and creatively problem-solve. In this context presence represents a period of focused attention that is instantiated by the interaction of empathy, altruism, and capacity. Other directed intentionality, an ability to care for the welfare of another (separate from empathy), and the cognitive, physical, experience, and knowledge base of capacity are all nurtured by the meaningful bidirectional theatrical encounter.

Conclusion

> The secret of reading is to close the book
>
> Brian Doerries [23, p. 34]

Thirty years ago, Susan Sontag famously wrote: 'Everyone who is born holds dual citizenship, in the kingdom of the well and the kingdom of the sick…Sooner or later each of us is obliged, at least for a spell, to identify ourselves as citizens of that other place' [49, p. 3].

Traditionally in medicine, as noted by Kleinman, physicians 'do their best to transfer chaotic human problems into close-ended practical puzzles meant to be managed by technology, which encases the patient in a peculiar exoskeleton, threatening their identity and agency' [50, pp. 209–227]. Without the creativity that enables the creation of meaning, it also encases the physician. Theatre promotes the privilege of stepping into that another's world to face the sentries which guard Sontag's frontier: ambiguity, shame, stigma, vulnerability, impaired empathy, and other challenges to our capacities as human beings and caregivers, including out authenticity and our autonomy [50].

The practice of medicine in this digitalized age of instant communication is challenged often by an unyielding pressure to deliver time-dependent cognitive expertise in diminishing aliquots of time. It is accompanied by narrowing expectations of what it means to be a physician or other health-care provider. The resulting lone silos of embodied expertise are burdened with an insularity that threatens the efficacy, connectedness, sense of community, and ability to comply with the moral imperative that we are to be companions with each other in the narrative of suffering, however that is defined.

Presence is not a one-way street. It is a cognitive experiential entity that requires time, focus, emotional energy, empathy, and altruism, calling upon courage and emotional muscle to fill in the gaps. It can only really be approximated in a lifelong journey, whether that of a health-care provider, of an arts professional, or of any work or interpersonal interaction in which we are called upon to recognize alterity, in all that that term implies. This is the journey that Kleinman challenges us to commit ourselves to.

The performing arts, herein exemplified by theatre, and the medical arts – both are lifelong challenges to engage empathy and presence in the experience of generous listening and informed critical thinking to help guide us into a future for humanity's journey as an integrative and collaborative endeavour that is sustainable in the service of living deliberately.[3]

[3] A portion of the text of the conclusion is excerpted from a presentation entitled 'The Quality of Mercy' presented by the author originally in a presentation at the University of Missouri-Kansas City School of Medicine (2018) and has not been published.

References

1. Auden WH. The art of healing. In: Bamforth I, editor. The body in the library: a literary anthology of modern medicine. London: Verso; 2015. p. 322–5.
2. Kleinman A, et al. Lancet. 2017;389:2466–7.
3. Johns J. Transitional object, space. In: De Mijolla A, editor. International dictionary of psychoanalysis. Farmington Hills: Thomson Gale [Macmillan Reference]; 2005.
4. Winnicott D. Transitional objects and transitional phenomenon. Int J Psychoanal. 1953;34:89.
5. Brannigan MK. The Buddhist noble truths, and presence. In: Goncalves J, editor. Presence in healthcare communication-implications for professional education, Niteroi. Brazil: Editora da UFF; 2013. p. 25–47.
6. Steuber K. Empathy. In: Stanford encyclopaedia of philosophy. Stanford: Stanford University Metaphysics Research Lab; 2017. p. 1–65 and 23–7.
7. Coplan A, Goldie P. Introduction. In: Coplan A, Goldie P, editors. Empathy: philosophical and psychological perspectives. New York: Oxford University Press; 2011. p. 24.
8. Klimecki O, Leiberg S, Ricard M, Singer T. Differential pattern of functional brain plasticity after compassion and empathy training. Soc Cogn Affect Neurosci. 2013;9(6):1–7.
9. Jamison L. The empathy exams. Minneapolis: Graywolf Press; 2014.
10. Jurecic A, Marenalik D. Examining empathy. Lancet. 2015;386(10004):1618. https://doi.org/10.1016/S0140-6736(15)00540-1.
11. Decety J, Cowell JM. The equivocal relationship between morality and empathy. In: Decety J, Wheatley T, editors. The moral brain: a multidisciplinary perspective. Cambridge: Massachusetts Institute of Technology Press; 2015. p. 279.
12. De Waal F. The antiquity of empathy. Science. 2012;336:874.
13. Decety J. Introduction. In: Decety J, Wheatley T, editors. The moral brain: a multidisciplinary perspective. Cambridge: Massachusetts Institute of Technology Press; 2015. p. vii.
14. McConachie B. Engaging audiences: a cognitive approach to spectating in the theatre. New York: Palgrave Macmillan; 2008.
15. Kidd DC, Castano E. Reading literary fiction improves theory of mind. Science. 2013;342(6156):372–80.
16. Bloom P. Against empathy: the case for rational compassion. New York: Harper Collins; 2016.
17. Reik T. Listening with the third ear. New York: Farrar, Strauss, and Giroux; 1948.
18. Poland W. The limits of empathy. Am Imago. 2007;64(1):87–93. & 87–8.
19. Amit R. Rule of sympathy: sentiment, race, and power. New York: Palgrave Macmillan; 2002.
20. Cummings L. Empathy as dialogue in theatre and performance. London: Palgrave Macmillan; 2016.
21. Coplan A. Understanding empathy: its features and effects. In: Coplan A, Goldie P, editors. Empathy: philosophical and psychological perspectives. New York: Oxford University Press; 2011. p. 5–6.
22. Schechner R. Performance studies: an introduction. 2nd ed. New York and London: Routledge; 2006.
23. Doerries B. The theatre of war: what ancient Greek tragedies can teach us today. New York: Alfred A. Knopf; 2015.
24. Butterworth J. The ferryman. London: Nick Hearn; 2017.
25. Wispe L. History of the concept of empathy. In: Eisenberg N, Strayer J, editors. Empathy and its development. Cambridge: Cambridge University Press; 1987.
26. Wood J. Foreword: entering into dialogue. In: Anderson R, and others, editors. Dialogue: theorizing difference in communication studies. London: Sage; 2004. p. 17.
27. Oliver K. Witnessing: beyond recognition. Minneapolis: University of Minnesota Press; 2001. p. 191.
28. Zahavi D. Self and other: exploring subjectivity, empathy, and shame. New York: Oxford University Press; 2014.
29. Roach J. It. Ann Arbor: University of Michigan Press; 2007. p. 8.

30. Popova Y. Performance and cognition: theatre studies and the cognitive turn. Mod Drama. 2008;51(3):426–8.
31. Cook A. Interplay: the method and potential of a cognitive scientific approach to theatre. Thea J. 2007;59:569–74, 580, 594.
32. Montrose L. The purpose of playing: Shakespeare and the cultural politics of the Elizabethan theatre. Chicago: University of Chicago Press; 1996. p. 40.
33. Halpern J. Clinical empathy in medical care. In: Decety J, editor. Empathy from bench to bedside. Cambridge: Massachusetts Institute of Technology Press; 2012. p. 43.
34. Shakespeare W. As you like it. In: Stanley WS, Taylor G, editors. William Shakespeare, the complete works. Compact edition. Oxford: Clarendon Press; 1988. Act 2, Scene 1.
35. West C, Dyrbye LN, Erwin PJ, Shanafelt TD. Interventions to prevent and reduce physician burnout: a systematic review and meta-analysis. Lancet. 2016;388(10057):2272–81.
36. Shanafelt T. Longitudinal study evaluating the association between physician burnout and changes in professional work effort. Mayo Clinic Proc. 2016;91(4):422–31. Elsevier.
37. Jager AJ, Tutty MA, Kao AC. Association between physician burnout and identification with medicine as a calling. Mayo Clinic Proc. 2017;92(3):415–22. Elsevier.
38. Levine R. The secret of care of the doctor is in caring for the doctor. Mayo Clinic Proc. 2016;91(4):408–10.
39. Faust D. Preface: the work of death. In: Drew GF, editor. This republic of suffering: death and the American civil war. New York: Vintage Books; 2008. p. 11.
40. Benjamin W, Arendt H, editors. Illuminations, essays and reflections. New York: Random House, Schocken Books; 1968. p. 94.
41. Eisenberg A, Rosenthal S, Schlussel YR. Medicine as a performing art: what can we learn about empathic communication from theatre arts. Acad Med. 2015;90(3):272–6.
42. Dow AW, Leong D, Anderson A, Wenzel RP. Using theatre to teach clinical medicine: a pilot study. J Gen Intern Med. 2007;22(8):1114–8.
43. Reilly JM, Trial J, Piver DE, Schaff PB. Using theatre to increase empathy training in medical students. J Learn Through Arts. 2012;8(1):n.1.
44. Watson K. Perspective: serious play: teaching medical students with improvisational medical techniques. Acad Med. 2011;86(10):1260–5.
45. Alexander M, Lenahan P, Pavlov A, editors. Cinemeducation: a comprehensive guide to using film in teaching medical students. Oxford: Radcliffe Publishing; 2005. p. 247.
46. Kontos P, Miller KL, Colantonio A, Cott C. Grief, anger, and relationality: the impact of a research-based theatre intervention on emotion work practices in brain injury rehabilitation. Eval Rev. 2014 Feb;38(1):29–67.
47. Gabriel J, Angevin E, Rosen T, Lerner MD. Use of theatrical techniques and elements as interventions for autism spectrum disorders. In: Theatre and cognitive neuroscience; 2016. p. 163–76.
48. Modugno N, Iaconelli S, Fiorlli M, et al. Active theatre as a complementary therapy for Parkinson's Disease rehabilitation. Sci World J. 2010;10:2301–13.
49. Sontag S. Illness as metaphor and aids and its metaphors. London: Penguin Press; 1991.
50. Kleinman A. The illness narratives: suffering, healing, and the human condition. New York: Basic Books; 1988. p. 209–27.

Chapter 3
The Best of Both Worlds: An Odyssey of Medicine and Music

William J. Dawson

Beginning the Journey

The seeds of a career, whether in medicine or the performing arts, often are sown early in life. A high percentage of musicians begin their art as young children. This is not surprising, since they have been exposed to musical sounds all their lives, even before birth. Studies [1] confirm that music can be perceived in utero and can elicit responses by the fetus. Newborns experience music from a variety of environmental sources; perhaps the most common one is listening to songs sung by their mothers. Reacting to pitch and rhythm also is a characteristic finding during the first 2 years of life [2], and mimicking sounds, tunes, and speech becomes a natural response to these stimuli.

For many children, exposure to and participation in music continues in the family environment, with parents or older siblings playing instruments or singing in groups while toddlers and other youngsters join in. Picking out melodies on a piano is often a child's first preliminary step to making instrumental music. With parental approval and encouragement, a few children will begin formal music lessons as early as age 4. In later years, participation in many forms of classroom music remains a staple of elementary education in most schools.

This introductory path is much the same as for medicine. Childhood play, complete with toy stethoscopes, bandages, and syringes, is common, and toy stores display a wide variety of offerings to facilitate this interest. Siblings and stuffed toy animals become the first "patients."

W. J. Dawson (✉)
Department of Orthopaedic Surgery, Feinberg School of Medicine, Northwestern University, Northbrook, IL, USA

Performing Arts Medicine Association, Northbrook, IL, USA
e-mail: w-dawson@northwestern.edu

S.-H. Lee et al. (eds.), *Perspectives in Performing Arts Medicine Practice*,
https://doi.org/10.1007/978-3-030-37480-8_3

Early play and personal and family experiences with health issues usually are the primary modes of familiarization with the world of medicine. Attempts at actual practice will, obviously, occur decades later for some, but learning first aid through Scouting or the Red Cross offers real-life experience and can begin as early as age 8 or 9. All this knowledge often leads to the desire "to be a doctor when I grow up," a commonly heard phrase among preschool and elementary students.

It's probably not surprising how often the worlds of music and medicine will combine in a person's life. In what proportions and how they are expressed are unique to each individual and may change with the passing years [3]. What follows is a series of observations about these two careers, how they can intersect and intermingle, and how they are affected by the maturing and aging process. These will be discussed in relation to a variety of studies and accompanied by some unabashedly autobiographical data from the writer's not-so-typical life embracing both the medical and musical worlds.

Priorities and Personal Progress

Arts before medicine is the norm for many physicians involved in both disciplines. Many healthcare professionals (HCP) developed a background in the arts as youngsters long before choosing a health-related line of work. Most commonly for musicians, their early experiences consist of taking lessons, playing piano or guitar, or singing. Early opportunities to participate are available in school programs and classes, religious activities, and/or private music programs and groups.

For many, musical activities remain an enjoyable childhood hobby or pastime. Others, however, take these early arts experiences much more seriously. Intensive lessons, performances, auditions, and competition opportunities abound for those with high motivation and supportive parents, and some students achieve exceptional levels of skill and competency while maintaining a full academic schedule. Some ultimately will become professional musicians through school or other tracks, whereas others choose a variety of occupations while keeping music in their lives as an avocation.

Much has been written about the positive effects of early music education on many facets of human development [4, 5]. What role such early training plays in the lives of those who choose a health professional career is, again, unique to the individual. For some, the choice may represent a detour from the path to becoming a professional musician. Other noneducational experiences arise, which can become determining factors. A few choose a career in the health professions because of prior personal medical problems which were associated with, or affected, their art; for these budding music professionals, medicine became an alternate career choice for them, with their music assuming a secondary role.

My own early musical experiences, fortunately, were positive, thanks to a combination of family interest, encouragement, and support, as well as my own personal desire. I began to take piano lessons at age 7; they continued for 3 years, until my teacher moved away. Clarinet lessons began in fourth grade through the school band system in my suburban community; group lessons were taught by our band director. A switch to bassoon occurred in eighth grade, partly to fill a band vacancy from graduation and partly because I liked the instrument's sound and it was a new musical challenge. Participation in school bands filled the elementary years, and I joined my church's youth choir at age 12. Both activities continued throughout high school, with opportunities arising to learn additional instruments (tuba, saxophones) on my own—no formal lessons, just picked it up and tried to make some music! Previous experiences played a major role in gaining facility; any artistry would have to come later. These years also provided a chance to participate in regional youth orchestras, solo and ensemble activities, and competitions. I began to think of a future career in music, thanks to my increasing competence on the bassoon.

Then, as a high-school sophomore, science entered my life. A general biology course began the process, thanks to a thoroughly engaging teacher who made the dryness of scientific words on a page come to life. This was followed immediately by a part-time job in the medical records department of the local hospital. This peripheral introduction into the world of medicine allowed me to observe many local physicians at work, to begin understanding the terminology of medical science, and to gain some insight into the medical lifestyle. The seeds were sown! By the beginning of my senior year, medicine had become a definite career choice. This decision was bolstered by a series of subsequent hospital jobs, from the menial (mopping floors) to the focused (scrubbing in for surgery as a technician and doing preoperative histories and physical examinations). These four hospital jobs lasted for 10 years, through the end of medical school, and introduced me to many more facets of the profession; even as a housekeeping employee, I was welcomed into the pathology lab to observe autopsies by doctors who knew of my interest in medicine as a career! The lockstep process of medical education continued through college premed studies, medical school, and internship (now known as first year residency).

Making music continued all the while. I played and sang throughout college, as well as during vacations from medical school. Ensembles included school and community bands and orchestras, as well as participation in the church choir and some ad hoc barbershop quartet work. Perhaps one of the most enjoyable ensemble experiences occurred during college, playing the saxophones, clarinet, and bass in a small "big band," or jazz band as it's known now. Additional involvement in music included being a classical music deejay for 4 years at my college radio station. Opportunities arose during this time to learn additional instruments (string bass, organ, and banjo), again without formal lessons but drawing on prior musical experience and theory that had accumulated over the years. This acquisition was not without problems, however. As a music teacher colleague reminded me many years later, "You had plenty of chances to develop bad habits." The years that followed certainly proved the truth and wisdom of his statement! Although performance on most of these instruments never reached the level of skill I had developed on bassoon, the enjoyment from playing them (coupled with a bit of income from occasional gigs) softened some of the academic stresses during those years.

A Balancing Act

Juggling two interests and talents as a part of pursuing a health professional's life is a major challenge! Not everyone can be successful in achieving an effective balance, and for a variety of reasons, the arts usually are relegated to second place; the profession—and paycheck—must come first! According to many members of the Association of Concert Bands, 95% of school musicians stop playing their instruments when they leave school [6]. Only some are able to return to their art in later years, and they do so at varying ages.

Many who enter the health professions must curtail their arts activity during their training years and the early stages of a career. Study time, hospital rotations, career responsibilities, and child-rearing all leave little free time! The interval away from music often is long, and when playing or singing is resumed, there must be a period devoted to regaining musical skills, also known as "rust removal" or "getting the chops back." Fingering patterns and flexibility must be regained, embouchure and vocal muscles must be strengthened, and the instruments themselves often require an overhaul after a long period of disuse [7]. The re-entry process into one's art form is unique to each healthcare professional; it will occur at different points in a career, with different opportunities, methods, and rates, as the musician/physician strives once again to attain some sort of life balance between these two often disparate worlds.

For an avocational adult musician, playing opportunities abound. A recent 20-minute search on Google netted an admittedly incomplete list of nine physician symphony orchestras—ranging from those affiliated with medical school organizations [8] to physicians in practice for many years and from local and national groups [9] to a worldwide organization of more than 1000 physician/musicians [10]. What was not included in this search are the myriad community bands and orchestras, as well as chamber, jazz, pop, and choral groups—all of whom welcome musicians of all ages, skills, and experiences.

My own musical activities followed this predictable pattern. There was no time to play during internship, the 4 years of residency, or the first 2 years in private practice. A fortuitous circumstance occurred between internship and residency, though: serving my compulsory 2 years in the US Army Medical Corps at a small Maryland post provided an opportunity for me (and four other officers) to play with the post band for many of its informal performances, something we all did with delight (and varying degrees of expertise). My conducting skills, honed since eighth grade with school pep and jazz bands, also were strengthened by conducting the army band in occasional rehearsals and concerts, plus leading the post-chorus.

My return to music-making during the early years of practice was one of dipping a toe tentatively into the water; it began by playing chamber music (mostly woodwind quintets) every 2–3 months, progressing some years later to also playing weekly with local chamber orchestras. As the rust was shed and I became reacquainted and comfortable with the vagaries and frustrations of bassoon reeds, the returning skills allowed participation in higher-level bands and, ultimately, with several major regional orchestras. The demands of a busy orthopedic and hand surgical practice limited the frequency of my playing during these years, but thanks to an expanding group practice, shared emergency call, and understanding partners, playing the bassoon occupied progressively more of my evenings and weekends. It's hard to remember now the number of rehearsals and concerts I played while wearing two long-range pagers on my belt (in silent mode, of course)! The re-entry process, though, was far from dramatic; indeed, this odyssey took more than 20 years.

Having the Best of Both Worlds

Few health professionals can be heavily involved in both music and medicine; one must take second place, and it usually is music. However, over the past 35 years, a medical specialty has developed which permits a combination of these two disciplines. This movement began in a small fashion, with a few interested physicians, and has developed into a multidisciplinary endeavor known as performing arts medicine (PAM). Combining loves and skills in both music and medicine is an excellent example of how parallel lives can intersect, as PAM not only provides benefits for performers but also helps maintain the musical interests of those treating them. This conjunction may occur sooner or later during a medical career and also can involve people with other artistic backgrounds, including dance and acting.

Using one's arts experiences in the practice of medicine or its related fields can provide significant benefits for the patient. However, it does require extra effort on the practitioner's part. Performers must be identified as such in medical records, and obtaining a useful performance history and physical examination requires developing special lines of questioning [11]. In many cases, additional time must be budgeted for evaluation. Examining a patient with her or his instrument is not only crucial but will demand from the practitioner a knowledge of specialized musical techniques, virtually all of which were never mentioned during medical and graduate training and so must be learned "on the job," as it were. Most PAM professionals become as much students as they are providers.

The average HCP who is involved in PAM, especially those in primary care, is likely to see a wide spectrum of performers; people of all ages, performance specialties, and levels of skill and experience (beginners to professionals) will arrive at the office or clinic. The variety and number of disorders seen will, in general, vary with the practitioner's specialty and area of arts interest. Many choose to concentrate on or limit the performing arts part of their practice to one type of performer; this often reflects their own life experiences and skills.

Knowing the terminology (aka jargon or slang) of the various arts disciplines is most helpful for HCPs when speaking to performers. Terms used in dance are markedly different from those used in music, and both actors and circus performers use yet different arrays of words and phrases to describe details of their own arts. These patients, however, are usually eager to explain the fine points of their profession, such as specifics of terminology and what makes up their special lives. For any HCP, this usually becomes an ongoing type of learning, and my personal experience has been that performers' answers to my many questions filled in large gaps in my personal knowledge base. This led to an improved quality of patient care, which is so dependent upon a full understanding of the patient and how the problem is related to the art.

Personal arts experiences were helpful in so many ways during my practice years. Especially beneficial was the knowledge gained from playing multiple instruments. An example of this involved a 12-year-old boy with an undisplaced wrist (radius) fracture who arrived in the emergency department while I was on call. He told me he needed to play his baritone saxophone in a competition later that day and was fearful that he could not. Being a baritone sax player myself, and knowing the hand/wrist position needed to play the instrument, my cast application was able to hold the wrist and forearm in the proper playing posture while providing appropriate treatment for his injury. He subsequently competed and did well; the fracture was only a nuisance to him that day and ultimately healed without incident.

For those wishing to be clinical researchers and writing or speaking about their arts medicine experiences, the importance of documenting the practice cannot be overstated. One difficulty in doing this is that our specialty is still too young to have developed any real standards for reporting clinical data. Even the definitions and use of terms such as "injury" or "overuse" will vary from one clinician to another [12]. Reporting one's data and comparing it with that of other practitioners requires an awareness of how others are acquiring and managing their data. Common ground is difficult to find. Each practitioner, depending on the nature and epidemiology of the practice, will devise his or her own methods, hopefully with some guidance from other's experiences.

Shifting Gears

When one career is over, life doesn't have to slow down (assuming adequate physical and mental health can be maintained). Certainly, life will—and must—change, and hopefully it will do so for the better. The old aphorism of retiring *from* one thing *to* another never held more true than in the practice of medicine, and the transition becomes much easier when one already has a second area of interest, experience, and/or skill. For many, the termination of a patient practice results in an abundance of unstructured time, ideal for expanding or returning to musical or other arts activities.

The new retiree (or perhaps I should say *transitioner*) has a wide variety of artistic pathways available to further the process; both instrumental and vocal opportunities abound in communities of all sizes, as mentioned earlier. Participating in local bands and orchestras, freelancing (paid or unpaid) for civic groups, and performing in other groups with a wide range of skill levels can satisfy an instrumentalist's desires, while choruses and choirs, as well as small ensemble singing, provide opportunities for vocalists. If medicine still exerts a firm hold on one's interests after patient practice ends, involvement in intersecting areas of medicine remains an option to fill some of the free time; medical education, writing and editing, and even some forms of research can help the years pass with accomplishment and satisfaction. A suggestion: if at all possible, look into some of these options *before* retirement, not after the transition, which usually will be much smoother.

The following is an example of one such transition. Keep in mind that the process of both beginning and ending a career will be unique to the individual. Following retirement from my suburban hand and orthopedic surgical practice, which emphasized treatment of instrumental musicians, I did not stop being a physician but merely changed my types of involvement. Performing arts medicine replaced hand surgery as the new professional emphasis. My orthopedic background was not sidelined, however, since so many musicians' problems involve the musculoskeletal system. Opportunities continued to arise for presenting lectures to physicians and therapists on a variety of arts medicine topics. Thanks to the off-site database of musician patients I developed during my practice years, I was able to write and have published a number of clinical papers. With documentation of nearly 1500 patients, the database proved to be a treasure trove of material, at least for the next 14 years until I ran out of ways to use it. During this time, I also took on the task of enlarging and maintaining the Performing Arts Medicine Association's (PAMA's) bibliography. This engendered an interest in studying and writing about the database itself, resulting in the publishing of several extensive bibliographic reviews [13]. Requests for reviewing and editing manuscripts for arts medicine and other journals provided yet another outlet for continuing my medical interests and kept me more or less up-to-date with current medical literature.

With writing came presentations, to both musical and medical audiences; additional lectures, clinics, and workshops for musicians, music students, and music teachers added to the "workload." Learning to write and speak to vastly different audiences as a scientifically grounded musician was a challenge of a much different kind. In general, musicians weren't (usually) scientists; they didn't understand "doc speak." It was "plain speak" they needed, everyday words and common terms. I had to adjust to using the active tense, not passive; writing and speaking conversationally; and—perhaps the ultimate challenge—doing what the comics call "stand-up": speaking from a bare podium without slides!

Decades of teaching medical and physical therapy students, residents, and military medical staff served as a springboard to becoming a medical consultant to musician organizations in which I already held membership. This was a role not involving diagnosis or treatment but rather acting as facilitator and occasional "booking agent," guiding musicians to sources of effective care, and discussing factors related to instruments I had played. Added to these duties were various administrative and leadership roles, especially with the newly formed PAMA, all of which were performed in a volunteer capacity.

Retirement from practice finally provided the opportunity to say "*NO*" more often to various vocational requests. What a joy it was to be able to set my personal schedule, staying as busy as I wanted to be at the activities I chose. There was time for more music-making in a variety of groups and on different instruments. Although the bassoon had been my first (and current) love, I became intrigued by other low-voiced double reeds. In short order, I added contrabassoon (the bassoon's big brother, which is twice as long and sounds an octave lower), orchestral tuba, and ultimately a legacy double reed instrument now long unused, the contrabass sarrusophone. The contrabassoon ultimately became my primary orchestral instrument, every symphony needs one from time to time, and players are relatively few, so being in demand has been a good thing. The sarrusophone found an occasional place in community concert bands, its deep, brash voice often substituting for tubas and its novelty leading to many surprised looks and comments from musicians and audiences alike.

Most importantly, retirement provided the time to take on a new role as an instrumental music teacher. What began as a favor to a local school band director/friend to mentor and teach one of his bassoon-playing students blossomed into an enjoyable and rewarding part-time job. The challenges of teaching middle- and high-school pupils were a far cry from working with orthopedic surgery residents, but this new role was equally challenging, and past teaching experiences proved most useful. This "second career" as a private teacher of low reed instruments has continued for the past 22 years.

Being able to speak as a music teacher with a significant medical background has made promoting musician health an easy transition away from the purely scientific domain. I incorporate elements of arts medicine into my bassoon lessons, hopefully for my students to gain an appreciation of the "structure and function" involved in making music and to learn preventative techniques that may help keep them playing healthy for a lifetime. So many playing-related problems in both students and older musicians are caused by technical and practice factors, and most physicians and therapists are not that familiar with the vagaries of low reed instruments. It is a blessing to be able to incorporate both musical and medical elements in my teaching.

Aging and the Performer

I've aged during this journey! Time affects us all, regardless of occupation, background, or gender. There are many ways to describe this process, but a useful definition is "the progressive accumulation over time of physical and mental changes that are associated with or responsible for the ever-increasing susceptibility to disease and death which accompanies advancing age" [14]. Most importantly, aging is natural for all of us.

Most people reach their peak functioning level around age 30; this is followed by a downhill course, increasing gradually with advancing years. The rate of progress is different for each of us, as is the sequence of body systems involved. How soon we notice age-related changes in stamina, strength, or sensory perception will vary, based on one's genetics, medical history, and personal health choices. Some age-related complaints are common, while other symptoms aren't caused by aging at all; examples of the latter are noise-induced hearing loss and post-injury degenerative changes [14]. Some common disorders are performance-related, while others are just age-related. Much has been written about performers and aging; PAMA's bibliography contains 110 listings prior to 2014 on this topic [15]!

Aging affects virtually all areas of our bodies.

- Vision: Presbyopia (requiring bifocals and trifocals to see properly), cataracts, macular degeneration, glaucoma.
- Cardiovascular: Stiffening of arterial walls produced by arteriosclerosis leads to, among other problems, decreased cardiac output and increased blood pressure; these changes create a propensity for strokes, heart attacks, and congestive failure.
- Respiratory: Alveoli stiffen; the decreased compliance results in impaired gas exchange, decreased vital capacity, and slower expiratory flow rates; ultimately, many will develop chronic obstructive pulmonary disease (COPD) or pulmonary fibrosis.
- Hearing: Presbyacusis (high-tone conductive hearing loss).
- Neurological: A variety of tremors, balance problems, and cognitive changes [16].
- Dental: Loss of bone support for teeth results in loosening, abnormal motion, and tooth loss; embouchure changes are also common.
- Musculoskeletal: Collagen begins to exhibit degenerative changes in the third decade of life, affecting the bone, cartilage, and other supporting tissues; degenerative joint disease is produced by physical wear and tear; decreased muscle mass results in more rigid and less toned muscles; loss of bone substance (osteoporosis) carries a greatly increased fracture risk [17].

Aging produces a variety of effects on artistic performance. Dance careers are relatively short, primarily due to musculoskeletal difficulties related to both overuse and acute trauma. This is especially true in classical ballet, whereas modern and jazz dancers often continue to perform into their 40s and 50s [18]. Instrumental and vocal careers generally last much longer, and it is not unusual to see high-level musicians performing into their 90s; recent examples of this include cellist Pablo Casals, trumpeter Doc Severinsen, and singer Tony Bennett. Studies confirm the belief that health problems increase with the number of birthdays we observe [19].

Aging affects career professionals and dedicated amateurs alike; in my case, both these categories apply. I began formally making music at age 7 and progressed to playing a variety of instruments, ultimately favoring those with low voice and large size. From college days onward, doubling on two or more instruments meant carrying or wheeling some very heavy loads. Several afflictions (music-related and otherwise) developed during my more than seven decades of playing.

- Hearing: noise-induced hearing loss, tinnitus, and presbyacusis
- Vision: using trifocals (including midrange correction to see the music stand), cataracts, macular degeneration
- Cardiorespiratory: bronchitis/emphysema/COPD; generalized arteriosclerosis
- Musculoskeletal: degenerative arthritis, especially of the hands (basal joint of the left thumb) and spine (spondylolysis and spinal stenosis); bilateral trigger digits and Dupuytren's contracture, a hand deformity characterized by cords and nodules of tissues under the skin

Conclusion

As we persist, we:

- Develop the experience and wisdom of increasing years (greater mileage); it's "not our first rodeo."
- Learn to adjust and compensate—to "make lemonade"—in ways unique to a given individual and his/her specific situation.
- Draw upon our own experiences to deal with our problems and then pass this information to performer patients and students, hopefully helping them develop prevention strategies.
- Recognize that mental exercise, in all forms, is beneficial for brain health, helping to stave off the "ravages of time." Making music, especially learning new material, is but one way to preserve cognitive and performance skills [20, 21]. Many forms of mental exercise are available, not just music; choose the one or a combination that's right for you.

Each person sets and travels his or her own path in life; the determinants of each differ not only among people but are unique to any individual. Some determinants derive from external sources, while others are internal; the result is always a combination of the two. Hopefully, it also will be positive in nature, providing feelings of accomplishment and satisfaction and resulting in some measure of success. Not everyone can claim the type of success Voltaire's *Candide* described as "the best of all possible worlds." However, for me, these intersecting and complementary lives in both music and medicine truly have made this phrase a reality!

References

1. Abrams RM, Griffith K, Huang X. Fetal music perception: the role of sound transmission. Music Percept. 1998;15:307–17.
2. Ilari B. Music and babies: a review of research with implications for music educators. Updat Appl Res Mus Educ. 2002;21(2):17–26. https://doi.org/10.1177/87551233020210020601.
3. Cesario SK, Cesario RJ, Cesario AR. Organized music instruction as a predictor of nursing student success. Nurse Educ. 2013;38:141–6.
4. Dawson WJ. Music lessons do much more than teach "do, re, mi"—their effects are widespread and lifelong. J Assoc Concert Bands. 2012;31(2):26–8.
5. Dawson WJ. Benefits of music training are widespread and lifelong: a bibliographic review of their non-musical effects. Med Probl Perform Art. 2014;29:57–63.
6. Dawson WJ. Rust removal (or, welcome back to the band). Assoc Concert Bands Adv. 2002;20:4–5.
7. Hogan N. Why children quit music. www.nikhilhogan.com. Accessed 5-9-2019.
8. Williams A. Students launch Northwestern Medical Orchestra. Northwestern Medicine News Center. 2018. https://news.feinberg.northwestern.edu/2018/03/students-launch-northwestern-medical-orchestra/. Accessed 20 June 2018.
9. Doctors Orchestral Society of New York. http://www.doctorsorchestra.org. 2018. Accessed 20 June 2018.

10. World Doctors Orchestra. https://www.world-doctors-orchestra.org. 2018. Accessed 14 July 2018.
11. Newmark J, Weinstein MS. A proposed standard music medicine history and physical examination form. Med Probl Perform Art. 1995;10:134–6.
12. Dawson WJ, Charness M, Goode DJ, Lederman RJ, Newmark J. What's in a name— terminologic issues in performing arts medicine. Med Probl Perform Art. 1998;13:45–50.
13. Dawson WJ. Wolfgang Amadeus Mozart – controversies regarding his illnesses and death. Med Probl Perform Art. 2010;25:49–53.
14. Harman D. The aging process. Proc Natl Acad Sci U S A. 1981;78:7124–8.
15. PAMA bibliography. 2018. http://www.artsmed.org/bibliography. Accessed 30 July 2018.
16. Bones O, Plack CJ. Losing the music: aging affects the perception and subcortical neural representation of musical harmony. J Neurosci. 2015;13:4071–80.
17. Boss GR, Seegmiller JE. Age-related physiological changes and their clinical significance. West J Med. 1981;135:434–40.
18. Greben SE. Career transitions in professional dancers. J Dance Med Sci. 2002;6:14–9.
19. Brandfonbrener AG. Old musicians never die: issues of aging in orchestral musicians. Med Probl Perform Art. 2003;18:135–6.
20. Balbag MA, Pedersen NL, Gatz M. Playing a musical instrument as a protective factor against dementia and cognitive impairment: a population-based twin study. Int J Alzheimers Dis. 2014;2014:836748. https://doi.org/10.1155/2014/836748.
21. Moussard A, Bermudez P, Alain C, Tays W, Moreno S. Life-long music practice and executive control in older adults: an event-related potential study. Brain Res. 2016;1642:146–53.

Chapter 4
Current Health Issues of Performing Artists: Implications for Health Promotion

Brandi S. Niemeier and Dawn Larsen

Introduction

Risks for disabling health conditions among professional performers are well-documented [1–16]. Instrumental musicians are at particular risk for physical injuries and playing-related musculoskeletal disorders [2, 8] due, in large part, to cumulative trauma or repetitive strain [9, 10]. Symptoms vary in type and severity, from sporadic tingling to pain and, ultimately, loss of function [10]. Pain is most frequently reported [11], with symptoms and severity differing between performers who play string vs. keyboard instruments [5, 12]. Physical conditions are often exacerbated when musicians perform while injured, and such activities lead to additional risk for chronic strain and permanent disability [12]. Risks for vocal disability and noise-induced hearing loss are also areas of concern and may affect the careers of performers [14, 15].

Health problems are not limited to physical injury, however. Performers may struggle with emotional issues related to anxiety and depression as well as environmental challenges to maintaining good health. In addition, the potential for disordered eating behaviors is elevated. This may be of particular concern among dancers who may be driven by body dissatisfaction and negative performance perception [13], but musicians are also vulnerable to disordered eating [7]. If not addressed, these issues can persist into professional life for not only performers but also teachers [16].

Though a number of the injuries and illnesses commonly experienced by performing artists can lead to disabling or career-ending conditions, many are

B. S. Niemeier (✉)
University of Wisconsin-Whitewater, Whitewater, WI, USA
e-mail: niemeieb@uww.edu

D. Larsen
Minnesota State University-Mankato, Mankato, MN, USA
e-mail: m-dawn.larsen@mnsu.edu

S.-H. Lee et al. (eds.), *Perspectives in Performing Arts Medicine Practice*,
https://doi.org/10.1007/978-3-030-37480-8_4

preventable if addressed early. The purpose of this report is to examine and summarize the current literature addressing the risk factors associated with preventable illnesses and injuries among performing artists. In addition, implications for future research and health promotion practice are considered.

Methods

Using EBSCO*host* and *Academic Search Premier*, we systematically collected peer-reviewed scientific publications, dated 1985–2017, that included empirical evidence of risk factors for preventable illnesses and injuries among performing artists. For the purposes of collecting and reviewing the literature, performing artists included music instrumentalists, vocalists, and dancers.

Primary publications providing experimental or comparative analyses of empirical data related to chronic or preventable illnesses and injuries, or the effectiveness of preventive measures, were retained. The articles were analyzed qualitatively to identify trends in behaviors and health issues among performers and to consider the effectiveness of prevention initiatives or curricular modifications in reducing performance-related health issues.

Results

A total of 24 publications [4, 7, 13–34] were retrieved and used in this review. Musculoskeletal pain and injury, heart disease, and mental and emotional health disorders were identified several times among various contexts of performance [4, 7, 13, 17–22, 24, 28–34]. Other health issues include hearing loss among music performers [14, 26, 27], gastrointestinal problems amid opera performers [15], and respiratory illness [25] and vocal injury among vocalists [16, 23]. Performance-related health issues typically surface when performers are students and may escalate to the point of compromising or ending professional careers. Although preventable or controllable, contributing variables perpetuate if not addressed.

Musculoskeletal Pain and Injury

Problems and pain in the neck and upper extremities regularly impact performers in British symphony orchestras [17], and not surprisingly, the locations of the injuries and pain are consistent with the demands placed on the specific related musculoskeletal areas (e.g., joints, muscles, and tendons primarily used for playing) [17]. Kaufman-Cohen and Ratzon [18] also report significant correlations between upper extremity injuries and the weight of the instrument held to play and the amount of time performing. In most cases, acute injuries are primarily caused by overuse, poor posture, and changes in the technique or intensity of playing [19]. While these injury risk factors are also significant for dancers, most dance injuries are attributed to faulty techniques [19]. Regardless of the type of performer, the extent of injuries is influenced by the length of warm-up times by performers [18, 19]. Tendencies to somaticize, or convert a mental state into physical symptoms, are associated significantly with pain and injury rates [17], although associations between performance anxiety and musculoskeletal problems are not significant [17, 20].

Heart Disease

Although musculoskeletal pain and injuries are well documented, there are other health concerns for performing artists, including elevated risk for chronic diseases [20, 21, 24, 28]. Among reports of heart disease prevalence for performing artists [20, 21, 24], the study by Iñesta et al. [21] provides empirical evidence with the use of heart rate monitors placed on participating performing musicians before, during, and after rehearsals and performances. The results are staggering, indicating that performing musicians experience substantial, even dangerous, increases in heart rates during performances. Further, the type of instrument played is a key contributing factor to the level of heart rate increases [21]. Performers of string instruments, for example, experienced heart rates of 137 beats per minute (bpm) for a sustained period of 12 minutes, on average. Those who played wind instruments had average heart rates of 151 bpm, sustained for 40.6 minutes. Pianists had average heart rates of 167 bpm for 27.5 minutes. The variations in the elevated heart rates and their durations are thought to be related to physical requirements for playing each type of instrument, the lengths of time each type of instrument is typically used during a performance, and whether the instrument is typically played solo or in a group. Musicians in this study had significantly lower heart rates during rehearsals, $p < 0.04$. Also, heart rates during concerts that had been previously performed by the artists were lower although not significantly [21]. The study by Iñesta et al. [21] is compelling but unique; therefore, further study using heart rate monitors is clearly warranted.

Mental and Emotional Health Disorders

Some health concerns and risk factors for performers are directly related to a combination of environmental factors and emotional well-being, according to the studies examined. For example, disordered eating behaviors have been attributed to myriad of factors in performers' training and lifestyle [7], including overly intensified training schedules, tendencies toward perfectionism, and unpredictable work schedules, employment, and income. Travelling performers are regularly faced with erratic routines and unfamiliar places, furthering their tendencies toward cycles of irregular, sometimes infrequent, and often unhealthy eating habits [4, 29, 30]. It has also been suggested that chronic weight loss behaviors in dancers are influenced significantly by body satisfaction regardless of BMI [13]. Furthermore, physical, emotional, and financial demands have been found to lead to loneliness, depression, anxiety, and substance abuse [7].

Other Health Concerns

Professional musicians are nearly four times as likely to develop noise-induced hearing loss as the general public [14]. According to Ginsborg et al., the United Kingdom Musicians Health and Well-Being Survey indicates that 47% of respondents suffered hearing changes. In addition, vocal disability appears to be a problem for 30–55% of young vocalists [23–25]. Although there is little evidence of causal relationships in the current literature, occupational conditions are thought to contribute to hearing loss for all musical performers [26, 27] and to vocal disability in vocalists [14–16, 28].

The presence of occupational hazards and resulting health problems among performers is established among the studies presented. Perhaps more concerning, additional evidence indicates that the problems surface in the early years, during college studies or, even earlier, during training in childhood. On average, 79% of university freshman performing arts students indicate pain each year [31], with up to 100% of students reporting pain among percussionists, followed by woodwinds and brass players (84–87%) and dancers (61%). Of all music students, 37% reported experiencing performance anxiety. Pain among student cellists was attributed to little health awareness, poor playing-related health behaviors, and negative attitudes about injuries [32]. These risk factors led to students avoiding medical attention, performing despite having pain, and, ultimately, furthering their musculoskeletal damage [32].

Spahn et al. [33] also concluded that playing-related health problems begin during college. They compared performance students to other university students and found that the performance students had higher levels of anxiety and more complaints that hampered performance, practice, or studying [33]. Consistent with studies by Brandfonbrener [31] and Rickert et al. [32], the students also had relatively high rates of physical symptoms and depression [33].

In children, playing-related musculoskeletal problems increase cumulatively for each year a young musician plays a particular instrument [34]. Irregular practice times, along with long practice durations, also increase risk [34]. Although relationships between performance anxiety and musculoskeletal problems were not established in adults [17, 20], in children, performance anxiety significantly contributes to musculoskeletal pain and injuries [34].

Discussion and Conclusions

It is apparent that performers' awareness of health issues and prevention practices has improved in the past 30 years, as evidenced by the recent recommendations on neuromusculoskeletal and vocal health, issued by the National Association of Schools of Music and the Performing Arts Medicine Association [28]. However, compromising behaviors persist among performing artists, and the predominant health-related outcomes include musculoskeletal pain and injury, chronic disease risk, and impaired emotional health. While risk factors for musculoskeletal pain and injury are documented consistently, more research is needed to better understand the specific causal relationships between performers' work conditions and health risks. Some studies suggest that the demands of performing, especially among those who travel, along with uncertainties about employment and income, are primary contributors. Although no other reports of studies of biometric measures during performance were available at the time of this current study, the report by Iñesta [21] of the remarkable heart rate elevations during performance provides insight to the suspected increases in chronic disease risk and impaired mental and emotional health. Performance demands, on top of erratic schedules, frequent travel, and job insecurities warrant further investigations of the chronic conditions.

Signs of injuries and illnesses typically develop early, while performers are engaged in formal training. Ginsborg et al. [22] observed that healthful changes in training for performing artists should be made from the earliest stages, so that students learn not only to prevent injuries and avoid other disorders but also to enhance their health and well-being. If appropriate education and support are available in the early years of training, many career-threatening injuries and disorders can be prevented or addressed before they become serious or debilitating. Several levels of prevention can be implemented [22]. Primary prevention involves intervening before the onset of symptoms or risk factors. Secondary *prevention* is focused on early awareness of performance-related problems so they can be addressed promptly and appropriately. If potential threats to overall health are identified early, it is likely that injuries could be reduced and careers extended [22]. Integrating health education and preventive practices into performers' training is, therefore, a strategic and prudent strategy to increase performers' longevity.

Zander et al. [35] illustrated success in integrating a curriculum that promoted positive health behaviors among university performing arts students, noting significant improvements in psychological health. Hackworth [36] attributed improved vocal health and performance successes among students following educational programs in vocal hygiene and behavior modification. Furthermore, Kava [37] found that a simple exercise intervention targeting the strength of the trunk muscles reduced injury risk and minimized pain among performers.

The development of professional training curricula in higher education to address issues specific to this target population is clearly warranted. Topics should include stress management and coping strategies, physical conditioning, strength training with emphasis on the torso muscles, proper recovery from injuries, and, perhaps the most important, integration of health promotion practices into professional schedules. Teachers should adapt curricula to the individual needs of students, realizing that performers often have unique learning styles and that effective teaching strategies may involve more than simply targeting knowledge and awareness. Learning and practicing positive behaviors depends largely on the personalities of students [38] and their frames of mind [35]. Performers who consistently demonstrate proactive approach-seeking behaviors, rather than reactive solution-seeking behaviors when addressing health issues, for example, have overall better health statuses and reduced injuries [35]. Social interactions, typically a top priority for performers, may be a gateway for reinforcing positive health behaviors [38]. Performing artists are, by nature, experiential learners [38]; therefore, teaching strategies should place greater emphasis on practical application and demonstrations of cause and effect relationships that influence health and career success.

Curriculum development and primary preventive strategies should involve multiple stakeholders, such as parents, educational institutions, mentors, and performance instructors [22]. Many music performing arts colleges and university departments recognize that it is important for health promotion to be prioritized within the curriculum. Chesky et al. [3] stressed that universities develop and offer undergraduate "occupational health" courses for performance majors or offer at least one undergraduate course covering occupational health concerns related to performers. Directors of health promotion and health-care resources such as student health centers, physical therapy services, speech and hearing centers, and mental health counseling centers should be aware that performance students may have unique and challenging health issues. Accordingly, students should be made aware that these resources are available and should be accessed if needed.

Frequently, teachers exert the strongest influence on performing arts students [39]. Faculty involved in music performance, education, pedagogy, and dance are extremely influential in determining or changing delivery of curricula. They can also be critical in providing a foundation for the beliefs, attitudes, and values that drive health-related behaviors [39]. Research has supported the value of involving teachers in the prevention of performance-related problems [34, 39–44]. Performance instructors are also uniquely placed to mitigate many of the previously cited risk factors related to musculoskeletal injuries, overuse, stress, fatigue, performance anxiety, and, to a certain extent, disordered eating behaviors. Schools of music should recognize that noise-induced hearing loss is a widespread and serious public health issue and that music is nearly always implicated as a causal factor [26, 27]. Frequently overlooked, this problem should be prioritized to inform students about the risks of hearing impairment. Although prevention strategies may vary by instrument, common strategies include use of ear monitors and avoiding practice or other loud noises (such as a lawnmower) for 16–18 hours after a concert [45].

Teachers can be equally as important in secondary prevention for performance students, noting signs of biomechanical or musculoskeletal injuries requiring early intervention. They may also serve as confidants and advisors for those struggling with anxiety or distress [24, 43, 46]. This dynamic can often help teachers observe early signs and symptoms of both physical and emotional threats to health [47, 48].

Consequently, it is critical that teachers receive guidance about how to react under these circumstances. Mentors and teachers can be fundamental in understanding the conditions under which students seek help and directing students to appropriate health specialists for assistance [42, 48].

References

1. Bosi B. The reality of injuries in a musician's career. Am Music Teach. 2017;67:16–20.
2. Buckley T, Manchester R. Overuse injuries among non-classical recreational instrumentalists. Med Probl Perform Art. 2006;21:80–7.
3. Chesky KS, Dawson WJ, Manchester R. Initial recommendations for schools of music. 2018. http://athletesandthearts.com/health-promotion-in-schools-of-music/. Accessed 20 Jan 2019.
4. Cizek E, Kelly P, Kress K, Mattfeldt-Beman M. Factors affecting healthful eating among touring popular musicians and singers. Med Probl Perform Art. 2016;31(2):63–8. https://doi.org/10.21091/mppa.2016.2013.
5. Davies J, Manginon S. Predictor of pain and other musculoskeletal symptoms among professional instrumental musicians: elucidating specific effect. Med Probl Perform Art. 2002;17:155–68.
6. Fishbein M, Middlestadt S, Ottai V, Straus S, Ellis A. Medical problems among ICSOM musicians: overview of a national survey. Med Probl Perform Art. 1988;3(3):1–8.
7. Kapsetaki ME, Easmon C. Eating disorders in musicians: a survey investigating self-reported eating disorders of musicians. Eat Weight Disord. 2017;24(3):541–9.
8. Abréu-Ramos A, Micheo W. Lifetime prevalence of upper-body musculoskeletal problems in a professional-level symphony orchestra: age, gender and instrument specific results. Med Probl Perform Art. 2007;22(3):97–104.
9. Sadeghi S, Kazemi B, Shooshtari SM. A high prevalence of cumulative trauma disorders in Iranian instrumentalists. BMC Musculoskelet Disord. 2004;5(35):1–5.
10. Fry H. Prevalence of overuse (injury) syndrome in Australian music schools. Br J Ind Med. 1987;44:35–40.
11. Antonopoulo MD, Alegaki AK, Hadjipavlou AG, Lionis CD. Studying the association between musculoskeletal disorders, quality of life and mental health: a primary care pilot study in rural Crete, Greece. BMC Musculoskelet Disord. 2009;10:143. https://doi.org/10.1186/1471-2474-10-143.
12. Kaufman-Cohen Y, Ratzon N. Correlation between risk factors and musculoskeletal disorders among classical musicians. J Occup Med. 2011;61(2):90–5.
13. Gearhart MG, Sugimoto D, Meehan WP III, Stracciolini A. Body satisfaction, performance perception, and weight loss behavior in young female dancers. Med Probs Perform Art. 2018;33(4):225. https://doi.org/10.21091/mppa.2018.4033.
14. Schink T, Kreutz G, Busch V, Pigeot I, Ahrens W. Incidence and relative risk of hearing disorders in professional musicians. Occup Environ Med. 2014;71:472–6.
15. Cammarota G, Mazala G, Cianci R. Reflux symptoms in professional opera choristers. Gastroenterology. 2007;132(3):890–8.
16. Sataloff RT, Hawkshaw MJ, Johnson JL, Ruel B, Wilhelm A, Lurie D. Prevalence of abnormal laryngeal findings in healthy singing teachers. J Voice. 2012;26(5):577–83.
17. Leaver R, Harris EC, Palmer KT. Musculoskeletal pain in elite professional musicians from British symphony orchestras. Occup Med. 2011;61:549–55. https://doi.org/10.1093/occmed/kqr129.
18. Kaufman-Cohen Y, Ratzon NZ. Correlation between risk factors and musculoskeletal disorders among classical musicians. Occup Med. 2011;61:90–5. https://doi.org/10.1093/occmed/kqq196.

19. Rietveld AB. Dancers' and musicians' injuries. Clin Rheumatol. 2013;32:425–34. https://doi.org/10.1007/s10067-013-2184-8.
20. Kenny D. The psychology of music performance anxiety. Oxford, UK: Oxford University Press; 2012.
21. Iñesta C, Terrados N, García D, Pérez JA. Heart rate in professional musicians. J Occup Med Toxicol. 2008;3:16. https://doi.org/10.1186/1745-6673-3-16.
22. Ginsborg J, Spahn C, Williamon A. Health promotion in higher music education. In: MacDonald R, Kreutz G, Mitchell L, editors. Music, health and well-being. Oxford: Oxford University Press; 2012. p. 356–66.
23. Donahue EN, LeBorgne WD, Brehm SB, Weinrich BD. Reported vocal habits of first-year undergraduate musical theatre majors in preprofessional training program: a 10-year retrospective study. J Voice. 2014;28(3):316–23.
24. Kwak PE, Stasney CR, Hathway J, Minard CG, Ongkasuwan J. Knowledge, experience, and anxieties of young classical singers in training. J Voice. 2014;28(2):191–5.
25. Zimmer-Nowicka J, Januszewska-Stanczyk H. Incidence and predisposing factors of common upper respiratory tract infections in vocal students during their professional training. J Voice. 2011;25(4):505–10.
26. Ivory R, Kane R, Diaz RC. Noise-induced hearing loss: a recreational noise perspective. Curr Opin Otolaryngol Head Neck Surg. 2014;22:394–8.
27. Pouryaghoub G, Mehrdad R, Pourhosein S. Noise-induced hearing loss among professional musicians. J Occup Health. 2017;59(1):33–7. https://doi.org/10.1539/joh.16-0217-OA.
28. National Association of Schools of Music & Performing Arts Medicine Association. Information and recommendations for administrators and faculty. 2014. https://nasm.arts-accredit.org/wp-content/uploads/sites/2/2016/02/1_NASM_PAMA_NMH-Admin_and_Faculty_June-2014.pdf. Accessed 27 Dec 2018.
29. Braun DL, Sunday SR, Halmi KA. Psychiatric comorbidity in patients with eating disorders. Psychol Med. 1994;24(4):859–67.
30. Tepas DI. Do eating and drinking habits interact with work schedule variables? Work Stress. 1990;4(3):203–11. https://doi.org/10.1080/02678379008256983.
31. Brandfonbrener AG. History of playing-related pain in 330 university freshman music students. Med Probl Perform Art. 2009;24(3):117–9.
32. Rickert DL, Barrett MS, Ackermann BJ. Are music students fit to play? A case study of health awareness and injury attitudes amongst tertiary student cellists. Int J Music Educ. 2015;33(4):426–41. https://doi.org/10.1177/0255761415582343.
33. Spahn C, Strukely S, Lehmann A. Health conditions, attitudes toward study, and attitudes toward health at the beginning of university study: music students in comparison with other student populations. Med Probs Perform Art. 2004;19(1):26–44.
34. Ranelli S, Smith A, Straker L. The association of music experience, pattern of practice and performance anxiety with playing-related musculoskeletal problems (PRMP) in children learning instrumental music. Int J Music Educ. 2015;33(4):390–412. https://doi.org/10.1177/0255761415597151.
35. Zander R, Voltmer E, Spahn C. Health promotion and prevention in higher music education: results of a longitudinal study. Med Probs Perform Art. 2010;25(2):54–65.
36. Hackworth RS. The effect of vocal hygiene and behavior modification instruction on the self-reported vocal health habits of public school music teachers. Int Soc Music Educ. 2007;25(1):20–30. https://doi.org/10.1177/0255761407074889.
37. Kava KS, Larson CA, Stiller CH, Maher SF. Trunk endurance exercise and the effect on instrumental performance: a preliminary study comparing Pilates exercise and a trunk and proximal upper extremity endurance exercise program. Music Perform Res. 2010;3(1):1–30. ISSN 1755-9219.
38. Schoeb V, Zosso A. You cannot perform music without taking care of your body: a qualitative study on musicians' representation of body and health. Med Probl Perform Art. 2012;27(3):129–36.

39. Guptill CA. The lived experience of professional musicians with playing-related injuries: a phenomenological inquiry. Med Probl Perform Art. 2011;1:84–95.
40. Guptill CA. Performing artists, part 2. Work. 2012;41(1):1–4.
41. Guptill CA, Zaza C. Injury prevention: what music teachers can do. Mus Educ J. 2010;96:28–34.
42. Palac J. Promoting musical health, enhancing musical performance: wellness for music students. Music Educ J. 2008;94:18–22.
43. Petty BE. Health information-seeking behaviours among classically trained singers. J Voice. 2012;26(3):330–5.
44. Ranelli S, Straker L, Smith A. Playing-related musculoskeletal problems in children learning instrumental music: the association between problem location and gender, age, and music exposure factors. Med Probl Perform Art. 2011;26(3):123–39.
45. Chasin M. Musicians and the prevention of hearing loss: an introduction. In: Audiology online. 2008 January. Available via the Articles Archive on http://www.audiologyonline.com.
46. Norton NC, Greasley AE. The BAPAM student advocate scheme: reflections on a health promotion initiative at the University of Leeds. BAPAM J. 2014;2:38–48.
47. Horvath KA. Adopting a healthy approach to instrumental music making. Music Educ J. 2008;94:30–6.
48. Wristen BG. Depression and anxiety in university music students. Updat App Res Music Educ. 2013;31(2):20–7.

Chapter 5
Exploring the Intersections of Arts and Medicine Through the Painters' Lens

Santo V. Nicosia

> ...painters demonstrate (the body) with all the forms of motion, which are infinite, with the shape of limbs, however subtle they may be, and even with the breath itself and the spiritual essence of sight; and that, for greater perfection in demonstrating not only the passion and emotions of the soul but also the events of the future ...
>
> – Giorgio Vasari. *The Lives of the Most Excellent Painters, Sculptors, and Architects* [1, p. xxxv]

Introduction

The relationship between arts and medicine is acknowledged and expressed in multiple ways. While some programs and initiatives focus upon applying arts-based methodologies and skills to medical practice and education, other initiatives focus upon heightening the social and emotional awareness of medical and health professionals through exposure to the arts, and still others aim to place trained artists in healthcare environments to support a patient's overall healthcare experience. Art therapy programs are yet another crossover, where trained therapists utilize arts-based experiences to attain specific therapeutic goals. Of specific relevance to this chapter is performing arts medicine, another distinct combination of arts and medicine, which aims to understand and address the healthcare needs of performing artists. The health conditions of visual and performing artists are customarily expressed, examined, and explained through a medical lens, producing one type of perspective. Instead, this chapter illuminates another dimension of arts and medicine intersections by highlighting the unique portrayal of visual and performing artists, with and without medical conditions, through the lens of a painter.

S. V. Nicosia (✉)
Department of Pathology and Cell Biology, University of South Florida
Morsani College of Medicine, Tampa, FL, USA
e-mail: snicosia@usf.edu

S.-H. Lee et al. (eds.), *Perspectives in Performing Arts Medicine Practice*,
https://doi.org/10.1007/978-3-030-37480-8_5

This exploration is limited to a selective sampling of paintings, classical and modern, and inclusive of primarily Western artists. A predominant focus is upon European artists.

Arts have been a part of human history since late geological times as revealed by prehistoric cave paintings of wild animals demonstrating an innate verve in our ancestors for visualizing life. Instances of medical iconography may be found later in Etruscan, Greek, Roman, Arab, and Byzantine times. These range from manuscript portraits of Hippocrates, Galen, and Avicenna to depictions of wound binding, bandaging, bone dislocations, analysis of urine, and surgical procedures including craniotomy and bladder stone lithotomy [2]. Facets of human reproduction, always a fascinating theme, including childbirth and ectopic pregnancy, have also been illustrated by painters and sculptors from different cultures and times [3].

A more realistic representation of a human body was promoted by the increasing interlinking of visual art and medicine during the Renaissance. The beautifully illustrated *De Humani Corporis Fabrica*, a classic treatise published in 1543, was in fact the result of a close collaboration between anatomist Andrea Vesalius and Titian's pupil Jan Steven van Calcar [4]. During the fifteenth and sixteenth centuries, the Italian polymath Leonardo da Vinci (1452–1519) also produced detailed and well-annotated anatomical drawings that were not discovered until the twentieth century. The painter, sculptor, and architect Michelangelo Buonarroti (1475–1564) experimented with fleshlike beeswax to create three-dimensional and lifelike representations of a human body. Building on anatomical discoveries, art schools of anatomical and pathological waxes flourished in eighteenth-century Florence and Bologna. Arguably, wax models afforded medical students and doctors a comprehension of typical and atypical conditions with a physical immediacy not afforded by fixed organs and tissues as, in addition to tridimensionality, they offered the dimension of color, an essential element to successful macroscopic diagnosis [4]. The contribution of Italian wax modelers to anatomy and pathology is undeniable and is a witness to the Italian genius at a time when participation in gross demonstrations was a proven tool that effectively complemented lectures and book readings [5].

Painting and wax modeling are visual arts and genres of humanities, which investigate human society and culture as well as enlighten the world of medicine [6]. In particular, the study of visual arts as well as performing arts is becoming part of medical and nursing curricula because of emerging evidence that it improves observational and listening skills, teamwork, reflection, and analytical thinking [7, 8]. Visual and performing arts experiences can indeed enhance the healthcare experience and make a better physician by improving observation, reflection, and empathy [9, 10]. Through visual cues from street murals, visual art may also offer opportunities in global health training by teaching medical students how caste, religion, gender, and socioeconomic status may influence human health in different countries [11].

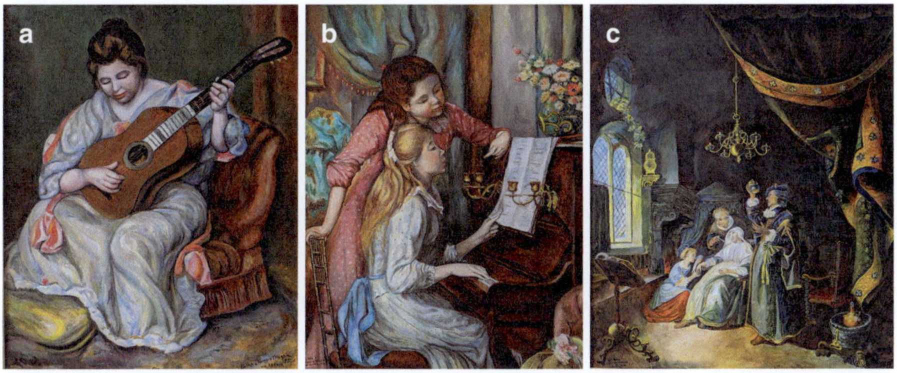

Fig. 5.1 Oil reproductions by Nunzio Nicosia of paintings on performing arts medicine (1995, 1996, 2004, Santo Nicosia private collection). Reproductions are from (**a**) *Woman Playing a Guitar*. (Pierre-Auguste Renoir, 1887, Musée des Beaux Arts, Lyon, France). (**b**) *Young girls at the Piano*. (Pierre-Auguste Renoir, 1892, Metropolitan Museum of Art, New York). (**c**) *The dropsical woman*. (Gerrit Dou, 1663, Louvre Museum, Paris). All figures are two-dimensional reproductions of works of art in the public domain

Henry A. Azar (1927–2008), a Renaissance-type of academic physician, introduced me in the late 1980s to the History of Pathology Society, an international medical organization dedicated to fostering interest in the social and cultural aspects of medicine and allied health sciences. Through many years of service in this society, I have learned how to better understand the human condition. Specifically, I have enjoyed appreciating the use of visual arts in medical pedagogy in eighteenth-century Italy and the artistic inclinations and societal contributions of famous physicians. As a diagnostic pathologist, I am frequently fascinated by the myriad of colorful patterns revealed by microscopy in normal and diseased human tissues. My interest in the intersections of arts and medicine was also kindled by my late father who, during his retirement, produced numerous oil paintings including some reproductions of performing artists and diagnostic physicians (Fig. 5.1a–c).

Depiction of Performing Arts in Paintings

Visual and performing arts create artistic responses to life experiences, the former traditionally interpreted as an extension of fine art and the latter as performances by various artists including dancers, musicians, vocalists, and theatrical actors and actresses [12].

In the context of performing arts, dance serves multiple purposes and functions on different levels from popular community activity (e.g., folk dance) to highly refined professional activity, as in classical ballet [13]. Although it is difficult to

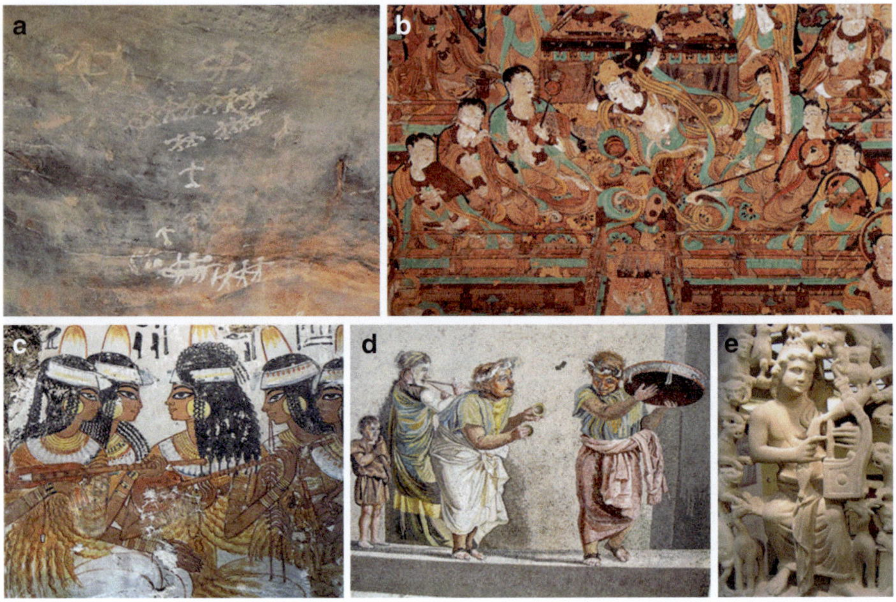

Fig. 5.2 Ancient illustrations of dancers and musical instruments. (**a**) *Mesolithic dancers*. (Bhimbetka rock shelter, Madhya Pradesh's Raisen District, India). (**b**) *Musicians*. (Dunhuang Cave 85, China, Min-Tang Dynasty, ninth century AD). (**c**) *Egyptian lute players*. (Tomb of Nebamun, Thebes, 1350 BC, British Museum, London). (**d**) *Musicians playing aulos, cymbal and tympanum*. (Villa of Cicerone, first century AD, Pompei, Italy). (**e**) *Orpheus with lyre*. (Fourth century AD, Byzantine and Christian Museum, Athens, Greece). All figures are two-dimensional reproductions of works of art in the public domain

pinpoint the exact origins of dance, historians suggest that it is likely to have been present in some form since the beginning of human history. Archeological findings have traced prehistoric dance artifacts from Indian Bhimbetka rock shelters to Egyptian tomb paintings (Fig. 5.2a) [14, p. 57; 15, pp. 39–62]. Europeans traveling to China along the Silk Road knew of dance artworks in the cave temples of China's Mogao at Dunhuang (Fig. 5.2b) [16, pp. 143–55]. Fast forward, dance was a popular performing art in fifteenth-century Italy. Indeed, the French word "ballet" originates from the Renaissance Italian word "balletto," which in turn etymologically derives from Latin "ballare" and Greek "βαλλίζω" (to dance or to jump). Later, France became the epicenter of ballet, while dance performances continued to blossom in Italy and were very successful in imperial Russia [17].

In regard to the performing art of music (from the Greek word "μουσική" for "art of the muse"), man began conveying emotions via the sound of various instruments thousands of years ago. Rudimental end-blown and notch-blown flutes were discovered in Paleolithic caves in the Swabian region of Germany, while conch trumpets and rock gongs were found in Southern France's Marsoulas Cave and in

Nigeria, respectively [18]. It is likely that string instruments, such as the musical bow, were developed in the early Mesolithic period when man also realized that amplification of sound could have been achieved by attaching and stretching strings over bows and boxes [18]. From a visual art viewpoint, paintings of bone and ivory flutes were created during the Upper Paleolithic era when early humans made their first appearance in Europe. Ensemble playing was later depicted in Mesopotamian and Egyptian iconographs (Fig. 5.2c) [18]. *Lyras* (lyres) and the more refined *kitharas* (guitars) were played in Greek and Roman times, and their renditions were depicted in epochal vases. Musical instrumentalist such as *auletes* or flute-players and *syrinx* (trumpet)-players also decorated Greek and Roman vases. Roman artists adorned the villas of wealthy Roman and Greek citizens with murals depicting wind, string, and percussion instruments (Fig. 5.2d, e). Devices (lutes, trumpets, chordophones, tambourines, violin-like instruments, and thumb pianos/lamellaphones or *kalimbas*) similar to modern musical instruments were illustrated in old African, Byzantine, Arabian, and Oriental documents [19]. Beginning with the dulcimer, a series of stringed instruments with an attached keyboard was developed in the early fourteenth century, leading ultimately to the 1789 invention by Bartolomeo Cristofori of the *gravicembalo col piano e forte* (liberally translatable as soft and loud keyboard instrument later called piano) in the Italian city of Padua [19]. Similar to other instruments, famous artworks have been inspired by a love for the piano including famous paintings by Boldini, van Gogh, Cézanne, Klimt, Picasso, and Dalí [20].

Dance and music share similar characteristics including rhythm, skilled precision, and spirituality. These and other features have been portrayed in visual artworks during classic, modern, and contemporary times. Edgar Degas (1834–1917), a member of a seminal group of French impressionists, is remembered for his extraordinary capacity to capture the spirit of dance and dancers' skills in coordinating their movements [21, 22]. These features are well illustrated in his *End of an Arabesque* where the interplay of light and shadows brings to evidence dancers reclining on the stage, floating and hovering atop their legs, outstretching arms, and, at the end of the position, balancing on their legs, one forward and the other behind (Fig. 5.3a).

In French fauvist Henry Matisse's *Dancers II*, the rhythm of dance comes alive. Dancers are performing here around an oval circle that represents the ever-renewing life and dance's eternal movement. The chromatic separation of red, blue, and green colors reinforces the dynamic movement of the dancers superimposed on the Mediterranean Sea and maritime pines. In depicting the dancers joining of hands, Matisse (1869–1954) suggested a common effort in sustaining their rhythmic movement [23].

The Music Lesson is a delightful painting by French Late Baroque "rococo" mannerist Jean-Honoré Fragonard (1732–1806) in which a young woman is seen playing a keyboard percussion instrument (harpsichord) while standing beside is a young man and on a nearby chair a string instrument, a viola (Fig. 5.3b). The

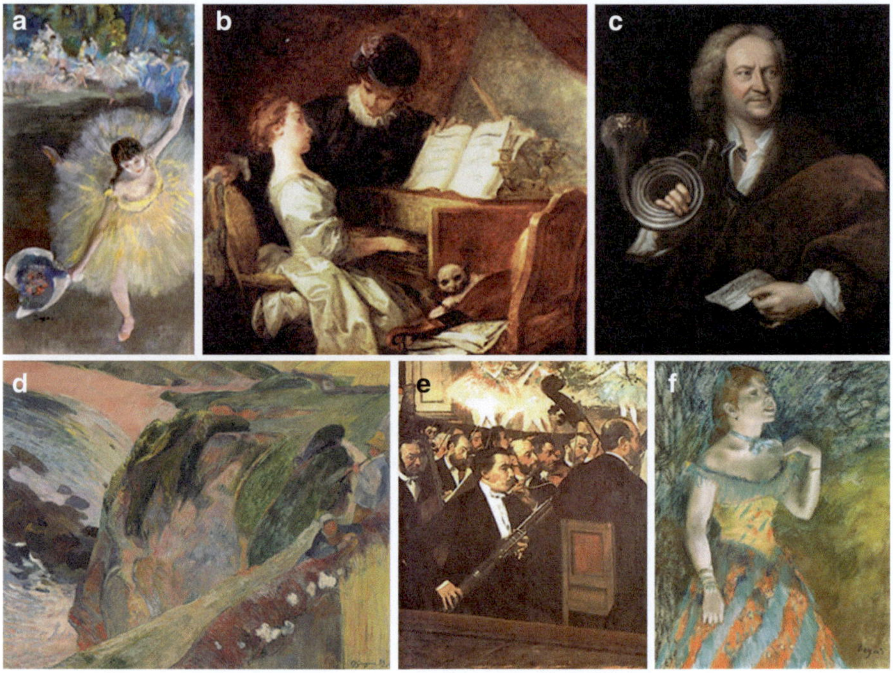

Fig. 5.3 (**a**) *End of an Arabesque*. (Edgar Degas, 1877, Orsay Museum, Paris, France). (**b**) *The Music Lesson*. (Jean-Honoré Fragonard, 1769, Louvre Museum, Paris). (**c**) *Trumpet player* Gottfried Reiche. (Elias Gottlob Haussmann, 1727, Stadtgeschichtliches Museum, Leipzig, Germany). (**d**) *The Flageolet Player on the Cliff*. (Paul Gauguin, 1889, Indianapolis Museum of Art). (**e**) *The Orchestra at the Opera*. (Edgar Degas, 1869, Orsay Museum, Paris). (**f**) *The Singer in Green*. (Edgar Degas, 1884, Metropolitan Museum of Art, New York). All figures are two-dimensional reproductions of works of art in the public domain

concentrated gaze of the woman on the music score suggests attention to musical precision and commitment to the craft. Taken together, the gaze and forward leaning of the man suggest attention to the charm of the woman rather than to her music performance [24].

A stringed instrument, a violin, is depicted by cubist/expressionist Marc Chagall (1887–1985) in *The Fiddler*. A violinist is represented on a rooftop of Chagall's native Russian village of Vitebsk. Color and other elements are utilized to signify the internal struggle of humankind. Of note, the image of a fiddler in a rustic village inspired the character of poor dairyman Tevye in the highly successful 1964 musical Fiddler on the Roof [25].

Wind instruments are portrayed in paintings of different eras. Two of these are by the baroque German painter Elias Gottlob Haussmann (1699–1754) and post-impressionist French painter Paul Gauguin (1848–1903). In the *Trumpet* player, Haussmann depicts Gottfried Reiche, a musician of great virtuosity and popularity in eighteenth-century Germany as surmised by the numerous trumpet parts written for and by him (Fig. 5.3c). The painting is of interest for portraying not only a coiled trumpet but also a sheet of a fanfare allegedly composed for Reiche himself by Johann Sebastian Bach [26]. In *The Flageolet Player on the Cliff*, a boy is playing a flute next to a farmer girl holding a scythe at the periphery of a Mediterranean landscape (Fig. 5.3d). Although peripheral to a dominating patchwork of field and seascape colors, one can almost hear the melody emanating from the flageolet (a French wind instrument member of the flute family). It is likely that in 1889 Gauguin used the sensation of music flowing from the instrument to symbolize his appreciation and love for the harmonies of Breton life [27].

A whole assembly of musicians and instruments (contrabassoon, viola, flute, harp, etc.) is depicted by Degas in *The Orchestra at the Opera* (Fig. 5.3e). His goal, accomplished here by dividing the painting into three segments with the orchestra pit dominating the audience and performers, was to highlight the musicians and not the dancers. In the second rendition of this painting a few years later, Degas expanded the canvas to show the entire bodies of the dancers reflecting an increasing interest in these performing artists [28].

In *The Singer in Green*, Degas exaggerates the vocalist's body features by inverting the normal patterns of light and shadow under her chin, along her neck, and below the collarbones in order to magnify the dynamic and music-driven movement of her body (Fig. 5.3f) [29].

While paintings of performing artists are arguably a predominant domain of French painters, the subject has not been ignored by other visual artists. In over 25 paintings, the Italian futurist Gino Severini (1883–1966) boldly illustrated the dynamic and energetic movements of dancers' legs, arms, and costumes [30]. Expression of energy in dance is also seen in *The Three Dancers* by Spanish futurist Pablo Picasso (1881–1973). Here, one of the dancers is hardly seen, while the other two display a sharply bent head or an abnormally stretched body. Besides conveying extreme movement and energy, the spiked forms of the dancers symbolize the artist's recollection of love, sex, and music [31]. In *The Musicians*, the Colombian figurative artist Fernando Botero (1932–) portrays five men and a woman playing different instruments or singing, respectively. The exaggerated body proportions are all in the style of the artist who likes to accentuate rounded body forms in all his paintings. All figures seem unaware of the sheets of music fallen on the floor; rather their expressions convey a sense of enthusiasm and passion for the entertainment they are creating [32].

Painters' Interpretations of Artists' Injuries

Injury in performing and visual artists can be a consequence of overuse of specific body parts (physical trauma) or to mental stress (emotional trauma). Ankle-foot injuries, including those affecting the Achilles tendon, are most common in dancers [33, 34]. Skin disorders, upper body musculoskeletal injuries, neurological complications, and arthritis are sources of disabilities in instrumental musicians [35, 36]. Oropharyngeal and vocal cord disorders are the source of vocal dysfunction in singers [33]. Emotional and psychological issues can also hinder the activity of artists [37]. Painters, especially during modern and contemporary times, have applied their creativity to illustrate injuries or situations interpretable as risk factors for injuries in performing and visual artists [38].

Dance

Dancers develop extraordinary athletic physical abilities through years of training and performance. The positions that they often assume (dancing in pointe shoes or *sur les pointes*, fifth position, *arabesque*, and *penchée* (among many others)) may, however, pose a risk for acute or chronic injuries. Predisposing factors for injury include improper training, faulty techniques, environmental hazards, foot deformities, and biomedical imbalances [34–37]. Painters of ballerinas have captured aspects of some of these challenging dance positions in their works. For instance, the anatomical feat of aligning both feet in parallel lines but in almost 180° opposite directions (fifth position) is well illustrated in Renoir's *The Dancer* (Fig. 5.4a). Besides the already cited elegant portrait by Degas (Fig. 5.3a), the balance-demanding aspect of the *arabesque en pointe* dance position is colorfully rendered by modern American impressionist Scott Mattlin in the painting *In Flight* (Fig. 5.4b) [39]. Although feet and arm movements are paused in time, both paintings vividly bring to attention the difficult task of balancing on one leg while extending back the other and keeping both arms elevated and stretched to various degrees. As the dynamic nature of this position could not be captured in a static portrait, the

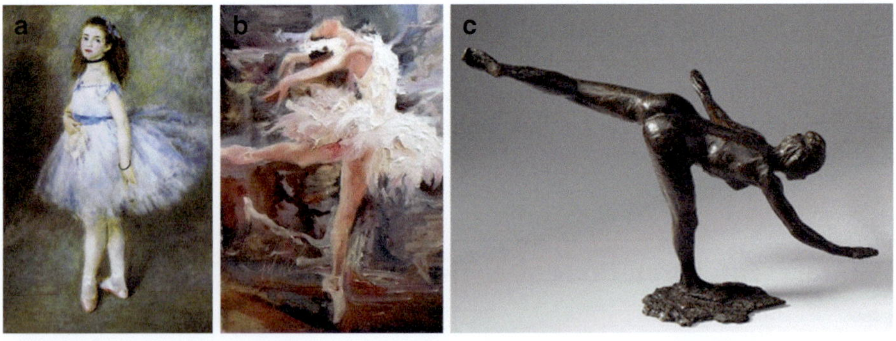

Fig. 5.4 (**a**) *The Dancer*. (Auguste-Pierre Renoir, 1874, Widener Collection, National Gallery of Art, Washington, D.C.) (**b**) *In Flight* (Scott Mattlin, 1955, Arts at Denver Gallery). (**c**) *Arabesque over the Right Leg, First Arabesque Penchée*. (Edgar Degas, 1889–1890), National Gallery of Art, Washington, D.C.). Figures **a** and **c** are two-dimensional reproductions of works of art in the public domain. (Permission to publish **b** has been granted by the artist)

resourceful Degas created wax sculptures of *arabesque*, which he could remodel in different positions using a supporting iron skeleton and cork stoppers for positional joint adjustments; the sculpture was later cast in bronze (Fig. 5.4c). This creative approach allowed for a more realistic demonstration of dexterity and limb motion in dance positions [21]. However, excessive leg stretching and leaning in dancers may excessively load posterior and inferior leg muscles and contribute to the development of related tendinopathies, including those involving hamstring and Achilles tendons. The latter tendon has evoked much curiosity in art and medicine, as detailed in the next section.

Achilles Tendon: Mythology and Pathology

The Achilles tendon is the largest and strongest tendon in the human body that connects the heel bone or calcaneus to the distal parts of the gastrocnemius and soleus muscles (Fig. 5.5a) [40]. Although it has the capacity to withstand weights of up to 2000 pounds during running or 12.5 times the body weight [41, 42], this tendinous structure can become acutely or chronically inflamed and rarely rupture. Rupture of this tendon is rare in dancers, but tendinopathies due to overuse, excessive stretching, or leaping are common in the dance community, especially in dancers with increased lower extremity displacements during takeoff in the *saut de chat* movement [43].

The tendon was described by Hippocrates, but the term "Achilles tendon" was probably assigned by the Flemish/Dutch anatomist Philip Verheyen in his 1693 book *Corporis Humani Anatomia* [44]. Rupture of the Achilles tendon was first described

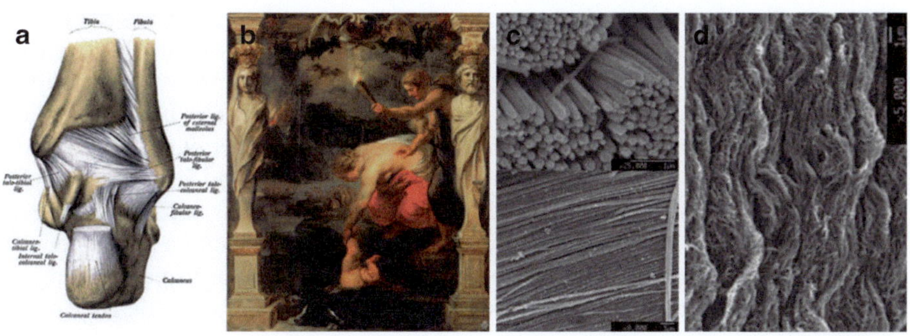

Fig. 5.5 Achilles tendon. (**a**) Anatomical aspects. The Achilles tendon emerges at the distal confluence of the gastrocnemius and soleus muscles and inserts into the calcaneus. (**b**) *Thetis dipping Achilles foot into the Styx river*. (Peter Paul Rubens, 1630–1635, Museum Boijmans Van Beuningen, Rotterdam, the Netherlands). (**c**) Longitudinal section of intact tendon. (**d**). Collagen tendon arrangement during healing. (**c–d**, scanning electron microscopy; 5000× magnification). Figures **a** and **b** are two-dimensional reproductions of works of art in the public domain. (Permission to publish **c**, **d** has been granted by the Oxford University Press)

in France by Ambroise Paré in 1649 [44]. The term "Achilles' heel" may have been first mentioned in the mid-nineteenth century to symbolize weakness or vulnerability based on the Homeric accounting of the modality of Achilles death [45]. Mythology tells us that Achilles' mother, the sea nymph Thetis, conscious of an ominous oracle predicting his son's death in a battle, immersed him in the miraculous waters of the river Styx in order to ensure invulnerability. Out of many pictorial renditions, a painting by the Flemish baroque artist Peter Paul Rubens (1577–1640) vividly visualizes this mythological story and the reason for Achilles' ultimate vulnerability to Paris' arrow at the end of the Trojan War. Here, a full-figured Thetis is seen holding Achilles by his left foot and ankle, while the Ades' ferryman Charon is portrayed in the foreground transporting the dead across the river (Fig. 5.5b) [46].

The mechanisms of human tendinopathies are still under investigational debate. Structurally, the Achilles tendon exhibits a hierarchical structure composed of collagen fascicles, fibers, and fibrils which are axially arranged in parallel arrays (Fig. 5.5c). Swollen and disorganized fibrils (Fig. 5.5d) return to their original fibrous axial arrangement after successful tissue repair [47]. Healing and repair are associated with significant changes in genes related to collagens, inflammation, proliferation, innervation, and tissue matrix remodeling [48].

Michelangelo's Hands

Osteoarthritis is not uncommon in instrumental musicians and dancers because of degenerative changes in the bones of wrist, fingers, and weight-bearing foot joints, respectively [33–36]. Prolonged overuse of hands and fingers can also lead to osteoarthritis in another group of artists traditionally not included in the category of performing artists [49], painters, and sculptors. For instance, a deformative type of injury was illustrated by the Italian mannerist Jacopino del Conte in his portrait of Michelangelo Buonarroti (Fig. 5.6) [50]. In later years, Michelangelo was aware of this condition based on a letter to a friend dated December 28, 1563, where the artist states "…I have received several letters from thee of late to which I have not replied because my hands refused to write" [51]. Although a definitive etiology has not been established (arthritis versus gout), the deformed knuckles and bony protrusions shown in del Conte's painting are likely be the result of arthritis secondary to damaged cartilage [49]. Michelangelo was not hindered by his condition and continued to work in his old age completing, a year before his death, the idealized Rondanini's Pietá and architectural plans for the Western end of Saint Peter's Basilica in Rome.

Emotional Issues

Psychological and emotional issues occur in performing artists and painters. These include anxiety, depression, dissociation, and shame [52]. In 1998, a survey by the International Conference of Symphony and Opera Musicians (ICSOM) reported

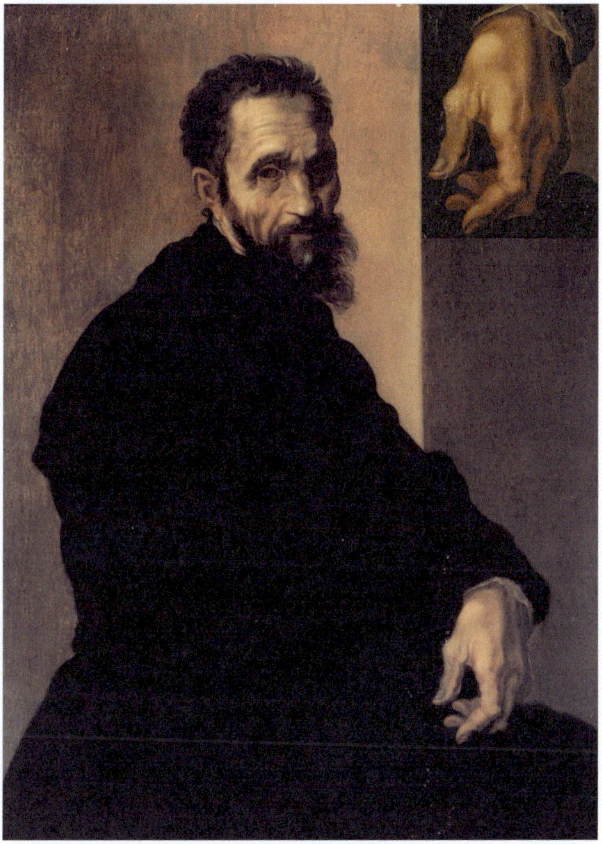

Fig. 5.6 *Michelangelo Buonarroti*. (Jacopino del Conte, ca. 1535, Metropolitan Museum of Art, New York). Portrait details the artist's arthritic hand. Figure is a two-dimensional reproduction of a work of art in the public domain

that 24% of over 2000 musicians suffered of stage fright, while 17% and 13% disclosed depression and acute anxiety, respectively [53]. A more recent Musician's Health Survey reported that over 60% of 447 study participants had experienced anxiety that definitively affected their performance work and that 70% of the ICSOM musicians used beta blockers for performance anxiety [54].

Portraying of emotional issues can also be found in the visual arts. Degas' pastel painting *Waiting* empathetically portrays a ballerina massaging her foot, seemingly exhausted and worried in anticipation of her upcoming stage performance. Next to her is probably her chaperone, an older former dancer herself, representing the saddening reality of a ballerina's career [55] (Fig. 5.7a). In a pastel drawing, *Dancer Stretching*, a ballerina is drawn extending her left arm, touching her forehead with the right hand, closing her eyes, and tilting her head back [56] (Fig. 5.7b). Beyond a literal definition of the drawing's title, such a body language suggests languor and stress from repetitive, perhaps not satisfactorily executed, exercise.

Emotional feelings are also depicted in *The Old Guitarist*, in which Pablo Picasso (1881–1973) exploits blue and other dark colors to signify sadness in an old artist

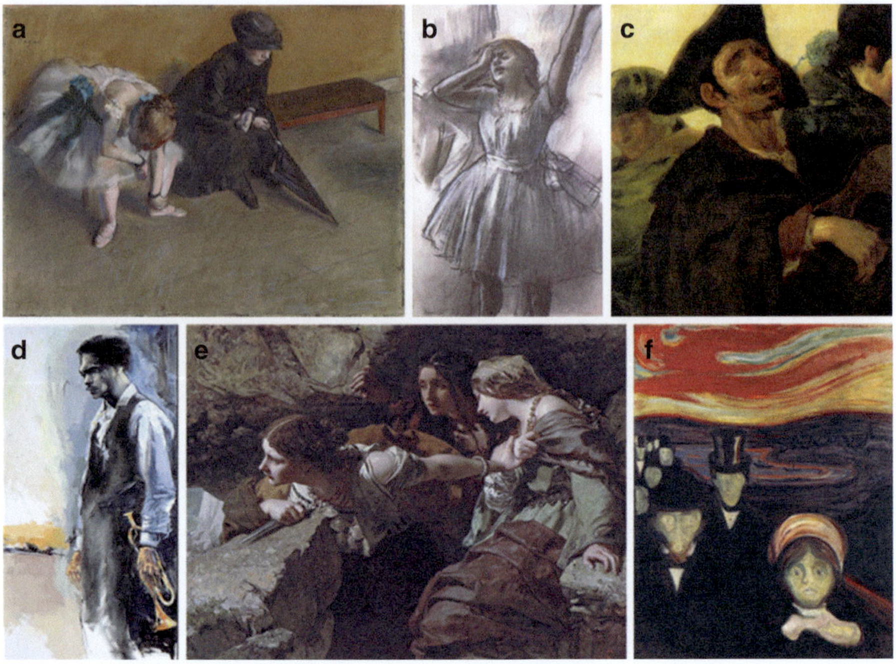

Fig. 5.7 (**a**). *Waiting*. (Edgar Degas, ca. 1882, Norton Simon Collection, J. Paul Getty Museum, Pasadena, Los Angeles). (**b**) *Dancer Stretching*. (Degas, 1882–1885, Kimbell Art Museum, Fort Worth, Texas). (**c**) *The Blind Guitarist*. (Detail from *El Ciego de la Guitarra*, Francisco Goya, 1778, Museo del Prado, Madrid). (**d**) *The Sound*. (Walter Marin, 2011, Pesaro Exhibition, Pesaro, Italy). (**e**) *Courage, Anxiety and Despair – Watching the Battle*. (James Sant, ca. 1850, private collection, England). (**f**) *Anxiety*. (Edvard Munch, 1894, Munch Museum, Oslo, Norway). Figures **a–c** and **e**, **f** are two-dimensional reproductions of works of art in the public domain. (Permission to publish **d** has been granted by the artist)

playing a stringed instrument, ostensibly without a strength to live. The hunched posture and the sagging hand of the guitarist signify a lifeless sense of weight and accentuate the psychological themes of human misery and alienation [57]. Goya's oil painting *The Blind Guitarist* also evokes sentiments of emotion and intense performance similar to those that may be observed in contemporary instrumentalists (Fig. 5.7c) [58].

The incidence of overuse disorders is rising in instrumental musicians [59]. Two major forces in the world of music have been pianists Leon Fleisher and Vladimir Horowitz. At the age of 35, Fleisher was forced to interrupt his piano career due to the fourth and fifth fingers on his right hand involuntarily curling into his palm, a classical presentation of focal dystonia [60]. In the 1940s, the virtuoso pianist Vladimir Horowitz begun to have his own share of problems (depression, alcoholism, memory lapses, and loss of physical control); these were managed with electroshock and other medical therapies but not always successfully, causing interruption of performances and eventual end of an otherwise dazzling career [61].

Vocal injuries are mostly secondary to excessive singing and comprise vocal hemorrhage, tears, bruises, vocal nodules, cysts, polyps, and granulomas [33]. Famous singers have been silenced, temporarily or permanently, from such pathologies. Vocal nodules affected Luciano Pavarotti, Frank Sinatra, and Elton John, whose voices became deeper after surgery. The singing career of Julie Andrews came to an end after unsuccessful surgery for throat nodules. The contemporary British singer Adele developed vocal cord hemorrhages causing tour cancelations before successful phonomicroscopy surgery [62, 63]. An anonymous cartoon illustrates the singer's drama through sets of irregular wheels abnormally rotating inside her windpipe [62].

Lip injuries, hypersensitivity pneumonitis, dystonia, overuse syndrome, depression, and substance abuse represent physical and psychological injuries that may affect wind instrumentalists [35, 36, 64]. A state of depression can be surmised in *The Sound*, a painting by contemporary Italian visual artists Walter Marin said to portray the great jazz protagonist Miles Davis (Fig. 5.7d) [65].

Life experience is a common theme in almost all paintings, sketches, and drawings of naïve-style Mexican visual artist Frida Kahlo (1907–1954) [66, 67]. The wreckage of her body after a terrifying traffic accident is portrayed in stark details in *The Broken Column*. To represent the effects of a piercing iron rod, the multiple bone fractures, and her recovery in a full body cast, here she portrays herself both as a complete and a broken woman with her body partially naked, split down the middle, her skin dotted, and her spine painted as a broken ornamental column [66].

Anxiety consists of an overwhelming sense of apprehensive uneasiness, frequently associated with physical changes, which can be observed in artists. This emotion has been portrayed in paintings not specifically associated with performing artists such as in *The Scream* and *Anxiety* by Norwegian painter Edvard Munch [68]. The latter painting depicts the mental state of an anxious artist and the alienation in people around him. In some artists, anxiety and mental illness may spawn creativity and without them art may indeed be diminished [69]. Anxiety is also portrayed in another *Anxiety* painting by the American figurative artist Mary Woronov, a contemporary actress, writer, and painter (1943–) [69]. It has been said that "…when it comes to mental health…the aesthetic elements of the (visual) art will never be diminished by the message, whether it is happiness, sadness, stress, or anger" [70]. Courage and despair are not commonly associated with anxiety, yet the coexistence of these three emotions is portrayed in James Sant's 1820 painting *Courage, Anxiety and Despair* by three women watching a battle. Here, the English artist seems to tell us that at some time point in human life strong-mindedness and resilience may represent hidden powers as also suggested by others in regard to anxious individuals [71].

Artworks by Artists with Disabilities

In contrast to "disability arts" in which disabilities represent the central theme, "disability in the arts" refers to artistic productions by people with disabilities [72, 73]. A classic example of the first concept is illustrated in *The Cripples*, a painting by sixteenth-century Flemish artist Pieter Bruegel the Elder (Fig. 5.8a). Here, disabled beggars are shown with crutch-like extensions against a background of green grass and red brick walls exposing human physical impairment [74]. A more modern (1994) representation of disability and an attestation of heightened cultural awareness toward people with disabilities are found in *Latino Woman Dancing in Wheelchair*, part of an extensive and colorful assembly of murals created by seven gifted female artists in a San Francisco's Mission District building that celebrates women's worldwide artistic contributions [75].

Artists with disabilities have willed to humanity the gift of their creativity in the face of their conditions [76–78]. The list is long and comprises musicians, vocalists, dancers, and visual artists. A few of them are briefly mentioned here before a discussion of works by representative visual artists. Ludwig van Beethoven wrote immortal music compositions throughout many years of hearing loss. Chuck Close painted while having quadriplegia and learning disabilities. Violinist Itzhak Perlman suavely played the violin while dealing with the sequelae of poliomyelitis. Blindness affected singers and piano players Ray Charles and Stevie Wonder. Mary Verdi-Fletcher, a woman born with spina bifida, practiced dance and founded Dancing Wheels, a premier physically integrated

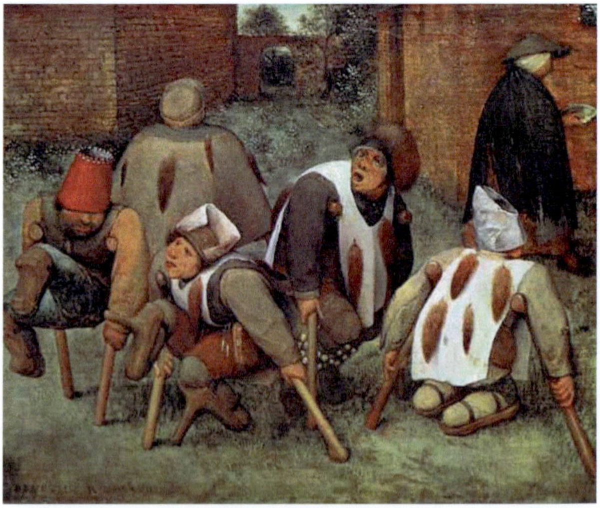

Fig. 5.8 Disability arts. *The Cripples*. (Pieter Bruegel the Elder, 1568, Louvre Museum, Paris). Figure is a two-dimensional reproduction of a work of art in the public domain

dance company [78]. Below-the-knee amputee Lisa Bufano performed many acclaimed dance choreographies before taking her own life at the age of 41. Besides arthritis in his later years, Michelangelo coped with bipolar disorder. Cataracts severely impaired the vision of Claude Monet. Pierre-Auguste Renoir and Vincent van Gogh continued to paint in spite of rheumatoid arthritis and severe auditory hallucinations, respectively. Edgar Degas, the iconic painter of ballerinas, dealt with progressive bilateral central visual loss and photophobia since his teen years which progressively worsened after his mid-30s. He commented on expecting to "...remain in the ranks of the infirm until I pass into the ranks of the blind," and his creative approach to address this limitation was to use less accurate pastels rather than oil, larger canvases to magnify his field of view, and empty areas at the periphery of paintings [79]. Blind visual artist have

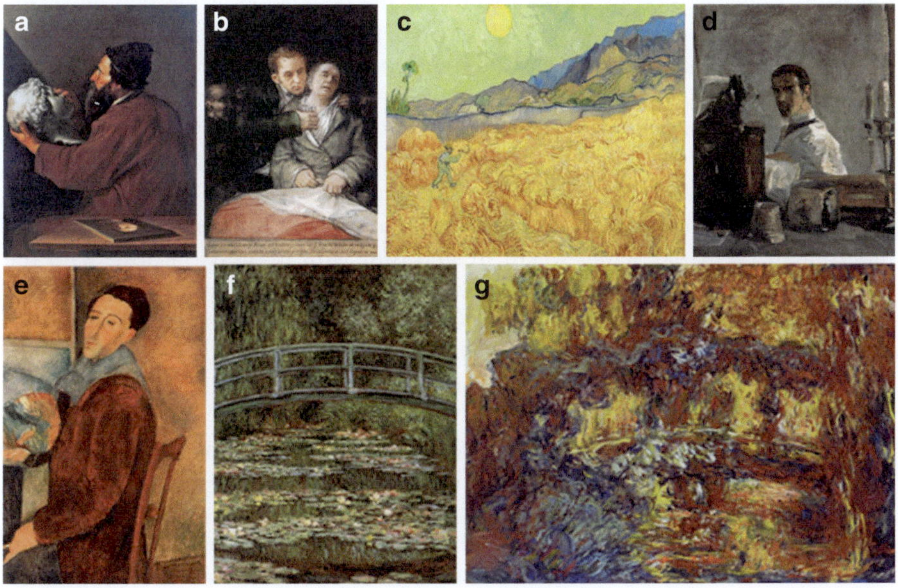

Fig. 5.9 Disabilities in the arts. (**a**) *The Sense of Touch* (portrait of Italian sculptor Giovanni Gonnelli by Jusepe de Ribera, ca. 1615–1616, the Norton Simon Foundation, Pasadena, California). (**b**) *Self-portrait with Dr. Arrieta* (Francisco Goya, 1820, Minneapolis Institute of Art, Minneapolis, MN). (**c**) *Wheatfield with Reaper* (Vincent van Gogh, 1889, Van Gogh Museum, Amsterdam, the Netherlands). (**d**) *Self-portrait in front of a mirror* (Henri de Toulouse-Lautrec, 1882–1883, Toulouse-Lautrec Museum, Albi, France). (**e**) *Self-portrait* (Amedeo Modigliani, 1919, Museum of Contemporary Arts, São Paulo, Brazil). (**f**) *The Japanese Footbridge* (Claude Monet, 1899, National Gallery of Art, Washington, D.C.). (**g**) *The Japanese Footbridge* (Claude Monet 1920–1922, Museum of Modern Art, New York). All figures are two-dimensional reproductions of works of art in the public domain

developed what is referred as a sixth sense that makes them capable of capturing surrounding realities and transferring into a visual medium. These gifted artists have never ceased to marvel and inspire from distant past to contemporary times. In 1630, José de Ribera's portrayed one of such artists, the sculptor Giovanni Gonnelli, in a painting from "The Four Senses" series [80]. Here, the blindman is shown while "feeling" the contours of a man's head as a preliminary step to painting his portrait (Fig. 5.9a).

The romantic painter Francisco Goya (1746–1828) experienced many conditions including dizziness and transient paralysis attributed by most experts to neurosyphilis and accompanied by general malaise and depression [81]. He was treated by Dr. Eugenio Garcia Arrieta to whom Goya dedicated *Self-portrait with Dr. Arrieta*, a painting where medical care, empathy, and gravity of illness are emphasized by the doctor standing behind and caringly administering a medication to the disheveled artist and by two grim female faces (Fig. 5.9b). The sensation of empathy is also underscored by Goya's words in the dedication at the bottom of the painting "Goya in gratitude to his friend Arrieta for the skill and great care with which he saved his life in his acute and dangerous illness, suffered at the end of 1819 at the age of 73 years" [81].

Post-impressionist Dutch painter Vincent van Gogh (1853–1890) experienced delusions, seizures secondary to temporal lobe epilepsy, and manic depressive mood and mental breakdowns aggravated by addiction to alcohol, smoking, and chemicals [82]. His creative, but tortured, life ended in suicide at the young age of 37. A physician treated him with digitalis, a drug with the disturbing side effect of seeing yellow spots. It has been speculated that this may have been the reason behind van Gogh' s predilection for the color yellow in his depictions of landscapes as in *Wheatfield with a Reaper* (Fig. 5.9c). Mental illness and creativity indeed converged in this quintessential and misunderstood artistic genius!

Henri de Toulouse-Lautrec (1864–1901), a post-impressionist French painter, bore skeletal defects whose etiology has been attributed to a rare autosomal recessive lysosomal storage bone disease (pycnodysostosis) associated with short legs, a normal trunk, pathologic bone fractures, and other abnormalities [83, 84]. He professed to be the life at the cafés of Montmartre where indeed he enjoyed the company of artists, dancers, and bohemians, but depression and alcohol addiction were not strangers to him. Because of comprehensible self-consciousness, no clue is given of his marred growth in *Self-portrait in front of a mirror* (Fig. 5.9d).

The Italian expressionist Amedeo Modigliani (1884–1920) abused hashish and absinthe, additions likely developed for alleviating pain and concealing his "great secret," the then incurable tuberculosis and cause of his early death [85]. In his *Self-portrait* (1919), Modigliani depicts himself pallid, with hollowed cheeks and sealed lips, all physical signs that unmask his disease and lifestyle (Fig. 5.9e). The striking hues of the portrait have also been interpreted as representative of Modigliani's tuberculous complexion [86].

Because of their characteristic and perhaps undefined style, artists of the impressionistic genre were thought to suffer from ocular ailments from myopia to cataract and even aphakia (absence of the eye's lens) [87]. The result of these conditions may be surmised in two paintings with similar titles, *The Japanese Footbridge*, but executed at distant times of Clause Monet's life. In the 1899 painting, a blue-green bridge over a flowery water garden is clearly defined, while, in a companion painting done 30 years later, thick swirls and indistinct strokes of various colors obscure the form of bridge and pond (Fig. 5.9e, f).

The naïf artist Frida Kahlo (1907–1954) developed poliomyelitis as a child and suffered a crippling and almost fatal bus accident during her teens that fractured her clavicle, ribs, spinal column, and pelvis [66]. These injuries necessitated the use of a body cast in normal life and while painting. Besides the artistic rendition of her painful moments in the already cited *The Broken Column* (section "Emotional Issues"), she produced over a hundred paintings revealing duality in personal identity, alienation, political ideology, strategy for alleviating pain, influence of photography, and pride in her indigenous heritage. All these sentiments pervade the painting titled *Self-portrait on the Border of Mexico and the United States* [88]. It may be useful to ponder on the actuality of this work in reference to current political issues between the two countries and their policies.

Painting provided a way to Lisa Fittipaldi (1948–) to find herself after losing the ability to see. She understood that painting her storehouse of memories was both a source of emotional nourishment and a way to keep her world alive. According to the artist, images in her mind's eye became clearer as her sight diminished; she asserted that "…by hearing or experiencing something, I can picture it in my head and paint it" [89]. She went on to develop in 1999 the Mind's Eye Foundation, a nonprofit charity educating the public and advocating for visually and hearing-impaired children [90]. Even if some perception of images may exist, it is remarkable how blind artists can maintain insight, probably through recollection of light and forms.

Inspired by Frida Kahlo, the living poet and painter Dilly Ward Bundy has created a series of paintings depicting her struggle with injured feet, torn Achilles tendon, and a marred spinal column requiring plaster corsets for support. As expressed by her, "tearing an Achilles tendon is no joke, particularly when trying to juggle life as wife, mother and art student" [91]. Images in her paintings project the pain and frustration resulting from an injured body and a sense of internment with "…ideas of the corseted body, my breast endeavoring to escape and the plastered foot hovering over my hidden but damaged heart" (Fig. 5.10a, b).

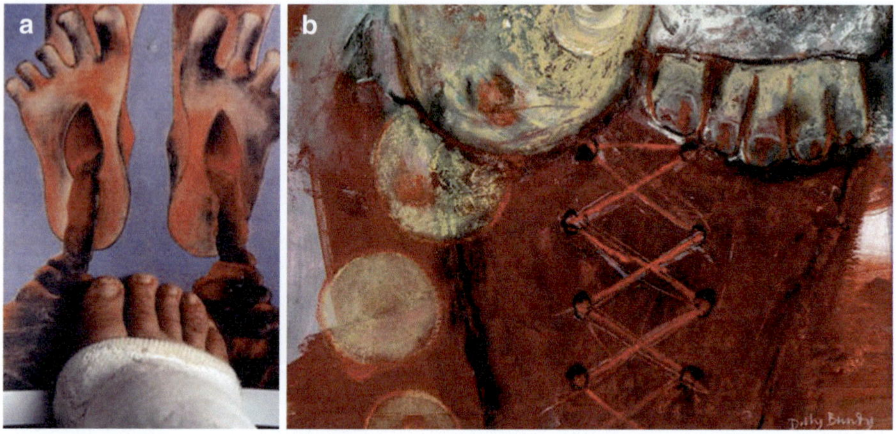

Fig. 5.10 Foot injury series. (**a**) *Pain and frustration associated with damaged foot and ankle*. (**b**) *Sense of confinement* (Dilly Ward Bundy, 1993, mixed media on paper, artist collection). (Permission to publish both figures has been granted by the artist)

Conclusions

As artists pursue their avocation, physical injury and mental strain can represent significant challenges [92]. Even so, injury is not always a hindering factor, thanks to the plasticity of physical and neurological body systems and their responsiveness to necessary therapeutic interventions as well as the creativity of the human spirit [93]. The agony and ecstasy of performing artists are indeed reflected in the words of renowned dancer Mikhail Baryshnikov commenting on the inevitability of injury and the road to recovery: "The more injuries you get, the smarter you get" and "Your body reminds you about your injuries as the body has a stronger memory than your mind" [94].

Navigating afflictions of various kinds is an inherently human endeavor drawn from the multitude and diversity of human experience. Addressing afflictions may be facilitated via the contemplation or even creation of provocative paintings that interpret experiences of artists in healthy and injury states [95, 96]. As the lives of many artists exemplify, the supposed "limitations" of these afflictions often promote new and otherwise unknown types of artistic creation, thoughtful content, and new possibilities.

Unlike a medical diagnosis, art can vividly capture the multifaceted dimensions of human health. This chapter has given a glimpse into the life experiences of visual and performing artists as portrayed through the lenses of different painters. The intersection of creative arts and health outcomes is under increasing investigation [12, pp. 317–18]. Further insight into the role of the arts in wellness and medical conditions will provide a complementary tool to therapeutics and set a unique holistic trajectory toward a healthier future.

Acknowledgments Images from Fig. 5.1a–c were obtained from the author's collection of painting reproductions inherited by his father. Other images are two-dimensional reproductions of works of art in the public domain except for Figs. 5.4b, 5.5c–d, 5.7d, and 5.10a, b. Permissions to publish these last images have been granted by Oxford University Press, License # 4607041200274, June 13, 2019, and authors' permissions (Mr. Scott Mattlin, email dated August 10, 2019; Mr. Walter Marin, email dated October 15, 2019; and Ms. Dilly Ward Bundy, email dated June 13, 2019), respectively. I am grateful to Professor Sang-Hie Lee for the invitation to participate, as co-editor and chapter contributor, to the making of this book. I am also indebted to Professor Merry Lynn Morris for insightful comments and constructive revision of this chapter.

References

1. Vasari G. The lives of the most excellent painters, sculptors, and architects (translated by Gaston du C. de Vere). New York: Modern Library, Random House Publishing Group; 2006. p. xxxv.
2. Antiqua Medicina – From Homer to Vesalius. Historical Collections at the Claude Moore Health Sciences of the University of Virginia, Charlottesville, VA. http://exhibits.hsl.virginia.edu/antiqua/instruments/. Accessed May 15, 2019.
3. Petraglia F, Bettini M. Human reproduction in art: from myths to history. Reprod Sci. 2010;17:711–7.
4. Nicosia SV. Anatomical waxes in 18th century Italy. History of pathology society companion meeting, 2006, Atlanta, USA. https://anatomiaitaliana.com/wp-content/uploads/2017/09/AnatomicalWaxes18thCentury.pdf. Accessed 23 Apr 2019.
5. Brandon AS. Artful Italy: the hidden treasures. Montpelier: Invisible Cities Press; 2002. p. 134–45.
6. Kaptein AA, Meulenberg F, Smyth JM. A breath of fresh air: images of respiratory illness, poems, films, music and paintings. J Health Psychol. 2015;20:246–58.
7. Bramstedt KA. The use of visual arts as a window to diagnosing medical pathologies. AMA J Ethics. 2016;18:843–54.
8. Fletcher KA, Bedwell WL, Voeller M, Coe D, Morris ML, Marsh B, Zambroski C. Art of critical thinking in nursing: a novel multi-modal humanities curriculum. Med Sci Educ. 2018;28:27–9.
9. Chambers M. Integrating arts planning into healthcare design. In: Lambert P, editor. Managing arts programs in healthcare. London: Routledge; 2016. p. 47–64.
10. Gowda D, Dubroff R, Willieme A, Swan-Sin A, Capello C. Arts as sanctuary: a four-year mixed-methods evaluation of a visual art course addressing uncertainty through reflection. Acad Med. 2018;93:S8–13.
11. Allison J, Mulay S, Kidd M. Life in unexpected places: employing visual thinking strategies in global health training. Educ Health. 2017;30:64–7.
12. Biggs M, Karlsson H. The Routledge companion to research in the arts. New York: Routledge Taylor & Francis Group; 2011. p. 317–8.
13. Mackrell J. "Dance". http://www.britannica.com/EBchecked/topic/150714/dance. Accessed 17 May 2019.
14. Varadpande ML. History of Indian theatre, vol. 1. New Delhi: Abhinav Publications; 1987. p. 57.
15. Kassing G. History of dance. 2nd ed. Champaign: Human Kinetics; 2017. p. 39–62.
16. Whitfield R, Whitfield S, Agnew N. Cave temples of Mogao at Dunhuang: art and history on the silk road. 2nd ed. Los Angeles: Getty Publications; 2015. p. 143–55.
17. Ballet in Italy. https://www.bvevents.com/Travel-And-Culture-News-From-Italy/Ballet-in-Italy-history-stars-etoiles/. Accessed 7 May 2019.

18. Montagu J. How music and instruments began: a brief overview of the origin and entire development of music, from is earliest stages. Front Sociol. 2017; https://doi.org/10.3389/fsoc.2017.00008. Accessed 23 June 2019.
19. Summers D, O'Rourke-Jones R. Music: the definitive visual history. London: Dorling Kindersley; 2015.
20. Iadanza S. The Piano – a common subject in famous paintings. 2018. https://simplymusic.com/piano-common-subject-famous-paintings/. Accessed 21 May 2019.
21. Edgar Degas. https://www.nga.gov/content/dam/ngaweb/Education/learning-resources/an-eye-for-art/AnEyeforArt-EdgarDegas.pdf. Accessed 24 Nov 2018.
22. Richman-Abdou K. Degas' dancers: how ballerinas inspired then iconic impressionist artist. Retrieved from https://mymodernmet.com/edgar-degas-dancers/.
23. Matisse H, Girard X. La Danse, Cahiers Henry Matisse, vol. 10. 1st ed: La Malmaison; 1993.
24. Sfetcu N. Louvre: Fragonard – the music lesson. https://www.setthings.com/en/lovre-fragonard-music-lesson/. Accessed 23 Oct 2018.
25. Blessing, J. Green violinist. Solomon R. Guggenheim museum. https://www.guggenheim.org/artwork/802. Accessed 29 Apr 2019.
26. Collins TA. Gottfried Reiche: a more complete biography. JSTOR. 1988;19:4–18.
27. The flageolet player on the cliff. https://en.wikipedia.org/w/index.php?title=The_Flageolet_Player_on_the_Cliff&oldid=847030170. Accessed 30 Apr 2019.
28. The Orchestra at the Opera by Degas. https://www.impressionists.org/the-orchestra-of-the-opera.jsp. Accessed 30 Apr 2019.
29. Tong D. How do the elements of color and light contribute into the portrayal of flesh. p. 1–17. http://theaaaartdept.com/A_Level_Personal_Studies_files/Colour%20Light%20Flesh.pdf. Accessed 16 June 2019.
30. How to draw and paint dancers. https://www.worlddanceheritage.org/how-to-draw-dancers/. Accessed 16 May 2019.
31. Tate Gallery – The three dancers. https://www.tate.org.uk/art/artworks/picasso-the-three-dancers-t00729. Accessed 6 May 2019.
32. Botero – the musicians. https://www.aaronartprints.org/botero-themusicians.php. Accessed 6 May 2019.
33. Ostwald PF, Baron BC, Byl NM, Wilson FR. Performing arts medicine. West I Med. 1994;160:48–52.
34. Bronner S, Brownstein B. Profile of dance injuries in a broadway show: a discussion of issues in dance medicine epidemiology. J Orthop Sports Phys Ther. 1997;126:87–94.
35. Kok LM, Huisstede BMA, Voo VM, Schoones JW, Nelissen RGH. The occurrence of musculoskeletal complaints among professional musicians: a systematic review. Int Arch Occup Environ Health. 2016;89:373–96.
36. Schaefer PT, Speier J. Common problems of instrumental athletes. Curr Sports Med Rep. 2012;11:316–22.
37. Russell JA. Preventing dance injuries: current perspectives. Open Access J Sports Med. 2013;4:199–210.
38. Kulasekara D. Representation of trauma in contemporary arts. Athens J Human Arts. 2017;4:35–60.
39. Scott Mattlin. 1955. https://www.tuttartpitturasculturapoesiamusica.com/2011/05/scott-mattlin.html. Accessed 25 May 2019.
40. Calcaneal tendon. https://ca.wikipedia.org/wiki/Tendó_d%27aquilles. Accessed 24 February 2020.
41. Doral MN, Alam M, Bozkurt M, Turhan E, Atay OA, Donmez G, Maffulli N. Functional anatomy of the Achilles tendon. Knee Surg Sports Traumatol Arthrosc. 2010;18:638–43.

42. Freedman BR, Gordon JA, Soslowsky LJ. The Achilles tendon: fundamental properties mechanisms governing healing. Muscles Ligaments Tendons J. 2014;4:245–55.
43. Kulig K, Loudon JK, Popovich JM, Pollard CD, Winder BR. Dancers with Achilles tendinopathy demonstrate altered lower extremity takeoff kinematics. J Orthoped Sports Phys Ther. 2011;41:606–13.
44. Suy R. Philip Verheyen and his corporis humani anatomia. Acta Chir Belg. 2007;107:343–54.
45. Klenerman. The early history of tendo Achillis and its rupture. J Bone Joint Surg Br. 2007;89:545–7.
46. Achilles' heel. https://en.wikipedia.org/wiki/Achilles%27_heel. Accessed 15 May 2019.
47. Sasaki K, Yamamoto N, Kiyosawa T, Sekido M. The role of collagen arrangement changes during tendon healing demonstrated by scanning electron microscopy. J Electron Microsc. (Tokyo). 2012;61:327–34.
48. Klatte-Shulz F, Minkwitz S, Schmock A, Bormann N, Kurtoglu A, Tsilonis S, Manegold S, Wildemann B. Different Achilles tendon pathologies show distinct histological and molecular characteristics. Int J Mol Sci. 2018;19:404–21.
49. Artists and arts workers in the United States: findings from the American Community Survey (2005–2009) and the Quarterly Census of Employment and Wages (2010). National Endowment for the Arts. NEA Research Note # 105, October 2011, p. 5.
50. Lazzeri D, Castello MF, Matuci-Cerinic M, Lippi D, Weisz G. Osteoarthritis in the hands of Michelangelo Buonarroti. J R Soc Med. 2016;109:180–3.
51. Ramsden EH. The letters of Michelangelo. Stanford University Press. 1963;2:153–211.
52. Thomson P, Jaque SV. Posttraumatic stress disorder and psychopathology in dancers. Posttraumatic stress disorder and psychopathology in dancers. Med Probl Perform Art. 2015;30:157–62.
53. Matei R, Ginsberg J. Music performance anxiety in classical musicians – what we know ow about what works. BJ Psych Int. 2017;14:33–5.
54. Beder J. The 2015 musicians' health survey results. Senza Sordino. 2017. https://www.icsom.org/senzasordino/2017/06/the-2015-musicians-health-survey-results/. Accessed 23 June 2019.
55. Thomson R. D Edward Degas: waiting (Getty Museum Studies on Art). J. Paul Getty Museum, 1995. ISBN 0-89236-285-5.
56. Edgar Degas' dancer stretching. https://www.kimbellart.org/collection/ap-196804. Accessed 15 Nov 2018.
57. "The Old Guitarist". The Art Institute of Chicago. https://www.artic.edu/artworks/28067/the-old-guitarist. Accessed 15 May 2019.
58. The Blind Guitarist. https://www.museodelprado.es/en/the-collection/art-work/the-blind-guitarist/. Accessed 24 February 2020.
59. Sheibani-Rad S, Wolfe S, Jupiter J. Hand disorders in musicians. The orthopedic surgeon role. Bone Joint J. 2013;95:146–50.
60. Garnett SE. Maestro Leon Fleisher uses "two hands" to thank NIH. The NIH Record. https://nihrecord.nih.gov/newsletters/2005/01_04_2005/story03.htm. Accessed 6 May 2019.
61. Glenn PG. Biography of Vladimir Horowitz. Quill United Kingdom: Macdonald; 1983. ISBN 0-356-09179-1ISB pp. 338, 387, 389.
62. Buia C, Morrill H. Meet music's top doctors who've saved the voices of Adele, Sam Smith and more. https://www.billboard.com/articles/news/magazine-feature/6738182/music-top-throat-doctors-adele-sam-smith-steven-tyler. Accessed 6 May 2019.
63. Zeitels SM. The art and craft of phonomicrosurgery in Grammy award-winning elite performers. Ann Otol Rhinol Laryngol. 2019;128:7S–24S.
64. Frucht SJ. Embouchure dystonia: portrait of a task-specific cranial dystonia. Mov Disord. 2009;24:1752–62.

65. Walter Marin Pittore. http://www.waltermarin.altervista.org/contatti.html. Accessed 22 May 2019.
66. Courtney CA, O'Hearn MA, Franck CC. Frida Kahlo: portrait of chronic pain. Phys Ther. 2017;97:90–6.
67. Weidemann C, Klier M. Fifty women artists you should know: Prestel Publishing; 2008. ISBN 3791339567 (ISBN13: 9783791339566).
68. Anxiety (painting). https://en.wikipedia.org/wiki/Anxiety_(painting). Accessed 24 Feb 2020.
69. Araujo S. The pain of crippling anxiety in 10 paintings. https://culturacolectiva.com/art/social-anxiety-paintings/. Accessed 26 May 2019.
70. Shawn T. The courage that comes with anxiety. 2018. https://psychcentral.com/blog/the-courage-that-comes-with-anxiety/. Accessed 24 Feb 2020.
71. James Sant – Courage, Anxiety and Despair – Watching the Battle. Wikimedia Commons, the free media repository. https://commons.wikimedia.org/wiki/File:James_Sant_-_Courage,_Anxiety_and_Despair_-_Watching_the_Battle.jpg. Accessed 24 Feb 2020.
72. Vasey S. Disability arts; A national perspective. Keynote speech at North West Disability Arts Forum, 1990. Liverpool.
73. Disability in the arts. https://en.wikipedia.org/w/index.php?title=Disability_in_the_arts&oldid=880922934. Accessed 6 May 2019.
74. The Beggars. https://en.wikipedia.org/wiki/The_Beggars.
75. Alicia J, Bergman M, Boone E, Cervantes S, Desai M, Littleton Y, Perez Y, Davis A. MaestraPeace. 2019. ISBN-13: 978-1597144834.
76. Emery AEH. Medicine, artists and their art. J R Coll Physicians Lond. 1997;31:450–5.
77. Wolf PL. The effects of diseases, drugs, and chemicals on the creativity and productivity of famous sculptors, classic painters, classic music composers, and authors. Arch Pathol Lab Med. 2005;129:1457–64.
78. Mackey A. Dancing against prejudice: a biography of Mary Verdi-Fletcher. Thesis. Cleveland State University, 1997.
79. Gruener A. Degas exercise of 'circumvention'. Brit J Gen Pract. 2014;64:246–7.
80. Giovanni Gonnelli. https://en.wikipedia.org/wiki/Giovanni_Gonnelli. Accessed 24 Feb 2020.
81. Mathiasen H. Empathic art: Goya and Dr. Arrieta Am J Med. 2008;121:355–6.
82. The wing of madness: the illness of Vincent van Gogh. Can J Psychiatr. 1993;38:480–4.
83. Ike JD. Henri de Toulouse-Lautrec: disability and art in *Fin-de-Siecle Paris*. JHR. 2017:1–7. http://journalofhumanitiesinrehabilitation.org. Accessed 26 May 2019.
84. Cawthorne T. President address – Toulouse Lautrec – triumph over infirmity. Proc R Soc Med. 1970;63:800–5.
85. Perciaccante A, Coralli A, Apenzeller O. Amedeo Modigliani and his "great secret": A brief history of medical and social aspects of tuberculosis in the nineteenth and early twentieth century. Infez Med. 2018;26:280–2.
86. Potter P. Amedeo Modigliani (1884-1920). Self-portrait, 1919 (about the cover). Emerg Infect Dis. 2002; 8.
87. Reich J. Were the impressionists myopic? www.mivision.com.au. Accessed 24 Feb 2020.
88. Ortiz Monasterio P. Frida Kahlo. Her photos. México: Ediciones RM; 2010. ISBN13: 9788492480753.
89. Lisa Fittipaldi blind artist. https://viola.bz/lisa-fittipaldi-blind-artist/. Accessed 11 May 2019.
90. Lisa Fittipaldi: The Mind's Eye Foundation. https://www.artbabyart.com/foa/lisa/fittipaldi.htm. Accessed 6 May 2019.
91. Poet Painter Dilly Ward Bundy. http://dillywardbundy.com/exhibitions%20.html. Accessed 11 Nov 2108.
92. Hamilton WG, Hamilton LH, Marshall P, Molnar MA. A profile of musculoskeletal characteristics of elite professional ballet dances. Am J Sports Med. 1992;30:267–73.

93. Petcu EB, Sherwood K, Popa-Wagner AM, Aceti L, Miroiu RH. Artistic skills recovery and compensation in visual artists after stroke. Front Neurol. 2016;13(7):76–88.
94. Mikhail Baryshnikov Quotes. https://www.brainyquote.com/authors/mikhail_baryshnikov. Accessed 6 May 2019.
95. Junck E, Richardson M, Dilgen F, Liederbach M. A retrospective assessment of return to function in dance after physical therapy for common dance injuries. J Dance Med Sci. 2017;21:156–67.
96. Stuifbergen AK, Morris M, Jung JH, Pierini D, Morgan S. Benefits of wellness interventions for persons with chronic and disabling conditions: a review of the evidence. Disabil Health J. 2010;3:133–45.

Part II
Research

Chapter 6
Development of an Exercise Program for the Prevention of Playing-Related Musculoskeletal Problems Among Violinists

Adedayo Tunde Ajidahun, Hellen Myezwa, Witness Mudzi, and Wendy-Ann Wood

Background

The art of making music is an occupational risk factor for health-related problems, especially in the upper extremity and trunk [1–3]. Musculoskeletal problems have proved to be the most common health problems experienced by musicians regardless of the level of professionalism, and the prevalence of musculoskeletal problems has been found to range from 37% to 77% [3–7]. Playing-related musculoskeletal disorder (PRMD) is a multi-symptomatic problem that includes pain, tingling, loss of flexibility, and weakness occurring in one or more regions of the body [1, 5]. Even though the anatomic body regions affected by PRMDs are mainly the upper extremities and the trunk [8–10], studies have revealed the existence of a direct relationship between the instrument played and the distribution of musculoskeletal problems in the body. Consequently, researchers have considered the demands made on the body when a specific instrument is played as major factors [5, 8, 11, 12].

The burden of musculoskeletal problems is higher among string instrumentalists than other instrumentalists, and string musicians are considered the most vulnerable to developing PRMDs [13, 14]. Playing a string instrument is demanding as it involves static postural adaptation to support and hold the instrument while the upper extremities are used repetitively in producing sound [11]. Injury prevention among musicians has received considerable attention over the past three decades around the world such as in Australia, Europe, and North America, by exploring injury prevention strategies to improve performance and reduce injury [15–17]. The exercise-based injury prevention program in these studies was focused on the injury pattern and the demands of performance in musicians in general. The pattern of

A. T. Ajidahun (✉) · H. Myezwa · W. Mudzi · W.-A. Wood
Department of Physiotherapy, Faculty of Health Sciences, University of the Witwatersrand, Johannesburg, South Africa
e-mail: hellen.myezwa@wits.ac.za; mudziw@ufs.ac.za

S.-H. Lee et al. (eds.), *Perspectives in Performing Arts Medicine Practice*,
https://doi.org/10.1007/978-3-030-37480-8_6

injury and the demands of performance vary for different musical instruments. In some studies, ergonomic adjustments, overall health promotion, and psychological support have been considered [18–20].

These injury prevention intervention programs have shown positive outcomes in reducing perceived exertion and eventual musculoskeletal injury in musicians. The components of the exercise programs are physiotherapy exercises for specific body regions that are usually involved in playing and performance [16, 17]. The focus of the exercise program is mainly to reduce perceived exertion, thereby reducing injuries, and not primarily to condition the musician to the demands of the profession [15–17]. A recent study that utilized an integrative intervention program comprised of health education, yoga, physical therapy exercises, and mental and improvisation training in college musicians reported positive outcomes in physical and mental efficacy [21]. Also, a specific physical activity program to manage perceived pain among clarinettists showed postural changes and reduction in self-report pain [22].

Despite these programs, musculoskeletal problems among string instrumentalists continue to be prevalent. As far as we know, there is no exercise-based injury prevention program specifically designed for string instrumentalists in the literature. Therefore, an instrument-specific exercise-based musculoskeletal injury prevention program focused on the pattern of injury and the biomechanical and postural demands of playing the violin would contribute toward strategies aimed at reducing the incidence of musculoskeletal problems among string instrumentalists.

The aim of this study was to develop an exercise-based injury prevention program for string instrumentalists. To achieve this aim, the study was conducted in two phases. The first phase of the study mapped out the commonly affected anatomic regions and identified biomechanical risk factors that predispose string players to musculoskeletal problems. The second phase of the study aimed to develop an exercise-based injury prevention program that would contribute toward the reduction of the burden of PRMDs and their associated disabilities among string instrumentalists. Our subjects are string players living in South Africa.

Theoretical Rationale

The integrated model for the theory of work-related musculoskeletal disorders by Karsh [23] outlined the interaction of four factors that could predispose the human body to work-related musculoskeletal disorders (WRMDs) – (1) individual factors, (2) psychological work demands, (3) physical work demands, and (4) work organization, the environment, and the social/cultural context. Figure 6.1 presents Karsh model of the interactions and relationships between the four factors.

As illustrated in Fig. 6.1, Karsh model asserts that the physical work demands of the job directly result in physical strain by increasing the load on contractile structures which would eventually result in physiological changes such as fatigue, overuse, and deformation. Similarly, the psychosocial demands of the job result in anxiety and stress which increase the likelihood of developing work-related symptomatic stressors, which would eventually result in a work-related musculoskeletal problem. The individual attributes of the worker such as gender, age, individual capacity, and

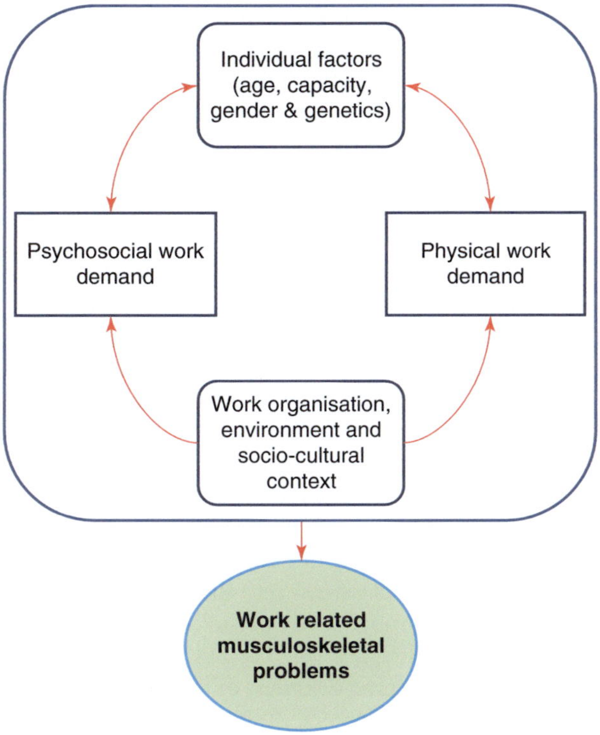

Fig. 6.1 Theoretical framework for work-related musculoskeletal disorders based on Karsh concept [23]

genetic factors modulate the risk of the worker to the psychosocial and physical demands of the work. The respective resultant effects of these individual factors, the psychosocial and physical work demands, or a combination of the three eventually affect the quality of the work performed [23]. We adopted the Karsh model of WRMD in analyzing the burden of PRMDs among instrumentalists associated with several risk factors and categorized the risk factors into four inter-related components, namely, individual factors, physical work demands, psychological work demands, and work organization, the environment, and socio-cultural factors.

Methodology

A mixed methods study design was used to achieve the stepwise objectives of this study. The mixed methods study design utilizes both quantitative and qualitative methods [24, 25]. The study was conducted in two phases; the aim of the first phase of the project was to establish the pattern of injury and determine possible risk factors that could predispose string players to playing-related musculoskeletal problems. The objectives of the first phase of the project were (1) to establish the prevalence, distribution, symptoms, and severity of musculoskeletal problems among string players and (2) to evaluate the biomechanical risk associated with playing the violin. The objective of the second phase of the project was to develop an exercise program for violinists based on the results of the first phase.

A cross-sectional study design was used to collect data on the prevalence, distribution, symptoms, and severity of musculoskeletal problems among string players (violinists, violists, cellists, and double bassists) using both online and paper-based survey. The eligibility criteria to participate in the study required the string players to be aged 18 and above and perform in an orchestra (youth and professional). A total of 16 orchestras (youth and professional) in all 9 provinces in South Africa were invited to participate in the study, and reminders were sent every 2 weeks for a period of 6 months. The overall data for this study was collected over a period of 1 year and 2 months from July 2014 to September 2015. Only 13 orchestras from 6 provinces and 62 violinists participated in this study.

The injury surveillance questionnaire was used to collect information on the lifetime and point prevalence, distribution, symptoms, and severity of PRMDs among instrumental musicians. The 17-item questionnaire was divided into 3 sections – demographics, playing experience, and occurrence of musculoskeletal injury. Disability was measured using the Quick Disability of the Arm, Shoulder, and Hand (DASH) questionnaire and the Neck Disability Index (NDI). The DASH is a Likert self-reported questionnaire with 30 items which measure physical functions and symptoms of people with musculoskeletal disorders in the upper limbs. The 11-item Quick DASH was classified into the 3 International Classification of Functioning (ICF) model constructs – activity limitation, impairment, and participation limitation using earlier studies [26, 27]. The DASH was developed as an outcome measure to evaluate region-specific disorders of the upper extremity, and it records symptoms as well as activity performance [28]. The Quick DASH is a reliable [29] and valid tool in measuring dysfunction of the upper extremity [30–32]. The Neck Disability Index is a self-administered instrument developed from the Oswestry Index for Back Pain and the Pain Disability Index [33]. It is used to assess neck pain complaints, and it is the most commonly used self-report instrument in evaluating neck pain in clinical research [34]. It has 10 sections, with a total of 5 possible scores for each section making a maximum total score of 50 which is then transformed to a percentage [33]. The NDI is a valid and reliable tool in measuring disability [35]. Descriptive statistics of median, interquartile range (IQR), and frequency were used to summarize the demographics, symptoms, distribution, and severity of PRMDs. Spearman correlation coefficient was used to determine the correlation between continuous variables number of anatomic regions affected and disability measure scores. Mann-Whitney U test was used to determine the significant difference in disability measures between violinists with PRMDs and violinists without PRMDs.

In the second phase of the project, the initial step was to conduct a scoping review of the literature to explore the content and structure of exercise-based intervention programs among musicians and in the general work population. In recent years, scoping reviews have been used to review evidence, identify gaps in research, and map out existing evidence about a topic and to explore the gray areas to provide answers to pertinent questions [36–38]. A scoping review was used to help map out the existing exercise-based intervention programs and to identify gaps that could assist in developing our exercise-based injury prevention program. Further, scoping review of a broad range of study helped clarify gray areas needed to address [39, 40].

The second step was to utilize data from phase 1 to develop an exercise-based intervention program for violinists based on clinical reasoning, and a draft of the program was content validated with physiotherapists and biokineticists. The exercise program was developed by integrating information from phase 1 which included pattern of injury, range of motion, muscle activity, and postural load with clinical and theoretical rationale of injury prevention. The biomechanical analysis results show that the joint positions of the neck, trunk, and shoulders put the violin player at risk of neck pain, low back pain, and impingement problems in the shoulder. Descriptive statistics of mean and standard deviation were used to summarize the muscle activity and joint angles of the participants. The stepwise methodology of the research is outlined in Table 6.1.

Table 6.1 Overview of methodology and procedure

Phase 1	
Objective 1	**To establish the prevalence, distribution, symptoms, and severity of musculoskeletal problems among violinists in South Africa**
Study design	Cross-sectional study
Population	62 violinists from 13 orchestras (youth and professional) in 6 of the 9 provinces, aged ≥18 years, participated in the study
Injury surveillance	Injury profile (prevalence, distribution, symptoms, and severity) questionnaire Disability – Neck Disability Index and the Quick Disability of the Arm, Shoulder, and Hand
Procedure	The survey was conducted using an online survey system and a paper-based questionnaire. Sixteen orchestra managers in South Africa were recruited; only 13 orchestras consented to participate in the study. A total of 129 string players completed the questionnaires, and only 114 string players met the age inclusion criteria with an overall response rate of 48.9%, out of which 62 were violinists. The overall data for this study was collected over a period of 1 year and 2 months from July 2014 to September 2015
Objective 2	**To evaluate the biomechanical risk associated with playing a violin**
Study design	Cross-sectional study
Population	Five violinists from Johannesburg, South Africa, with the competence to play the first movement of the Eine Kleine Nachtmusik, aged ≥18 years, participated in the study
Outcome measures	Joint range of motion in the shoulder, elbow, wrist, *cervical* and lumbar was measured using the inertial motion sensor using MVN BIOMECH® Muscle activity in the large muscles of the upper extremity (right and left middle fiber of the deltoid, right and left elbow extensors, right and left elbow flexors, right and left wrist extensors, right and left wrist flexors trunk (right and left upper trapezius and erector spinae) Postural load using the Rapid Upper Limb Assessment. Subjective and objective musculoskeletal assessment of the participants was conducted to assess for shoulder impingement, scapular dyskinesia, scapular stabilization, postural problems, and joint hypermobility.
Procedure	Five violinists volunteered for the biomechanical assessment. Subjective and objective musculoskeletal assessment was conducted in the biomechanical laboratory at Wits University, and violinist's injury history and playing experience were recorded. The volunteers were set up in the Xsens BIOMECH suit, and the wireless electrode to measure muscle activity was attached to the selected muscles of the upper extremity and trunk. Prior to recording, the violinists were required to practice and get comfortable in the clothes. During performance, muscle activity, postural load, and the joint range of motion were recorded

Table 6.1 (continued)

Phase 2	
Objective 1	**To extract reproducible exercise programs from literature**
Study design	Scoping review
Eligibility criteria	Studies focused on upper extremity, neck, and trunk work-related problems among musicians and the general population were reviewed. A total of 86 studies were reviewed, in the general population (*n* = 74) and among musicians (*n* = 12)
Extracted focus of exercise programs	Region-specific exercise programs for the management and/or prevention of musculoskeletal problems Rationale for the exercise program Implementation process of the exercise program
Procedure	**The methodology of the scoping review involved five steps, namely:** *Identifying research questions and relevant studies*: the research question in this study was, what are the exercise-based intervention programs that have been used and/or developed for the management of musculoskeletal problems among musicians and the general work population? *Study selection*: Databases were searched using various combination of key words such as "musicians," "instrumentalists," "musculoskeletal," "injury," "rehabilitation," and "exercise" matched with the following anatomical regions – neck, elbow, shoulder, hand, and trunk *Charting of data*: the extracted exercise programs were charted into the specific regions of interest – cervical and shoulder, forearm and wrist, and lumbar region *Summarizing and collating results*: the results were summarized into exercise components with the rationale and justification for each of the exercise programs
Objective 2	**To develop an exercise-based injury prevention program for violinists**
Study design	Clinical reasoning/content validation
Population	A total of ten experts (seven sports physiotherapists and three biokineticists) with an average 10.8 ± 6.7 years of experience using the snowball method was used to recruit participants
Procedure	The extracted exercise programs from the scoping review were categorized into components according to the anatomic regions into stretching, stabilization, strengthening, and endurance exercises. Also, the pattern of musculoskeletal problems was used in categorizing the exercises. The developed exercise program was validated for content with experts (sports physiotherapists and biokineticists). The developed exercise program was sent via emails to the experts with the justification for the inclusion of the exercise program per region
Objective 3	**To explore possible implementation strategies of the developed program in South Africa**
Study design	Focus group discussion
Participants	Music educators and instructors at 2 music schools in Johannesburg, South Africa, and a total of 11 music educators with an average year of teaching/playing experience of 12.4 ± 3.8 participated in the focus group discussion
Procedure	The rationale and aim of the study and the exercise development procedure were explained to the participants prior to their opinion on the potential usefulness of the exercise program and implementation strategies. The participants were approached to participate in the study. The focus group discussion (FGD) was conducted at the convenience of the participants, and the discussion was facilitated using an interview guide. The focus group discussions were conducted at the workplace (music) of the participants (music schools). Focus group discussion continued till there were no emerging themes. The discussions were audio-taped, field notes were taken, and the researcher facilitated the discussions

Results

Musculoskeletal Problems Among Violinists in South Africa

A total of 62 violinists with an average age of 29.5 (22.75–42.5) years completed the questionnaires. Majority (72.6%) of the violinists were females and played the violin for an average of 18.5 years (12.75–36). The period prevalence (past 12 months) and point prevalence (past 7 days) of musculoskeletal problems among the violinists were 54.8% and 32.8%, respectively. The result of this study is consistent with other studies that have reported a high period (past 12 months) prevalence of musculoskeletal problems among string instrumentalists [41, 42]. Over a 12-month period, 79% of string instrumentalists reported PRMDs [42]. In the study by Abreu Ramos and Micheo [41], 68% of string instrumentalists reported symptoms of PRMDs. In this study, females reported a higher prevalence of musculoskeletal problems than males. An increased prevalence of musculoskeletal problems among female string instrumentalists is similar to previous studies [43]. Female string instrumentalists are generally more prone to musculoskeletal injuries than their male counterparts; body frame and the adaptation of the body structure of the females have been suggested as possible predisposing factors. Risk factors such as joint laxity [44], hormonal differences [45], and smaller body frame [46] have been identified in literature as contributing factors to the higher injury reported in females than males. It has been reported that females are more predisposed to reporting illnesses when compared to males [47, 48].

In our study, impairments associated with playing the violinists were predominantly in the left shoulder (50%), neck (48.4%), upper back (48.4%), low back (43.5%), and right shoulder (40.3%) (Fig. 6.2). These reported body locations are

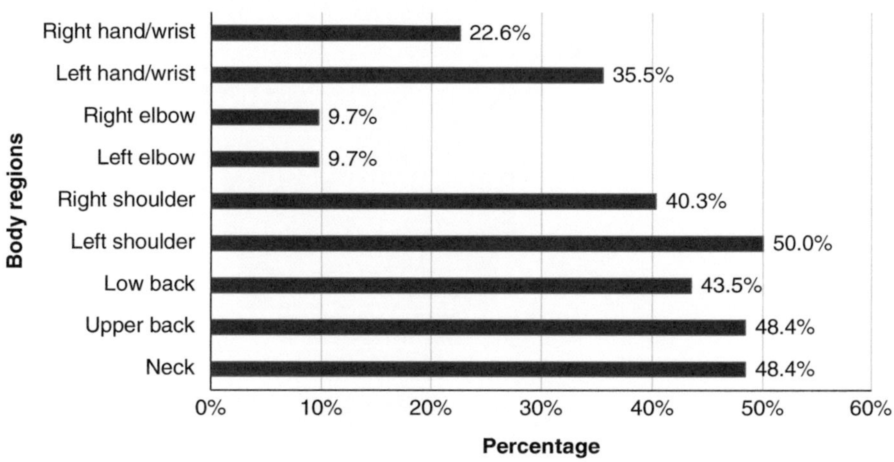

Fig. 6.2 Distribution of musculoskeletal problems in the nine anatomic regions in violinists ($n = 62$)

similar to what has been established before [7, 10]. It therefore follows that the body regions commonly used in playing the musical instrument are the most injured anatomical regions. The physical demands of playing a violin predispose the player to musculoskeletal problems and impairments [49]. During violin playing, the left upper extremity is usually used for support and fingering, the right upper extremity is the bowing and/or the plucking arm, and the trunk is usually the major postural support region [7, 11]. It is therefore not surprising that musculoskeletal problems are common in these anatomical regions.

Violinists with a history of playing-related musculoskeletal problems majorly described their symptoms as aching (58.8%), soreness (50%), and tingling (47.1%) (Fig. 6.3). The symptoms of musculoskeletal problems among violinists in this study are consistent with the common symptoms of overuse injuries in other studies [50]. Overuse injuries are the most common musculoskeletal problem of instrumental musicians, and they are normally due to a direct consistent loading of the neuromusculoskeletal structures involved in performing an activity [51].

The severity of musculoskeletal problems in the affected anatomical regions was majorly reported as mild to moderate, although some violinists reported severe pain intensity in the upper back and left shoulder (Fig. 6.4).

The increased pain severity in the upper back and left shoulder is consistent with the posture assumed in supporting the violin during performance [7, 11]. Steinmetz [14] showed similar results among professional orchestra musicians, and the average pain score using the numeric pain rating score in the affected body regions was between 3.9 and 4.7. It is noteworthy to highlight the relatively higher severity of

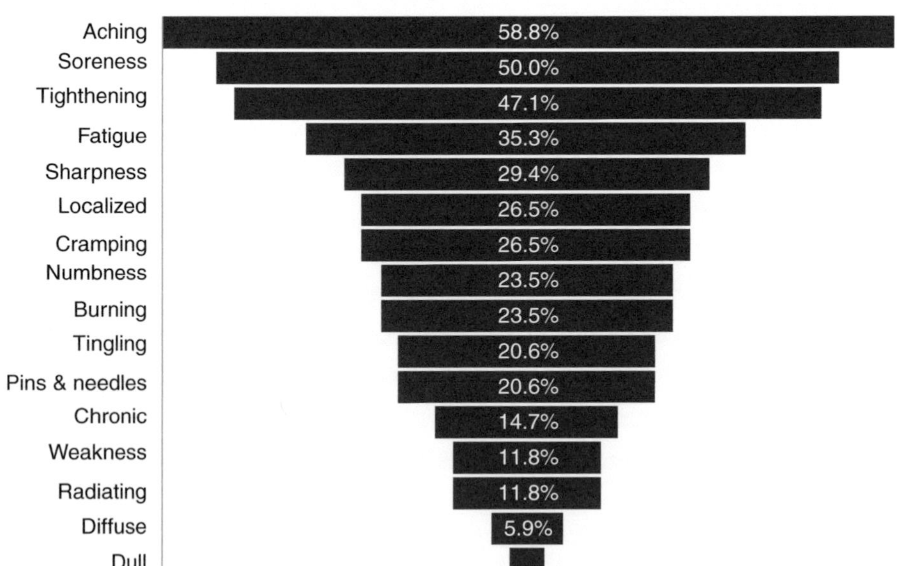

Fig. 6.3 Symptoms of playing-related musculoskeletal problems among violinists ($n = 34$)

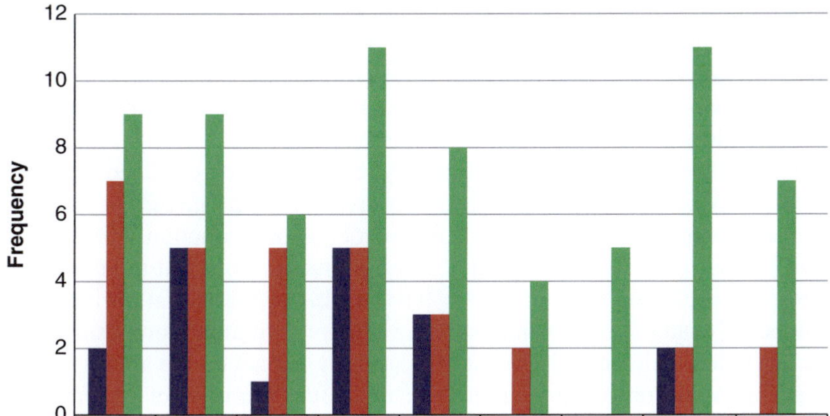

	Neck	Upper back	Low back	Left shoulder	Right shoulder	Left elbow	Right elbow	Left hand/wrist	Right hand/wrist
■ Severe	2	5	1	5	3	0	0	2	0
■ Moderate	7	5	5	5	3	2	0	2	2
■ Mild	9	9	6	11	8	4	5	11	7

Fig. 6.4 Pain severity among violinists ($n = 34$)

musculoskeletal problems in the upper back and left shoulder when compared to the other affected anatomical regions. Prolonged neck flexion and the static abnormal posture of the left shoulder could be responsible for the increased severity in the upper trunk and left shoulder [11]. Playing the violin requires an intermittent lateral flexion of the neck to support and hold the instrument [11]. The postural adaptation increases the likelihood of developing neck and upper back complications with time [11]. The results of this study are consistent with earlier studies which have shown that postural imbalance is common among string instrumentalists and that postural structures are often the most injured body regions in the string instrumentalist [11, 52]. The implication is that correct ergonomics could be an important factor in reducing musculoskeletal problems among violinists. It therefore follows that an understanding of the demands on these structures could help proffer solutions to reducing the presence and severity of musculoskeletal problems and resultant disability emanating from the regions affected. Disability is defined using the ICF and is an interaction between impairment, activity limitation, and participation restriction [53]. As such disability was measured in this study using the Quick DASH and the NDI.

In this study, the disability score (Quick DASH) was 50% significantly higher among violinists with PRMDs compared to those without PRMDs. The Neck Disability Index score showed no significant difference in violinists with or without PRMDs. This is not surprising as PRMD is a multi-symptomatic disorder that usually affects more than one anatomic region [1, 3]. In this study 76.5% of the violinists reported symptoms in two or more anatomic regions, and disability scores were increased proportionately with an increase in the number of affected body regions. The median Quick DASH disability score of 13.63 (2.44–31.02) in this study is slightly higher to the mean DASH score in the study by Barton et al. [54] with college string players reporting a mean DASH score of 11.8 (11.7). The presence of musculoskeletal problems is often associated with an increase in Quick DASH disability scores [32, 55]. In our study, there was a significant positive correlation between the number of anatomic regions affected and the disability score (rs = 0.351, p-value = 0.045). An increase in disability scores is often associated with morbidity of musculoskeletal problems [56], and this is reflected in the further analysis of the ICF subthemes – activity limitation and participation restriction. There was significant positive correlation between activity limitation score and the number of anatomic sites affected ($r_s = 0.35$, $p = 0.043$). This suggests that an increase in the number of anatomic sites would increase activity limitation score resulting in activity limitation which could eventually negatively impact on the ability to earn a living. This is not surprising as an increase in dysfunction in more anatomical regions will increase activity and participation limitation and eventual disability [57]. Musculoskeletal problems of instrumental musicians usually affect more than one anatomic region [1]. It is therefore important to explore injury prevention strategies to reduce disability associated with playing the musical instrument and other activities of daily living. Other studies have only reported disability associated with playing a musical instrument [54, 58]. This study was the first study to explore the relationship between PRMDs and the components of the ICF model for disability – activity limitation and participation restriction.

It can be concluded that there is a burden of PRMDs among violinists in South Africa with associated disability which impacts negatively on activities of daily living. Therefore, reducing the incidence of PRMDs among violinists may reduce activity limitation and participation restriction which would possibly result in an improved quality of life.

Biomechanical Analysis and Justification for Exercise Intervention Components

A cross-sectional study design was used to collect data on muscle activity, joint range of motion, postural load, and shoulder dysfunction. Joint range of motion of the upper extremities (shoulders, elbows, and wrists) and trunk (cervical, thoracic, and lumbar) which are the commonly reported sites of PRMDs among violinists was measured using the inertial motion unit (IMU) sensor using the MVN BIOMECH® (Xsens Technologies BV, Enschede, the Netherlands). Muscle activity of the large muscles of the upper extremity (elbow flexors and extensors, upper trapezius, wrist flexors and extensors, middle deltoid, and the trunk (erector spinae)) was measured using the eight-channel wireless electrode. Postural load demands of performance were evaluated by using the RULA. The upper extremity, neck, and trunk were evaluated based on the postural demands during performance, and the score is calculated as a sum of the posture, muscle, and force used in performing the activity in the upper limbs, neck, trunk, and legs [59]. The RULA is a valid tool in measuring postural load during work [59]. Musculoskeletal assessment of the participants was conducted prior to the biomechanical analysis. EMG electrodes and inertial motion sensors were attached to the participants. Data was collected on postural load, muscle activity, and range of motion during the musical performance of the first movement of the Eine Kleine Nachtmusik (by Mozart).

Five violinists with an average age and years of experience of 27.2 (4.02) years and 15 (9.12) years, respectively, volunteered for the study. Two of the five participants reported musculoskeletal problems. Subjective postural abnormalities (forward head posture and increased thoracic kyphosis) were present in two of the violinists. Objective assessment of shoulder impingement syndrome was positive in 4/5 violinists. Rapid Upper Limb Assessment score was 4–5 in all the participants in the right and 3–5 in the left.

Cervical region The results of this study showed that the cervical region is static in an awkward position during the music performance in flexion and left lateral bending with a mean joint angle of 17.45 ± 1.43 degrees and 3.17 ± 2.12 degrees, respectively. Work-related neck flexion has been reported to be a risk factor for neck pain in a working population [60]. During performance, the neck position can be sustained in this direction (neck flexion with lateral flexion) for a prolonged time. Out of the five violinists in the biomechanical analysis study, subjective postural evaluation showed forward head posture in two of the participants. The static asymmetry position of the neck sustains muscle activity in the muscles stretched in neck flexion especially the upper trapezius and the sternocleidomastoid (SCM). Sustained muscle activity has been hypothesized to result in muscle damage [61]. Muscle activation in painful major muscles is reduced, and this results in increased muscle activation in the accessory neck muscles by a compensatory mechanism [62]. The increased muscle activity in the accessory muscles would result in symptoms of overuse injuries [62]. The result of the descriptors of PRMDs in the cross-sectional study is consistent with the common symptoms of overuse injuries. Therefore, stretching exercises with the aim of improving muscle compliance and relaxation would be beneficial in reducing the risk of overuse injuries.

Violinists in this study showed an increased muscle activity in the upper trapezius (right = 10.89 ± 9.09 and left = 5.8 ± 3.89) (Fig. 6.5). Postural asymmetry and increased muscle activity in the neck muscles are predisposing factors to neck pain [60, 63]. The demand of playing the violin and viola requires the sustained asymmetric position; however, endurance and strength training of the deep neck flexors could reduce the onset of muscle fatigue and subsequently prevent the forward head posture. Likewise, stretching of the neck muscles (SCM, upper trapezius, levator scapulae) could reduce muscle activity and improve muscle compliance. From the extracted exercises, endurance exercises of the deep neck flexors (longus capitis, longus colli, rectus capitis anterior and lateralis) [64] and stretching exercise of the upper trapezius and pectoralis would be beneficial in preventing musculoskeletal problems associated with string instrument playing [65]. The deep neck flexor

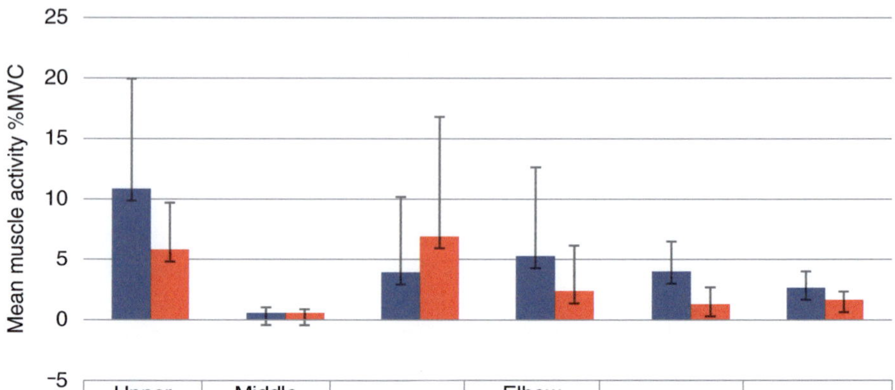

	Upper trapezius	Middle deltoid	Elbow flexors	Elbow extensors	Wrist flexors	Erector spinae
Right	10.87	0.58	3.93	5.28	4	2.68
Left	5.81	0.57	6.93	2.37	1.31	1.65

Fig. 6.5 Muscle activity using EMG of violinists ($n = 5$)

endurance exercises and stretching exercises showed significant positive outcomes in the management of neck pain [64, 65].

Lumbar region Muscle activity in the erector spinae reported % RMS MVC of 2.68 ± 1.33 and 1.65 ± 0.70, respectively (Fig. 6.5). This suggests that the muscle activity in the lumbar region is reduced in comparison to the amplitude of muscle activity in the upper trapezius. The upper thoracic region and the lumbar region are normally support structures for the whole musculature during performance [49]. From the results of cross-sectional survey, the prevalence of the musculoskeletal problems in the upper back and the lumbar region in violinists was 48.4% and 43.5%, respectively (Fig. 6.2). Low back pain is a common problem in the general population, and musicians are not exempt from the activities of daily living that predisposes people to back problems [66]. Additionally, postural problems associated with playing a string instrument can predispose the string player to back problems [67–69].

The result of the biomechanical analysis showed that only one violinist had weak core stabilizers. The role of the core stabilizers in maintaining posture is important in injury prevention according to several studies [70]. The core stabilizers have been explored in several studies as a major contributor to the stabilization of the lumbar region [71–74].

This study measured trunk movement and position associated with performance. The mean range of motion at the lumbosacral junction was 9.43 ± 6.43 degrees flexion and 0.1 ± 3.44 degrees left lateral bending and axial rotation of −1.19 ± 6.1 degrees (Fig. 6.6). This implies that the trunk position was not in the neutral position throughout the music performance. Neutral position when sitting in a correct ergonomic posture would reduce the risk of back pain [75]. Several injury preven-

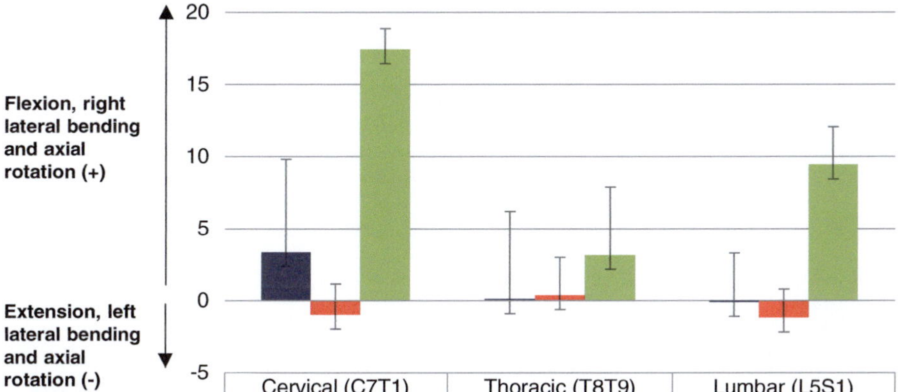

	Cervical (C7T1)	Thoracic (T8T9)	Lumbar (L5S1)
■ Lateral bending	3.37	0.09	-0.1
■ Axial rotation	-0.97	0.38	-1.19
■ Flexion - extension	17.45	3.17	9.43

Fig. 6.6 Cervical, thoracic, and lumbar range of motion of violinists

tion programs have identified the importance of trunk training; however, the movement pattern associated with trunk performance is not well reported in the literature [15, 76–78].

Our scoping review concludes that strength, endurance, or core stabilization exercises would be effective in the management of low back pain. However, feed forward activation of the stabilizers has a prophylactic effect in anticipating movement which has been suggested to reduce the risk of lumbar pain [79, 80]. Therefore, stabilization exercises of the lumbar region would be effective in reducing the risk of low back pain among string players. Core stabilization exercise described by Inani and Selkar [81] and general lumbar stabilization exercises were adopted and included in our exercise program.

Shoulder region The left shoulder functions mainly to support the instrument and the right, in bowing action in violin and viola players [49]. Our survey data showed the prevalence of musculoskeletal problems in the left and right shoulder was 50% and 40.3%, respectively, among violinists (Fig. 6.2). The results of the biomechanics analysis in our study using the inertial motion unit sensor measured movement in the shoulder and the scapula-thoracic joints (C7 shoulder) showed that in the right upper extremity, there was considerable movement in the shoulder joints in the coronal, sagittal, and transverse planes. The right shoulder averaged 17.09 ± 14.4 degrees of abduction, 16.17 ± 9.53 degrees of internal rotation, and 21.43 ± 16.23 degrees of flexion (Fig. 6.7), while the left shoulder averaged 4.21 ± 8.33 degrees of abduction, 13.24 ± 14.14 degrees of internal rotation, and 23.23 ± 22.8 degrees of flexion during violin performance (Fig. 6.8).

The demands of the bowing arm (right arm) require repetition of quick movements which predisposes the string instrumentalists to overuse and possibly shoul-

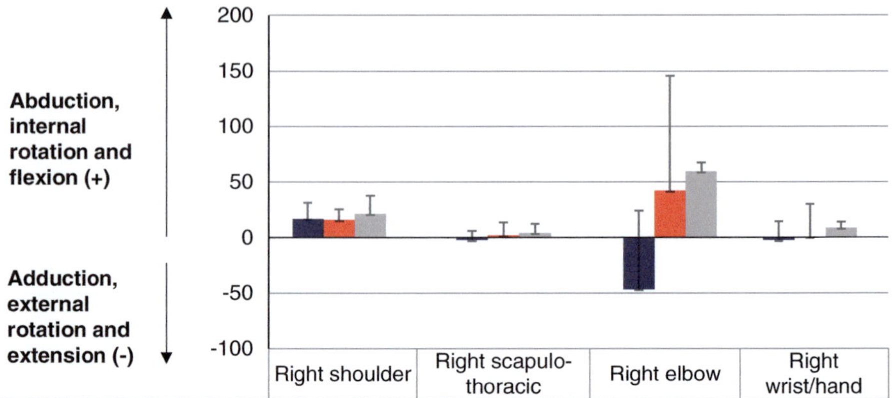

	Right shoulder	Right scapulo-thoracic	Right elbow	Right wrist/hand
■ Abduction - adduction	17.09	-2.17	-46.75	-2.65
■ Internal - external rotation	16.17	2.14	42.2	0.23
■ Flexion - extension	21.43	4.28	59.43	8.87

Fig. 6.7 Right upper extremity joint range of motion of violinists

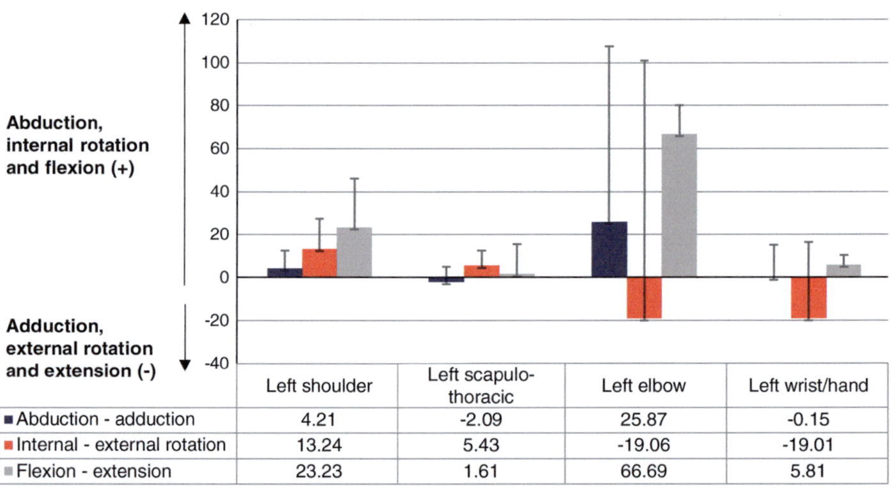

	Left shoulder	Left scapulo-thoracic	Left elbow	Left wrist/hand
■ Abduction - adduction	4.21	-2.09	25.87	-0.15
■ Internal - external rotation	13.24	5.43	-19.06	-19.01
■ Flexion - extension	23.23	1.61	66.69	5.81

Fig. 6.8 Left extremity joint range of motion of violinists

der impingement syndrome [82]. The bowing arm (right) was averagely positioned in about 16.17 ± 9.53 degrees of shoulder internal rotation which puts a strain on the internal rotators and could result into impingement syndrome [82]. Unlike the right shoulder joint, the left shoulder joint was held in a static position for the violinists in 4.21 ± 8.33 degrees abduction, 13.24 ± 14.14 degrees internal rotation, and 23.23 ± 22.84 degrees flexion (Fig. 6.8). This static position is usually held throughout the duration of performance which results into constant contraction of the muscles involved in abduction, internal rotation, and flexion. Shoulder impingement

Region	Cervical	Lumbar	Shoulder	Elbow/wrist
Results summary	Prevalence: Neck – 48.4% and Upper back – 48.4% Static neck flexion ↑ muscle activity in the upper trapezius	Prevalence: 43.5% Upper thoracic rotation Postural load: 4.2 (0.8)	Prevalence: Left: 50% and Right: 40.3% Static internal rotation of the left shoulder and repetition of specific movements Positive signs of shoulder impingement syndrome	Prevalence: Left and right elbow 9.7% Movement at the right elbow was mainly pronation, internal rotation and flexion while the left elbow was static mainly in supination, external rotation and flexion.
Implications	Static neck flexion would result in fatigue and subsequent muscle pain and ↑ muscle activation of accessory muscle would compensate for the muscle pain	Upper thoracic rotation would result in pain due to the sustained awkward posture in the region which could result in asymmetry and eventual back dysfunction.	The static position of the left shoulder as well as the repetitive movement of the right shoulder predisposes the violinist to shoulder impingement syndrome.	The postural position can result into musculo-tendinous strains which are common in playing related musculoskeletal injury of musicians.
Exercise intervention programme	Stretching – Sternocleidomastoir muscles, levator scapulae and upper trapezius Neuro-mobilization exercises Strength and endurance training of the deep neck flexors Thoracic rotation exercises	Lumbo-pelvic stabilization exercises Core stabilization exercises	Stretching – posterior capsule stretch, pectoralis stretch, biceps and triceps stretch Strengthening exercises – resistance exercises incorporated with proprioceptive neuromuscular diagonal patterns Shoulder range of motion exercises	Forearm stretches Strengthening exercises incorporated with incorporated with proprioceptive neuromuscular diagonal patterns Intrinsic hand muscle exercises.

Overview of the rationale for the developed exercise program

dysfunction has been reported as a common musculoskeletal problem among string players, and the repetition of movement and static position has been reported to be risk factors [82, 83]. In our data, four out of the five participants showed positive Hawkins and Kennedy test, an objective assessment used to evaluate shoulder dysfunction [84]. Positive tests indicate early signs of nerve impingement syndrome in the participants. Maintaining the integrity of the rotator cuff muscles should be an important component of the exercise-based injury prevention strategy. Smooth shoulder movement is often accompanied with scapula-thoracic movements [85, 86]. Therefore, scapular stabilization exercises to improve stability and ensure smooth shoulder movements would be important in maintaining the integrity of shoulder movements.

The average range of motion in the left upper extremity in this study using the inertial motion sensors showed a reduced range of motion in all the segments measured when compared with the study by Shan and Visentin [87]. This study showed an increased joint angles in the left shoulder joints when compared to the study by Shan and Visentin [87].

In the right shoulder, the study by Shan and Visentin [87] could not be directly compared with this study because the joint angle was reported with respect to the string played unlike this study where the mean of the joint angle irrespective of the string played was reported. However, Shan and Visentin [87] reported that the joint angles in flexion-extension, abduction-adduction, and rotation when playing on the G-string are higher than when playing on the E-string. This is not surprising because the position of the G-string on the violin requires the right upper extremity to move across the body during bowing [88]. The left wrist position in this study is similar to the study by Shan and Visentin [87], as this position during performance was at supination, flexion, and adduction with mean joint angles of 29, 8, and 0 degrees, respectively. However, discrepancies have been reported between Xsens and a camera-based system (Optotrak) in the lower limbs which could be responsible for the differences observed [89]. Also, the variation in joint angles can be attributed to interindividual differences in skills and performance [90]. An analysis of postural flaws of violinists during a musical performance showed that all violinists measured in the study had postural flaws during performance especially in the wrist and neck [90]. Individual violinists often adjust and adapt their own pattern of play to the most suitable pattern, and this usually results in interindividual differences among violinists [91].

In our scoping study, we learned that scapular stabilization exercises of the scapula retractors were found to reduce pain intensity in participants with impingement syndrome [92]. Posterior shoulder and pectoralis minor stretch as a component of an overall exercise-based program was effective in the prevention of shoulder disorders among construction workers [93]. Strengthening exercises (front raise, lateral raise, reverse flys, and shrugs) of the shoulder muscles [94–97] and serratus anterior [98] showed significant positive outcome in the management of shoulder dysfunction. Therefore, strengthening and endurance exercises of the shoulder muscles in the sagittal, coronal, and transverse planes would reduce the incidence of overuse-related injuries in the shoulders. Scapular stabilization exercises to improve support would improve endurance, and stretching exercises of the rotator cuffs could reduce the strain on the rotator cuffs.

Forearm and wrists In our study, the wrist joint is mainly positioned in 19.01 ± 35.41 degrees external rotation and 5.81 ± 4.57 degrees flexion. It is important to note that violinist's right forearm functions mainly in determining the force applied to the bow in sound generation and it works synchronously with the left hand [88]. The right wrist functions mainly in holding the bow. Therefore, biomechanically, violinist's movement at the right elbow is mainly in pronation, internal rotation, and flexion, while the position of the left elbow was static mainly in supination, external rotation, and flexion in the violinists. This position can result in musculo-tendinous strains which are a common injury of musicians. Hence, strengthening and stretching exercises would improve endurance and relaxation, respectively, in the forearm. In the elbow, the range of motion left elbow 66.69 ± 13.47 degrees was higher than in the right elbow 59.43 ± 7.80 degrees. The results of this study can be compared to the findings by Shan and Visentin [87] which measured arm kinematics in violin performance by using a nine-camera motion capture system.

Evaluation and Validation of Exercise Program

A total of 10 exercise experts with mean experience of 10.8 ± 6.7 years participated in the study. It comprised five males and five females and seven physiotherapists and three biokineticists. Three of the physiotherapists have experience in the management of neuromusculoskeletal system problems in the upper extremity, neck, lower limbs, and back. One of the sports physiotherapists also plays the violin and has experienced playing-related injury management. The other two sports physiotherapists are mainly involved in the treatment of soccer-related injuries in both the acute and the rehabilitation stages. The three biokineticists are involved in the exercise-based rehabilitation of musculoskeletal injuries.

The exercise experts considered the exercise program relevant and useful in the prevention of PRMDs among violin players. Further recommendations and suggestions based on theory and logical argument of the causative factors of PRMDs among violinists were considered. We modified the program adopting some of the recommendations and suggestions of the participants. The recommended exercises were included and categorized based on the anatomic region. The procedure of the exercises used TheraBand(s) instead of dumbbells for resistance due to easy availability and portability. The dosage of the various exercises was suggested to be in line with the basic principles of exercises prescription [99].

The exercise regimen was divided into three main categories which included warm up, general exercises, and cool down (Table 6.2). Specific anatomical regions were also addressed: cervical/thoracic region, shoulder, elbow and wrist, and lum-

Table 6.2 Modified exercise program for violinists

Exercise category	Specific exercises
Warm up and cool down exercises/ breaks	Upper trapezius stretches Bicep and triceps stretch Fingers clenched and unclenched Wrist rotations Oppositional finger wrist press Hand/finger extensions Posterior capsule stretch Rotatory shoulder shrugs Hold and relax exercises of the upper trapezius (PNF) Pendulum arc exercises
General exercises	General active mobilization exercise of the neck, trunk, shoulder, elbow, wrist, and fingers to the end of range should be performed prior to the specific exercises Postural education – proper posture as a component of activities of daily living
Cervical/thoracic region	Stretching – SCM, levator scapulae, upper trapezius Neuro-mobilization – upper neural tension exercises *Strength and endurance training* of the *deep neck flexors* *Thoracic rotation exercises*
Shoulder	Stretching – posterior capsule stretch, pectoralis stretch, biceps and triceps stretch Strengthening exercises – resistance exercises with TheraBand incorporated with proprioceptive neuromuscular diagonal patterns Scapular stabilization exercises – serratus anterior, rhomboids, middle and lower trapezius Scapular strengthening exercises Shoulder shrugs – rotatory shrugs Pendulum arm exercises Rotator cuff exercises – thumbs up and down
Elbow/wrist	Stretch – *forearm* stretch Strengthening exercises – resistance exercises with TheraBand incorporated with proprioceptive neuromuscular patterns Intrinsic hand muscle exercises – clench and unclench exercises and resistance against rubber band
Lumbar region	Lumbo-pelvic stabilization exercises Core stabilization exercises Bird dog exercises

bar region. Additional exercise was also recommended, and these included proprioceptive neuromuscular facilitation (PNF), neuro-mobilization exercises, general mobilization, stabilization exercises, stretching, and thoracic rotation exercises.

Proprioceptive neuromuscular facilitation (PNF) Proprioceptive neuromuscular facilitation was suggested to be included in the exercise program for shoulder exercises. The strength training exercise programs were suggested to be performed putting into consideration the PNF patterns of shoulder movements. PNF has been recommended as a component of injury prevention programs in sports [100, 101]. A recent exercise program developed for musicians also included proprioceptive training as a part of injury prevention program developed generally for musicians irrespective of the instrument played [76].

Neuro-mobilization exercises Neuro-mobilization exercises of the median, radial, and ulnar nerve were proposed to be included as part of the exercise program. The rationale of the inclusion was due to the static position of the cervical region in holding and supporting the upper string instruments could result into compression of the nerve roots of the brachial plexus. Therefore, the integrity of the neural structures using neuro-mobilization exercises could be important in reducing nerve irritations and musculoskeletal injuries associated with compression neuropathy. Compressive neuropathy has been reported as a common problem among musicians [102].

General mobilization An inclusion of general mobilization exercises of the upper extremity and trunk to ensure full range of motion was also suggested. To maintain the physiological joint integrity, full range of motion is important.

Stabilization exercises The adapted exercise program was focused on stabilization of the scapular stabilizers (serratus anterior) and the core stabilizers. Stabilization exercises of the rhomboids were suggested to be included in the exercise program. The scapular is important in supporting the violin and in the excursion of shoulder movement. The shoulder is a complex joint, and the integrity of the each of the joints that made up the shoulder complex is important in ensuring smooth movements.

Stretching The adapted exercise program was focused on stretching the upper trapezius in the cervical region. The experts suggested gentle stretch exercises of the sternocleidomastoid. The rotation movement and position of the cervical region in holding the violin/viola could result into a strain on the right side and shortening on the left side. Therefore, the rationale of stretching of the sternocleidomastoid could be important in reducing cervical problems in the cervical region.

Thoracic rotation exercises The prevalence of musculoskeletal problems in the thoracic region (upper back) was relatively high in the population studied. However, there were no exercises of the thoracic region extracted from literature. The experts in this study suggested thoracic rotation exercises as well as progressive strengthening exercises of the thoracic region. The rationale for the inclusion was due to the trunk rotation associated with playing the string instrument and the high prevalence of musculoskeletal problems in the upper thoracic region.

Implementation of the Developed Exercise Program

The final step in this phase was to explore the possible implementation strategies of the developed exercise program. A focus group of 11 professional musicians met twice to discuss implementation of the exercises. The mean age and the mean years of experience of the participants were 28.2 ± 6 years and 12.4 ± 3.8 years, respectively. The participants comprised two females and nine males. Eight of the participants play one of the string instruments, while four play other instruments and teach music. Several themes emerged from the focus group discussions.

Usefulness of the exercise program The focus group thought the exercise program would be beneficial in reducing musculoskeletal injuries:

> I think it is going to benefit us a lot. I suffer from back and shoulder pain. I know it is a struggle for me to play, especially when we have a lot of work, concerts and tour. I get muscle spasm, it is a struggle to work and play. I definitely would be open to learn and teach the exercises

Intervention strategies The focus group would be willing to adopt the exercise program, and the participants suggested that the intervention should be introduced to the musicians at the early stage when they are still acquiring motor skills needed to play a string instrument.

Adherence to an exercise program is important to the effectiveness of the program in management and injury prevention [77, 103], and exercises designed for the work place were more effective than exercises performed at home [104]. Therefore, supervision of the exercises and the group therapy effect could be responsible for the better adherence to the program and eventual reduction in pain as one of the music tutors commented:

> It is beneficial to everyone, we might have to make arrangements and probably teach the students in batches and that way everybody gets a chance to learn the exercises. We can create time

Duration of an exercise program must be considered to ensure adherence. An intervention program for strength training implemented with four different groups showed that the group with 7 minutes of training three times a week showed significant improvement when compared to other groups which had longer duration [105]. The longer the exercise program, the less likely participants would be to adhere to the program.

Time constraints in implementing the program were a major point of discussion. Implementing the exercise program in a more structured setting – music schools, youth orchestra, and professional orchestra – might be more effective. Compliance and adherence with the exercise program can be ensured by the music tutors and management.

The exercise-based injury prevention program for string players was generally considered important in preventing injury among string players, and the participants showed willingness in understanding the components of the exercise program as well as looking forward to implementing the program. Due to the experience of playing-related musculoskeletal problems experienced by several of the participants, a preventative approach to their injuries was considered a good intervention.

Discussion

The aim of this study was to develop an exercise-based injury prevention program for violinists. The research occurred in two phases. Based on the theoretical approach of injury prevention, the extracted exercise program was adapted for violinists. The face and content validity of the exercise program was conducted with ten exercise experts, and implementation strategies were discussed in a focus group comprised of music tutors.

The exercises were developed based on the physical demands of performance for each affected region in violin playing. The components of the exercise program focused on improving strength and endurance in the cervical region, shoulder strengthening and stabilization exercises, core stabilization exercises, and strengthening and stretching exercises.

Our exercise experts panel suggested additional exercises including proprioceptive neuromuscular facilitation, neuro-mobilization, thoracic mobilization, general mobilization exercises, rhomboids stabilization exercises, and additional stretching exercises. Proprioceptive neuromuscular facilitation was suggested as an important component of the left and right shoulder exercises based on the pattern and demands of the bowing arm especially. Thoracic rotation exercises as well as progressive strengthening exercises of the thoracic region were included as a part of the exercise program. The rationale for the inclusion was due to the trunk rotation associated with playing the string instrument and the high prevalence of musculoskeletal problems in the upper thoracic region. Stabilization exercises of the rhomboids were recommended for inclusion in the exercise program as well. The scapula muscles are important in supporting the violin and in the excursion of shoulder movement. The shoulder is a complex joint, and the integrity of each of the joints that make up the shoulder complex is important in ensuring smooth movements. General mobilization exercises of the upper extremity and trunk to ensure full range of motion aimed at maintaining the physiological joint integrity is suggested.

The components of the current exercise program are similar to the exercise program developed for musicians by Chan et al. [76], especially the shoulder proprioceptive neuromuscular facilitation exercises, deep neck flexor exercises, and core stabilization exercises. In this study, the developed exercise program is more preventive than rehabilitative, focusing on warm up, main exercises, cool down, and exercises during breaks. Stretching during breaks has been shown to reduce perceived discomfort and eventual musculoskeletal injury in string instrumentalists [106].

The inclusion of neuro-mobilization exercises in this program is important as one of the most common symptoms of PRMDs is tingling sensation. The position of the cervical region during violin performance can cause a possible nerve compression of the median, radial, or ulnar nerve, triggering tingling [1]. Specific exercises to improve neuro-mobilization and lessen nerve compression could reduce the incidence of PRMDs. Unfortunately, most studies have overlooked nerve compression in the cervical region as a possible risk factor for PRMDs [15, 17, 76]. Clearly, the consistent static position of the neck during violin performance could result in nerve compression at the C5, C6, C7, C8, and T1 nerve roots.

An exercise-based injury prevention program was first reported in literature two decades ago [17]. Evidence on the components and the effectiveness of exercise as an injury prevention and management for musicians has been explored and evaluated in several studies [15, 17, 76]. Chan et al. study was the first to develop an exercise-based injury prevention program for orchestral musicians using the patho-anatomical pathway of injury and the demands of performance [76]. The anatomic regions commonly affected are synonymous to the demands of performance. Therefore, the biomechanical demands of performance were evaluated as a primary risk factor for the development of PRMDs. The exercise program developed in this study was specific to violin players as an injury prevention strategy. Injury prevention in performing artists has progressed from only surveillance to prevention over the last three decades. Earlier exercise-based injury prevention studies were focused on the overall management of musicians without consideration of the different demands required to play a specific musical instrument [15, 17, 76]. The current research followed the Chan et al. model and developed an instrument-specific exercise-based injury prevention program. A trend in exercise-based injury prevention could be established whereby the specific biomechanical demands of playing the various instruments are evaluated in the exercise development process. Specific exercise-based injury prevention could result in a significant reduction in the problems associated with playing the musical instrument.

Another novelty of this exercise program is having neuro-mobilization included as a component of the exercise program due to the static left lateral bending position of the neck in supporting the violin during performance. The experts in this study suggested a likelihood of nerve compression in the nerve roots of C7–T1 as a result of the awkward position. The results of the cross-sectional study showed that pins/needles and tingling were reported in 15.8% and 13.2% of the string instrumentalists surveyed. We included thoracic mobilization exercise as a component of the exercise program during exercise validation phase due to the mean joint angle results of the thoracic region. The upper thoracic region mean joint angle was in 3.26 (1.91) degrees during violin performance, and the upper back was commonly reported as the site of musculoskeletal problems in 44.7% of violinists. Thoracic mobilization exercise could reduce the discomfort associated with posture among violinists.

In conclusion, this new exercise program emphasizes prevention of musculoskeletal injury among violin players and is focused on improving strength and endurance in the commonly affected anatomic regions. The implementation strategy, emerging from the focus group discussions among music tutors and string players, emphasized educating both the instructors and the students. The instructors also suggested that monitoring and implementation of the exercise program can be done by them. Comments such as "we can follow up on the kids and ensure compliance and adherence" and "we are open to learn the exercise program and teach the program" were shared by the music instructors during the focus group discussion.

Recommendations

The novel exercise program developed specific to violin playing should be piloted among violinists and possibly modified for other string instrumentalists. A longitudinal intervention study to test the effect of the specific program in the prevention of PRMDs among violinists could be conducted. Subsequently, further research related to the biomechanical analysis (physical demands) of playing the cello and double bass would be important in such an adaptation of this program. A process of face and content validation of the adapted program would be important. The specific effect of each exercise on the anatomic region should be evaluated. Furthermore, the education of musicians in South Africa on the associated risk factors and health promotion programs should be integrated as a component in music education training in South Africa.

Finally, compliance and adherence to an exercise program is a challenge. The cultural beliefs of musicians, for example, not having enough time, many repertoires to learn in short time, etc., could be an impediment to the implementation of the program. Therefore, it would be important to approach through a holistic health promotion program involving health education on risk factors, injury prevention and management.

Strengths and Limitations of Study

In developing an exercise-based injury prevention program specific to violinists, the biomechanical demand of playing the violin was evaluated, and the clinical reasoning approach was used to address the symptoms of PRMDs in the anatomic regions commonly affected. The strength of this new exercise program remedies the weaknesses of early exercise programs which have focused on the basic demands of playing a musical instrument overall instead of being instrument specific. The new exercise program developed in this study was modified specifically to meet the demands of violin performance.

This study integrated the biomechanical demands and the pathoanatomical pathway to develop an exercise-based injury prevention program. However, the study has its limitations. The selected experts for validation did not have experience in managing musicians; therefore, the developed exercise program could have been biased toward a more general preventative approach although the experts were provided with the results of the biomechanical demands of performance. Also, significant differences between injured and uninjured violinists could have further evaluated the impact of PRMDs on the bio-kinematic results reported. Despite these limitations, the developed exercise program could be adapted for other string instrumentalists and implemented, although the developed exercise program is best suited for violinists.

Acknowledgments We would like to acknowledge the contribution of the University of the Witwatersrand's Financial Aid Office for the funding provided for this study.

References

1. Bragge P, Bialocerkowski A, McMeeken J. A systematic review of prevalence and risk factors associated with playing-related musculoskeletal disorders in pianists. Occup Med. 2006;56(1):28–38.
2. Ramazzini B. De morbis artificum diatriba [diseases of workers]. Am J Public Health. 2001;91(9):1380–2.
3. Zaza C. Playing-related musculoskeletal disorders in musicians: a systematic review of incidence and prevalence. Can Med Assoc J. 1998;158(8):1019–25.
4. Barnes R, Attwood H, Blom J, Jankielsohn S, Janse van Rensburg W, Smith T, Van Ede L, Nel M. Injury profile of musicians in the Bloemfontein-based Free State symphony orchestra: a short report. S Afr J Physiother. 2011;67(2):41–4.
5. Brusky P. The high prevalence of injury among female bassoonists. Med Probl Perform Art. 2010;25(3):120–5.
6. Fotiadis DG, Fotiadou EG, Kokaridas DG, Mylonas AC. Prevalence of musculoskeletal disorders in professional symphony orchestra musicians in Greece: a pilot study concerning age, gender, and instrument-specific results. Med Probl Perform Art. 2013;28(2):91–5.
7. Paarup HM, Baelum J, Holm JW, Manniche C, Wedderkopp N. Prevalence and consequences of musculoskeletal symptoms in symphony orchestra musicians vary by gender: a cross-sectional study. BMC Musculoskelet Disord. 2011;12(1):1–14.
8. Allsop L, Ackland T. The prevalence of playing-related musculoskeletal disorders in relation to piano players' playing techniques and practising strategies. Music Perform Res. 2010;3(1):61–78.
9. De Sousa CMG, Greten HJ. The prevalence of playing-related musculoskeletal disorders (PRMSD) among professional orchestra players. Rev Musica Hodie. 2015;14(2):111–21.
10. Leaver R, Harris EC, Palmer KT. Musculoskeletal pain in elite professional musicians from British symphony orchestras. Occup Med. 2011;61(8):549–55.
11. Moraes GF, Antunes AP. Musculoskeletal disorders in professional violinists and violists: systematic review. Acta Ortop Bras. 2012;20(1):43–7.
12. Rigg JL, Marrinan R, Thomas MA. Playing-related injury in guitarists playing popular music. Med Probl Perform Art. 2003;18(4):150–2.
13. Kivimäki M, Jokinen M. Job perceptions and well-being among symphony orchestra musicians: a comparison with other occupational groups. Med Probl Perform Art. 1994;9(3):73–6.
14. Steinmetz AS, Scheffer I, Esmer E, Delank KS, Peroz I. Frequency, severity and predictors of playing-related musculoskeletal pain in professional orchestral musicians in Germany. Clin Rheumatol. 2015;34(5):965–73.
15. Ackermann B, Adams R, Marshall E. Strength or endurance training for undergraduate music majors at a university? Med Probl Perform Art. 2002;17(1):33–41.

16. De Greef M, van Wijck R, Reynders K, Toussaint J, Hesseling R. Impact of the Groningen exercise therapy for symphony orchestra musicians program on perceived physical competence and playing-related musculoskeletal disorders of professional musicians. Med Probl Perform Art. 2003;18(4):156–61.
17. Brandfonbrener AG. Orchestral injury prevention intervention study. Med Probl Perform Art. 1997;12(1):9–14.
18. Ackermann B, Adams R, Marshall E. The effect of scapula taping on electromyographic activity and musical performance in professional violinists. Aust J Physiother. 2002;48(3):197–203.
19. Burin AB, Osório FDL. Interventions for music performance anxiety: results from a systematic literature review. Rev Psiquiatr Clin. 2016;43(5):116–31.
20. Zander MF, Voltmer E, Spahn C. Health promotion and prevention in higher music education. Med Probl Perform Art. 2010;25(2):54–65.
21. Lee S-H, Carey S, Lazinski M, Kim ES. An integrative intervention program for college musicians and kinematics in cello playing. Eur J Integr Med. 2019;25:34–40.
22. Cerveró CG, Ruiz JM, Sanchis LR, Ros CR. Pain perception in clarinetists with playing-related pain after implementing a specific exercise program. Med Probl Perform Art. 2018;33(4):238.
23. Karsh B-T. Theories of work-related musculoskeletal disorders: Implications for ergonomic interventions. Theor Issues Ergon Sci. 2006;7(1):71–88.
24. Creswell JW. Research design: qualitative, quantitative, and mixed methods approaches. London, United Kingdom: Sage Publications; 2013.
25. Johnson RB, Onwuegbuzie AJ, Turner LA. Toward a definition of mixed methods research. J Mixed Methods Res. 2007;1(2):112–33.
26. Dixon D, Johnston M, McQueen M. The Disabilities of the Arm, Shoulder and Hand Questionnaire (DASH) can measure the impairment, activity limitations and participation restriction constructs from the International Classification of Functioning, Disability and Health (ICF). BMC Musculoskelet Disord. 2008;9:1–6.
27. Drummond AS, Sampaio RF, Mancini MC, Kirkwood RN, Stamm TA. Linking the disabilities of arm, shoulder, and hand to the international classification of functioning, disability, and health. J Hand Ther. 2007;20(4):336–44.
28. Hudak PL, Amadio PC, Bombardier C. Development of an upper extremity outcome measure: the DASH. Am J Ind Med. 1996;29(6):602–8.
29. Gummesson C, Ward MM, Atroshi I. The shortened disabilities of the arm, shoulder and hand questionnaire (QuickDASH): validity and reliability based on responses within the full-length DASH. BMC Musculoskelet Disord. 2006;7(1):1–7.
30. Angst F, Schwyzer HK, Aeschlimann A, Simmen BR, Goldhahn J. Measures of adult shoulder function: Disabilities of the Arm, Shoulder, and Hand Questionnaire (DASH) and its short version (QuickDASH), Shoulder Pain and Disability Index (SPADI), American Shoulder and Elbow Surgeons (ASES) Society standardized shoulder assessment form, Constant (Murley) Score (CS), Simple Shoulder Test (SST), Oxford Shoulder Score (OSS), Shoulder Disability Questionnaire (SDQ), and Western Ontario Shoulder Instability Index (WOSI). Arthritis Care Res (Hoboken). 2011;63(S11):S174–S88.
31. Wu A, Edgar D, Wood F. The QuickDASH is an appropriate tool for measuring the quality of recovery after upper limb burn injury. Burns. 2007;33(7):843–9.
32. Fan ZJ, Smith CK, Silverstein BA. Assessing validity of the QuickDASH and SF-12 as surveillance tools among workers with neck or upper extremity musculoskeletal disorders. J Hand Ther. 2008;21(4):354–65.
33. Vernon H, Mior S. The Neck Disability Index: a study of reliability and validity. J Manipulative Physiol Ther. 1991;14(7):409–15.
34. Pietrobon R, Coeytaux RR, Carey TS, Richardson WJ, DeVellis RF. Standard scales for measurement of functional outcome for cervical pain or dysfunction: a systematic review. Spine. 2002;27(5):515–22.
35. Cleland JA, Childs JD, Whitman JM. Psychometric properties of the Neck Disability Index and Numeric Pain Rating Scale in patients with mechanical neck pain. Arch Phys Med Rehabil. 2008;89(1):69–74.

36. Crooks VA, Kingsbury P, Snyder J, Johnston R. What is known about the patient's experience of medical tourism? A scoping review. BMC Health Serv Res. 2010;10(1):266.
37. Hanass-Hancock J, Regondi I, Van Egeraat L, Nixon S. HIV-related disability in HIV hyper-endemic countries: a scoping review. World J AIDS. 2013;3(3):1–23.
38. O'Flaherty J, Phillips C. The use of flipped classrooms in higher education: a scoping review. Internet High Educ. 2015;25:85–95.
39. Dijkers M. What is a scoping review. KT Update. 2015;4(1):1–4.
40. Levac D, Colquhoun H, O'Brien KK. Scoping studies: advancing the methodology. Implement Sci. 2010;5(1):1–9.
41. Abreu Ramos AM, Micheo WF. Lifetime prevalence of upper-body musculoskeletal problems in a professional-level symphony orchestra. Med Probl Perform Art. 2007;22(3):97–104.
42. Chan RF, C-y C, Lee GP, To L-k, Tsang XY, Yeung SS, Yeung EW. Self-perceived exertion level and objective evaluation of neuromuscular fatigue in a training session of orchestral violin players. Appl Ergon. 2000;31(4):335–41.
43. Davies J, Mangion S. Predictors of pain and other musculoskeletal symptoms among professional instrumental musicians: elucidating specific effects. Med Probl Perform Art. 2002;17(4):155–69.
44. Brandfonbrener AG. Joint laxity and arm pain in a large clinical sample of musicians. Med Probl Perform Art. 2002;17(3):113–5.
45. Anderson AF, Dome DC, Gautam S, Awh MH, Rennirt GW. Correlation of anthropometric measurements, strength, anterior cruciate ligament size, and intercondylar notch characteristics to sex differences in anterior cruciate ligament tear rates. Am J Sports Med. 2001;29(1):58–66.
46. Ekman A, Andersson A, Hagberg M, Hjelm E. Gender differences in musculoskeletal health of computer and mouse users in the Swedish workforce. Occup Med. 2000;50(8):608–13.
47. Barsky AJ, Peekna HM, Borus JF. Somatic symptom reporting in women and men. J Gen Intern Med. 2001;16(4):266–75.
48. Van Wijk CMG, Kolk AM. Sex differences in physical symptoms: the contribution of symptom perception theory. Soc Sci Med. 1997;45(2):231–46.
49. Wilke C, Priebus J, Biallas B, Froböse I. Motor activity as a way of preventing musculoskeletal problems in string musicians. Med Probl Perform Art. 2011;26(1):24–9.
50. Dawson WJ. Upper extremity overuse in instrumentalists. Med Probl Perform Art. 2001;16(2):66–71.
51. Hawkins D, Metheny J. Overuse injuries in youth sports: biomechanical considerations. Med Sci Sports Exerc. 2001;33(10):1701–7.
52. Barczyk-Pawelec K, Sipko T, Demczuk-Włodarczyk E, Boczar A. Anterioposterior spinal curvatures and magnitude of asymmetry in the trunk in musicians playing the violin compared with nonmusicians. J Manipulative Physiol Ther. 2012;35(4):319–26.
53. World Health Organisation. World Health Organisation: international classification of functioning, disability and health. Geneva: World Health Organisation; 2001.
54. Barton R, Killian C, Bushee M, Callen J, Cupp T, Ochs B, Sharp M, Tetrault K. Occupational performance issues and predictors of dysfunction in college instrumentalists. Med Probl Perform Art. 2008;23(2):72–9.
55. Niekel MC, Lindenhovius AL, Watson JB, Vranceanu A-M, Ring D. Correlation of DASH and QuickDASH with measures of psychological distress.J. Hand Surg. 2009;34(8):1499–505.
56. Wong JY, Fung BK, Chu MM, Chan RK. The use of Disabilities of the Arm, Shoulder, and Hand Questionnaire in rehabilitation after acute traumatic hand injuries. J Hand Ther. 2007;20(1):49–56.
57. Am K, Tennant A, Fear J, Emery P, Conaghan PG. Impact of multiple joint problems on daily living tasks in people in the community over age fifty-five. Arthritis Care Res. 2006;55(5):757–64.
58. Kaufman-Cohen Y, Ratzon N. Correlation between risk factors and musculoskeletal disorders among classical musicians. Occup Med. 2011;61(2):90–5.
59. McAtamney L, Corlett EN. RULA: a survey method for the investigation of work-related upper limb disorders. Appl Ergon. 1993;24(2):91–9.

60. Ariëns G, Bongers P, Douwes M, Miedema M, Hoogendoorn W, van der Wal G, Bouter L, van Mechelen W. Are neck flexion, neck rotation, and sitting at work risk factors for neck pain? Results of a prospective cohort study. Occup Environ Med. 2001;58(3):200–7.
61. Visser B, van Dieën JH. Pathophysiology of upper extremity muscle disorders. J Electromyogr Kinesiol. 2006;16(1):1–16.
62. Falla D, Bilenkij G, Jull G. Patients with chronic neck pain demonstrate altered patterns of muscle activation during performance of a functional upper limb task. Spine. 2004;29(13):1436–40.
63. Yip CHT, Chiu TTW, Poon ATK. The relationship between head posture and severity and disability of patients with neck pain. Man Ther. 2008;13(2):148–54.
64. Abdel-aziem AA, Draz AH. Efficacy of deep neck flexor exercise for neck pain: a randomized controlled study. Turk J Phys Med Rehabil. 2016;62(2):107–15.
65. Sihawong R, Janwantanakul P, Jiamjarasrangsi W. Effects of an exercise programme on preventing neck pain among office workers: a 12-month cluster-randomised controlled trial. Occup Environ Med. 2013;71(1):63–70.
66. Van Tulder M, Malmivaara A, Esmail R, Koes B. Exercise therapy for low back pain: a systematic review within the framework of the cochrane collaboration back review group. Spine. 2000;25(21):2784–96.
67. Eijsden-Besseling M, Kuijers M, Kap B, Stam H, Terpstra-Lindeman E. Differences in posture and postural disorders between music and medical students. Med Probl Perform Art. 1993;8(3):110–4.
68. Ramella M, Fronte F, Converti R. Postural disorders in conservatory students: the Diesis project. Med Probl Perform Art. 2014;29(1):19–22.
69. Steinmetz A, Seidel W, Muche B. Impairment of postural stabilization systems in musicians with playing-related musculoskeletal disorders. J Manipulative Physiol Ther. 2010;33(8):603–11.
70. Lederman E. The myth of core stability. J Bodyw Mov Ther. 2010;14(1):84–98.
71. Brandt Y, Currier L, Plante TW, Schubert Kabban CM, Tvaryanas AP. A randomized controlled trial of core strengthening exercises in helicopter crewmembers with low back pain. Aerosp Med Hum Perform. 2015;86(10):889–94.
72. Peate W, Bates G, Lunda K, Francis S, Bellamy K. Core strength: a new model for injury prediction and prevention. J Occup Med Toxicol. 2007;2(3):1–9.
73. Willson JD, Dougherty CP, Ireland ML, Davis IM. Core stability and its relationship to lower extremity function and injury. J Am Acad Orthop Surg. 2005;13(5):316–25.
74. Yang EJ, Park W-B, Shin H-I, Lim J-Y. The effect of back school integrated with core strengthening in patients with chronic low-back pain. Am J Phys Med Rehabil. 2010;89(9):744–54.
75. Vergara M, Page A. Relationship between comfort and back posture and mobility in sitting-posture. Appl Ergon. 2002;33(1):1–8.
76. Chan C, Driscoll T, Ackermann B. Development of a specific exercise programme for professional orchestral musicians. Inj Prev. 2013;19(4):257–63.
77. Chan C, Driscoll T, Ackermann BJ. Effect of a musicians' exercise intervention on performance-related musculoskeletal disorders [AGB award 2014]. Med Probl Perform Art. 2014;29(4):23–30.
78. Kava KS, Larson CA, Stiller CH, Maher SF. Trunk endurance exercise and the effect in instrumental performance: a preliminary study comparing Pilates exercise and a trunk and proximal upper extremity endurance exercise program. Music Perform Res. 2010;3(1):1–30.
79. Smith CE, Nyland J, Caudill P, Brosky J, Caborn DN. Dynamic trunk stabilization: a conceptual back injury prevention program for volleyball athletes. J Orthop Sports Phys Ther. 2008;38(11):703–20.
80. Griffin LYE. Neuromuscular training and injury prevention in sports. Clin Orthop Relat Res. 2003;409:53–60.
81. Inani SB, Selkar SP. Effect of core stabilization exercises versus conventional exercises on pain and functional status in patients with non-specific low back pain: a randomized clinical trial. J Back Musculoskelet Rehabil. 2013;26(1):37–43.

82. Moore M, DeHaan L, Ehrenberg T, Gross L, Magembe C. Clinical assessment of shoulder impingement factors in violin and viola players. Med Probl Perform Art. 2008;23(4):155–64.
83. Rickert D, Barrett M, Halaki M, Driscoll T, Ackermann B. A study of right shoulder injury in collegiate and professional orchestral cellists: an investigation using questionnaires and physical assessment. Med Probl Perform Art. 2012;27(2):65–73.
84. MacDonald PB, Clark P, Sutherland K. An analysis of the diagnostic accuracy of the Hawkins and Neer subacromial impingement signs. J Shoulder Elbow Surg. 2000;9(4):299–301.
85. Phadke V, Camargo P, Ludewig P. Scapular and rotator cuff muscle activity during arm elevation: a review of normal function and alterations with shoulder impingement. Braz J Phys Ther. 2009;13(1):1–9.
86. Struyf F, Nijs J, Baeyens JP, Mottram S, Meeusen R. Scapular positioning and movement in unimpaired shoulders, shoulder impingement syndrome, and glenohumeral instability. Scand J Med Sci Sports. 2011;21(3):352–8.
87. Shan G, Visentin P. A quantitative three-dimensional analysis of arm kinematics in violin performance. Med Probl Perform Art. 2003;18(1):3–10.
88. Rolland P, Mutchler M, Hellebrandt F. The teaching of action in string playing. Illinois, USA: Illinois String Research Associates; 1986. 61801 p.
89. Zhang J-T, Novak AC, Brouwer B, Li Q. Concurrent validation of Xsens MVN measurement of lower limb joint angular kinematics. Physiol Meas. 2013;34(8):N63–N9.
90. de Araújo NCK, Gatto Cardia MC, Másculo FS, Gomes Lucena NM. Analysis of the frequency of postural flaws during violin performance. Med Probl Perform Art. 2009;24(3):108–12.
91. Ericsson KA, Krampe RT, Tesch-Römer C. The role of deliberate practice in the acquisition of expert performance. Psychol Rev. 1993;100(3):363.
92. Bernhardsson S, Klintberg IH, Wendt GK. Evaluation of an exercise concept focusing on eccentric strength training of the rotator cuff for patients with subacromial impingement syndrome. Clin Rehabil. 2011;25(1):69–78.
93. Ludewig P, Borstad J. Effects of a home exercise programme on shoulder pain and functional status in construction workers. Occup Environ Med. 2003;60(11):841–9.
94. Zebis MK, Andersen CH, Sundstrup E, Pedersen MT, Sjøgaard G, Andersen LL. Time-wise change in neck pain in response to rehabilitation with specific resistance training: implications for exercise prescription. PLoS One. 2014;9(4):1–6.
95. Andersen CH, Andersen LL, Gram B, Pedersen MT, Mortensen OS, Zebis MK, Sjøgaard G. Influence of frequency and duration of strength training for effective management of neck and shoulder pain: a randomised controlled trial. Br J Sports Med. 2012;46(14):1004–10.
96. Häkkinen A, Kautiainen H, Hannonen P, Ylinen J. Strength training and stretching versus stretching only in the treatment of patients with chronic neck pain: a randomized one-year follow-up study. Clin Rehabil. 2008;22(7):592–600.
97. Andersen LL, Jorgensen MB, Blangsted AK, Pedersen MT, Hansen EA, Sjogaard G. A randomized controlled intervention trial to relieve and prevent neck/shoulder pain. Med Sci Sports Exerc. 2008;40(6):983–90.
98. Borstad JD, Buetow B, Deppe E, Kyllonen J, Liekhus M, Cieminski CJ, Ludewig PM. A longitudinal analysis of the effects of a preventive exercise programme on the factors that predict shoulder pain in construction apprentices. Ergonomics. 2009;52(2):232–44.
99. American College of Sports Medicine. In: Pescatello L, editor. ACSM's Guidelines for exercise testing and prescription. 9th ed. Philadelphia: Lippincott Williams and Wilkins; 2014.
100. Steffen KM, Willem H, Romiti M, Kang J, McKay C, Bizzini M, Dvorak J, Finch C, Myklebust G, Emery CA. Evaluation of how different implementation strategies of an injury prevention programme (FIFA 11+) impact team adherence and injury risk in Canadian female youth football players: a cluster-randomised trial. Br J Sports Med. 2013:1–9.
101. Soligard T, Myklebust G, Steffen K, Holme I, Silvers H, Bizzini M, Junge A, Dvorak J, Bahr R, Andersen TE. Comprehensive warm-up programme to prevent injuries in young female footballers: cluster randomised controlled trial. Br Med J. 2008;337:95–9.

102. Lederman RJ. Entrapment neuropathies in instrumental musicians. Med Probl Perform Art. 1993;8(2):35–9.
103. Chan C, Driscoll T, Ackermann B. Exercise DVD effect on musculoskeletal disorders in professional orchestral musicians. Occup Med. 2013;64(1):23–30.
104. Jakobsen MD, Sundstrup E, Brandt M, Jay K, Aagaard P, Andersen LL. Effect of workplace- versus home-based physical exercise on musculoskeletal pain among healthcare workers: a cluster randomized controlled trial. Scand J Work Environ Health. 2015;41(2):153–63.
105. Dalager T, Bredahl TG, Pedersen MT, Boyle E, Andersen LL, Sjøgaard G. Does training frequency and supervision affect compliance, performance and muscular health? A cluster randomized controlled trial. Man Ther. 2015;20(5):657–65.
106. Cooper SC, Hamann DL, Frost R. The effects of stretching exercises during rehearsals on string students' self-reported perceptions of discomfort. Update Univ D C Dep Music. 2012;30(2):71–6.

Chapter 7
Nikolai Bernstein's Theory of Movement Construction as a Foundation of Flow in Piano Technique

Evgeny Chugunov

Introduction

Pianists, after even the most successful performance in concert, competition, or exam, will ask themselves: why did I periodically lose my connection with the instrument? Why didn't some passages sound natural enough? Why didn't hands and fingers cooperate with the flexible and purposeful line of the musical phrase? In the simplest possible terms, why didn't it just *flow*?

In most specialized forms of skilled physical training, be it dance, sport, or musical performance, experts have been trying for decades to understand, describe, achieve, and maintain a state of flow. Flow involves coordinated and balanced actions on all levels of the motor system: neural, musculoskeletal, kinetic, spatial, etc. Different fields of research call this state of flow by different names, but the descriptions of it often are similar. It is a physical and mental state, a "special zone," in which the performer is fully immersed in a feeling of energized focus and involvement [1]. The question, therefore, is how to achieve this state of flow, this sense of perfect control over movements, and this moment of transformation of body and mind into the motion itself.

Theoretical Framework

The idea of the flow as an *optimal experience* was developed in detail by Mihaly Csikszentmihalyi [1]. As he describes it, this optimal experience emerges as a result

E. Chugunov (✉)
Department of Music, Lakehead University, Thunder Bay, ON, Canada
e-mail: etchougo@lakeheadu.ca

S.-H. Lee et al. (eds.), *Perspectives in Performing Arts Medicine Practice*,
https://doi.org/10.1007/978-3-030-37480-8_7

of dealing with challenging, yet creative situations. It is a state that enables a person to transform the authentically challenging practice and achieve a qualitatively superior, more complex, and finely organized performance. The "optimal experience" brings with it a sense of satisfaction, energy, and enjoyment of the immediate experience [1]. This notion of optimal experience broadly overlaps with Bernstein's state of readiness, the skillfully trained movement conceived as a living and goal-directed action, dynamically cooperating with its environment [2].

Dominance and Readiness

The notion of state of readiness is described as a specific functional psychophysiological state or *functional organ*, which we can witness in movements, actions, perceptions, memories, knowledge, consciousness, emotions, and many other entities according to Ukhtomsky's classification [3]. A. Ukhtomsky's vision of functional organs played a key role in the formation of Bernstein's physiology of activity. These functional organs evolve in two phases: (1) initial development leading to maturation and (2) plateau, an eventual background state favoring professional improvement and personal growth of the pianist. By defining performance motion as an active, goal-oriented, and hierarchically organized functional organ, it may well be possible for us to move significantly closer toward that desirable yet elusive state of flow [4].

Another useful concept of Ukhtomsky's, which largely anticipated the current vision of the flow, is dominance, a psychological or physiological governing center of a person's functional organ, or a unique functional state. Once achieved as the result of an optimally organized training, dominance becomes a background "state of readiness," able to engage and co-opt various mental and physiological mechanisms to perform a specific action.

Bernstein also explored this state of readiness in considerable detail within the psychophysiology of movement construction. He saw readiness as *tonus*, not defined as elasticity but rather as a *pre-condition to an effect* [2]. Essential features of this psychological and physiological state include as follows: (1) the high level of excitability and concomitant stability; (2) the capacity to summate its own excitation states; (3) the ability to inhibit weaker centers of activity; and (4) inertia, which sustains the psychological and physiological dominant over time. All of these contribute to enhancing the dominant center [5].

Performance Readiness

Csikszentmihalyi's theory of flow pointed out that optimal experience brings someone to an entirely new level of functioning, with a greater sense of control over actions, decreasing awareness of self and of time passing [1]. Similarly,

Ukhtomsky's dominance also describes the functional state as a dominant center capable of involving the entirety of the body to perform a specific task, suppressing weaker centers or co-opting them to achieve a precise goal. Hence, setting a clear and achievable goal, establishing a dominant center, and providing immediate feedback are the essential conditions for the successful achievement of Csikszentmihalyi's flow, Ukhtomsky's functional organs, and Bernstein's performance of movement. However, each of these theories contributes a different perspective. Csikszentmihalyi goes on to describe flow as an *autotelic* experience, while Bernstein refers to the achievement of the "model of the required future" [1, 5]. Bernstein's model of the required future includes two interrelated processes: one of them is a probabilistic prognosis based on a perceived current situation and the other a procedure of programming an action whose goal is to bring about the realization of the desired future [5].

Music performance, much like sports and physical education, shares a common idea of "ready position." This position requires a larger base of support, which is the entire space formed by the points of contact with a resistive surface (the keyboard in our case) that provides reaction forces. It is called ready position because the pianist is prepared to move in any direction quickly and absorb impact from different forces more effectively. Also, changing the size, shape, and direction of the base of support as well as lowering the center of gravity can significantly contribute to increased dynamic stability and balance of the pianistic apparatus, which provides continuous control of equilibrium and coordination.

Within the state of performance readiness, a much broader concept than either flow or performing movement is necessary; motor control is essential. The understanding of motor control was profoundly influenced by Nikolai Bernstein's hierarchical theory of motor coordination, discussed below. The purpose of this chapter is to explicate Bernstein's levels of movement construction as they apply toward achieving flow and readiness in piano technique.

Bernstein's Levels of Movement Construction

By studying a hierarchical inventory of motions, Bernstein formulated general concepts of the structure and function of the motor control system. He postulated that the motor control system is comprised of a number of structural-functional levels. Every level operates within a certain area of the human brain [6][1].

[1] On the Construction of Movements, 1947. In Russian. Still not fully available in translation, Bernstein was one of the premier intellectuals of the twentieth century. His work pioneered the field of motor control, to which he dedicated most of his life. His broad scientific legacy was celebrated in the international conference, *Bernstein's Traditions in Motor Control*, at Pennsylvania State University in 1996.

Subcortical Levels of Movement Construction

Level A The first level, A, is the lowest in the hierarchy of movement construction. It is also called the *paleokinetic* level, or the *rubrospinal* level. It is governed by a part of the spinal cord and lower parts of the brain stem. This level is assisted by its own afferent group of nerves that deliver signals on the amplitude and direction of muscle tension and efforts, on the position of body parts with respect to each other and to the space and gravitational field. Pure level A movement is involuntary, for example, shivering, teeth chattering, or flinching. Level A movement regulation begins in the first weeks of a child's life, but it functions properly only when a child can sit down and keep a straight neck. Pathological dysfunction at level A is seen in dystonic symptoms in adults [7].

In pianistic movement, the right muscle tonus support is essential to be able to use Bernstein's functional levels. Level A generates and maintains the necessary level of muscle tension, supplying those muscles with suitable tonus. Level A also maintains proper posture – always a priority – and helps the performer to keep all the body parts involved in piano playing well aligned. This alignment allows the shoulder, upper arm, forearm, wrist, hand, and fingers to work in coordination as a continuous unit. Such efficient coordinated movement has been described in details by Otto Ortmann [8] and highlighted in the Taubman Approach [9]. Ortmann devoted his research to investigating multiple physiological aspects of pianistic movements, such as the mechanics of muscular action, alignment, coordination, relaxation, and weight transfer. He viewed the proper organization of the pianistic apparatus as an efficient collaboration, resulting in a middle range of motion by multiple levers: fingers, hands, and arms, with the joints of the hands, elbows, and shoulders operating as fulcrums [8].

The Taubman Approach, largely inspired by the ideas of Otto Ortmann, taught efficient and safe coordination with practical insights. Here, the proper alignment of the pianistic apparatus is critical in two ways: first, it creates the feeling of connection with the instrument; second, it keeps that connection stable and consistent during performance [10]. The action of holding something, like a particular key in piano, is another significant function of level A. Level A allows the performer to press a key down as long as necessary, even as other movements change the weight applied to a key or the position of the finger holding it.

Attention to the development of level A motions should be teachers' priority, especially with beginners. Teachers should pay special attention to maintaining the alignment of bones and joints in the hand. It is important to note that the bones of the hand are arranged in three arches: the proximal transverse arch which passes through the distal carpus and is relatively fixed, the distal transverse arch which passes through the metacarpal heads and is more mobile, and the longitudinal arch which connects the other two [11]. The intrinsic muscles of the hand are generally responsible for supporting the shape of the three arches, and collapse, especially in the distal transverse arch (metacarpophalangeal joint), will result in extensive tension, a shift of the center of gravity, loss of control, and, possibly, future injury.

However, forcing a student to keep the "correct" hand position at a young age, without gradually developing the sense of muscular tonus and joints' support, especially in the MCP joint, might develop focal dystonia later on.

With muscle strength gained through practice, the student should be gradually able to create a state of equilibrium and stability. The different aspects of motion control need to be introduced, such as force of gravity, center of gravity, base of support, equilibrium, balance, directional stability, etc. It is important to note that level A is responsible for providing the *ready position* in which a pianist is ready to move in any direction quickly and absorb forces in the most efficient way.

Level B This is the level of synergies and patterns (or models); it is also called the *thalamo-pallidar* level. This level occurs in subcortex layers and the cerebellum. Level B receptors transfer information about muscle angles, speeds, pressure, and directions and process it to form a complete image of the body in any position, not unlike snapping an X-ray. Level B has three essential characteristics for the construction of movement: First, it governs a wide range of motions involving a large group of coordinated muscles. Second, it performs a movement set in time with extraordinary precision and reproducibility. Third, it allows rhythmic movements to be precise not only in time but also in space. The body receives limited information from the outside, so there are very few independent movements carried out by level B. Indeed, level B acquires data mostly from the actions of the body itself. Bernstein compares level B to a flight mechanic rather than a pilot or navigator [7]. Level B handles all the minute internal details of compound movements.

In piano playing, level B is responsible for coordination (including rhythmic) between alternating motions or different playing apparatus parts involved in the movement such as rotation, shaping motions, repeated octaves or chords, etc. Level B also ensures consistency in the shape of a movement by providing rotational equilibrium and rotational stability. Rotational stability is closely related to the position of the center of gravity, and if this center of gravity is in the middle of the base of support, then the hand is in rotational equilibrium. The pianist is able to increase the rotational stability by widening the base of support or by lowering the center of gravity. This type of stability is essential when the pianist plays a passage within the hand position which requires smooth and consistent shape in small rotational movements. When the motion goes beyond the comfortable space of the hand position, a pianist should be ready for the sudden change from a stable to an unstable position in a short time, and at that moment, level C will take control of their movements.

Cortical Levels of Movement Construction

Level C Bernstein called level C the spatial field and considered it to be one of the most important levels of movement construction. Anatomically, it is on the border between the ancient (subcortical) and the modern (cortical) structures of the human brain. Also called *pyramido-striatal* level, level C has two sublevels: C1, striatal or extrapyramidal, and C2, pyramidal. Level C has five characteristics: First, it is linked to the outside world and is governed by external stimuli, unlike levels A and B, which are all about the internal sensations of the body. Second, it is served by receptors which widen and amplify incoming information from external sources in both volume and quality. Third, level C is immobile, i.e., the world beyond the body remains motionless. To quote Bernstein directly, "the spatial field for level C is extensive, unwavering and homogeneous. When we walk, climb stairs, when we turn, not only do we know, but we also feel with great clarity and immediacy that we move, while the space in which we are moving is filled with motionless objects, all receptors tell us the reverse" [7]. Fourth, level C is geometrical, with precise measurements of distances and shapes to allow accurate movement. The final characteristic arises from the preceding four: movement originating from level C is always purposeful and always gives a concrete and observable result. For example, we hit a nail, we move a chair, we turn a page, we hit a key [7].

Level C has two sublevels, as mentioned, and both are significant in piano playing. Sublevel C1 adapts motion in space, and sublevel C2 uses this adaptability to reach the goals of adjustments for precision and accuracy. Mastering the C sublevels is crucial to the development of piano skills. Sublevel C1 is like tightrope walking, where trusting your body in space is essential. This sublevel is closely connected with level B and, in turn, adds directional stability for movement at the piano by widening the base of support in the direction of the line of action. In piano, the performer needs to sense the space with the palms, before incorporating sight control. In developing that ability to sense space, the pianist often switches sight off, because there is no need for compelling sight for performing some part of the musical texture that fits within a hand position. Sight control can then be reserved for leaps when moving outside or in between the hand positions.

Sublevel C2, with the help of sight control, changes the situation dramatically in a short time. To execute a leap or to move in between hand positions, a previously stable condition becomes a highly mobile and unstable position. The base of support is now formed only by contact of a single finger with a key or fingers playing simultaneously an interval or a chord with a few keys, whereas before, it included the entire palm area of the hand. The pianist is in a mobile or highly unstable position because the base of support has been minimized and the center of gravity is outside of the base of support. This change causes an unbalanced force, which in turn allows a rapid acceleration of motion. Level C always works in close collaboration with the following level D in Bernstein's classification.

Level D is the level of actions (object actions, meaningful actions), or the *parietal-premotor* level. Level D measures topology and chronology, i.e., top, bottom, between, under, above the key surface, as well as before and after touch [7]. Level D is concerned more directly with real space, surface, and distance, and it plays a major part in assisting the highly mobile work of level C. Consequently, it also performs the critical distinction of actions by the right and left hands, a difference less marked in levels A, B, and C. Level D movements become formalized much later in human development, at about 7 years of age, with obvious implications for early piano training.

For piano practice, the musician needs to be aware of such specifics as keyboard topology, the distance between the keys, forces used to depress the keys, and more. The white and black keys are on different planes, requiring adjustments into the black key area, especially with the shorter 1st and 5th fingers, and out of the black key area with the longer 2nd, 3rd, and 4th fingers. It is also important to consider under shaping and over shaping motions, to minimize the size and number of those very motions. Level D is also responsible for controlling weight application and the speed of attack of that specific part of the key descent so-called the point of sound that triggers the double escapement mechanism. The double escapement mechanism lies at the heart of piano technique: it has the potential not only to transform tone production but also to contribute significantly to developing a sense of connection, a feeling that the piano is an extension of the performer's body. Controlling the speed of attack and weight application onto the point of sound of the key is a crucial step toward adjusting tone production and, eventually, achieving flow.

Level E is the level of symbolic, highly coordinated actions such as speech, writing, dancing, instrumental performance, etc. It is based on the highest cortical control, the last and highest of Bernstein's theory of movement construction. It is concerned with intellectual motor behavior. It contributes primarily to speech and writing movements, including symbolic or coded speech such as sign language or Morse code. On level E, abstract verbal meanings establish movement, rather than by subject [7]. In musical performance, level E motivates motor action, makes all necessary adaptations, and brings about a sound to fulfill a musical intention created by the initial "model of the required future," which in turn provides a necessary direction for every musical movement [12]. There is no musical phrase possible if the goal and the direction are not defined prior to its execution. The definite purpose or direction is crystallized after thorough practicing, but the initial draft of the movement must pre-exist. One of the most frequent problems in musical practice that can perpetuate bad habits is the absence of direction or a goal in the model of the required future.

A Novel Scheme for Injury-Free Piano Technique Development

Automation Phase

It is now possible to develop an overview of the development of performance skills adopting Bernstein's theory. After the pianist determines the concept of the desired sound, motion construction starts at levels A and B with auxiliary functions such as providing muscle tonus, maintaining posture, and supporting locomotor and autonomous movements of the whole body over time. Further development relies on the voluntary actions of sublevels C1 and C2. Mastering an instrument occurs with level D, and providing the symbolic meaning of music occurs through level E. Every type of movement is dominated by one particular level, while the others perform supporting functions. All levels, therefore, play their strictly defined roles, whether primary or secondary. In many situations, levels in supporting roles must consciously be trained in order to reach ease of automation. That, in turn, will free up the player to focus levels D and E, attending to immediate musical tasks.

Stabilization Phase

After an initial analysis of the structure of the composition to be played, much as a theatre director would cast leading and supporting roles, it becomes possible to create the desired movements, ensuring successful connection between the "real performance situation" and its constant changes. At the very moment of external creation, stabilization of developing piano skills begins. The new motion will face interaction between different internal and external forces, such as a reaction force where even small changes in muscle activity will produce a reaction or force capable of changing the position and tonus of other body parts [13]. These will inevitably result in changes in the position and movement of muscles, nerves, joints, and other body parts. Some of the most common solutions to these external forces are for the student to minimize reaction to them, but this leads inevitably to energy-wasting tensions in the facial muscles, jaw, tongue, neck, and shoulders. Ideally, the pianist should gradually harness those forces to achieve engaged, conscious artistry and, eventually, create a sense of *flow*.

Despite all these caveats, developing flow, along with other technical skills, is possible by seeking a dynamic (i.e., constantly adapting) equilibrium. Stability and balance in this context would be produced by perfect coordination of levels A and B and more unstable or mobile equilibrium by active collaboration of levels C and D. In the case of a pianist, level B activates an immediate response right after the fingertip lands on the surface of a key. That reaction force in the opposite direction, provided by the entire playing apparatus preventing the finger from compressing or sinking into the key, is a level D motion. Level A then provides small vibrating motions to maintain the tonus required for alignment of pianistic apparatus as well as the arch in the hand. Again, after a pianist creates the concept of required sound, the initial training of movement starts with lower levels and works toward the upper levels; once the development of the lower levels is complete, the stabilization phase works from higher levels down. In this process, control is initiated exclusively from the highest level, i.e., in the cortical part of the brain [7].

Ultimately, the pianist must strive to maintain a state of *equilibrium* during practice as the foundation of *dynamic stability*. Dynamic stability releases rather than constrains freedom of motion, and it minimizes muscular effort and saves energy. The resulting feeling of relaxation is indeed one of the highest forms of coordination, where inactive muscles relax and do not impede the perfectly balanced work of active muscles. In dynamic but resilient equilibrium, all planes of movements are unused except the ones required to maintain the smooth curvilinear shape of motions originated as a response to the reaction forces mentioned above. In other words, the work of muscles has been economized, as have been the CNS's effectors. Moreover, once the movement reaches that state, it runs like a train on rails, without the need of an operator for the steering wheel.

Conclusion

This argument began with a discussion of applications of flow in musical performance. A well-coordinated pianistic motion and the state of equilibrium and dynamic stability can be compared to bobsleigh technique, where two or four teammates make timed runs down narrow, twisted ice tracks in a gravity-powered sleigh. First, a sleigh is made of light but solid metal to allow dynamic positioning of mass through the turns of the course. The pianist's playing apparatus should feel this lightness and at the same time maintain a coordinated alignment within a solid structure of unlocked and freely moving stabilized joints and fingers. The success in bobsleigh technique then depends on the remarkably synchronized work of teammates (lower levels A, B, and C) and very subtle steering adjustments made by a pilot (leading levels D and E). The shape of the track walls also triggers the involvement of different forces, particularly the reaction forces which are essential elements in the attainment of flow. Virtuosity and the development of injury-free piano technique largely depend on the further understanding of these principles of multilevel movement coordination both on their own and in interactions between them and multiple external and internal forces.

References

1. Csikszentmihalyi M. Flow: the psychology of optimal experience. New York: Harper; 1990.
2. Chugunov E. Phenomenon of performer's readiness in the theory and practice of music training [Феномен исполнительской готовности в теории и практике обучения музыке]. Ph.D. [dissertation]. Moscow, Russia: Moscow State Pedagogical University; 2001.
3. Ukhtomsky AA. Selected works [Избранные труды]. Leningrad: Leningrad University Publisher; 1978.
4. Kolesnikov VN. Lectures on the psychology of individuality [Лекции по психологии индивидуальности]. Moscow: Institute of Psychology of RAS; 1996.
5. Zueva EY, Zuev KB. The concept of dominance by A.A. Ukhtomsky and Anticipation. New York: Springer International Publishing; 2015.
6. Latash ML. Progress in motor control – Bernstein's traditions in movement studies, vol. 1. Champaign: Human Kinetics Publishers; 1998.
7. Bernstein NA. On the construction of movements [О построении движений]. Moscow: Medgiz; 1947.

8. Ortmann O. The physiological mechanics of piano technique: an experimental study of the nature of muscular action as used in piano playing, and of the effects thereof upon the piano key and the piano tone. New York: Da Capo Press; 1981.
9. Taubman D, Golandsky E, Bloomfield J, Yagupsky A. Virtuosity in a box: the Taubman techniques [DVD]. New York: Taubman Institute, The Golandsky Institute; 2005. Disc 1.
10. Chugunov E. Motor control in piano technique. Doctor of music [Thesis]. Montreal, QC: Université de Montréal; 2006.
11. Bejjani FJ, Landsmeer JMF. Biomechanics of the hand – basic biomechanics of the musculoskeletal system. Philadelphia, London: Lea & Febiger; 1989.
12. Feigenberg IM. To see – to foresee – to act. Nauka (in Russian): Moscow; 1986.
13. Feldman AG, Meijer OG. Bernstein's heritage. Discovering the right questions in motor control: movements (1929). Motor Control. Human Kinetics Publishers, Inc. 1999;3:105–34.

Chapter 8
Breathing Techniques in Collegiate Vocalists: The Effects of the Mind-Body Integrated Exercise Program on Singers' Posture, Tension, Efficacy, and Respiratory Function

Emily Lopez, Sang-Hie Lee, Ruth Bahr, Stephanie L. Carey, Brittany Mott, Ashleigh Fults, Matthew Lazinski, and Eun Sook Kim

Introduction

The act of efficient vocalization for collegiate singers is physically and mentally demanding as they engage in rigorous training to prepare for a professional singing career. Course work in this field requires additional components in building daily wellness habits along with the ability to learn and memorize music quickly. In reality, voice students tend to take shortcuts during practice, cut back on sleeping

E. Lopez (✉)
School of Music, University of South Florida, Tampa, FL, USA

University of Florida, College of Pharmacy, Department of Medicinal Chemistry, Gainesville, FL, USA
e-mail: emily.lopez@ufl.edu

S.-H. Lee
School of Music, College of the Arts, University of South Florida, Tampa, FL, USA
e-mail: slee@usf.edu

R. Bahr
Office of Graduate Studies & Department of Communication Sciences and Disorders, Tampa, FL, USA
e-mail: rbahr@usf.edu

S. L. Carey · B. Mott · A. Fults
Department of Mechanical Engineering, Center for Assistive, Rehabilitation & Robotics Technologies (CARRT), University of South Florida, Tampa, FL, USA
e-mail: scarey@usf.edu; britanny.e.mott@nasa.gov; alf3@mail.usf.edu

M. Lazinski
School of Physical Therapy and Rehabilitation Sciences, USF, Tampa, FL, USA
e-mail: mlazinsk@health.usf.edu

E. S. Kim
Department of Measurement and Evaluation, College of Education, USF, Tampa, FL, USA
e-mail: ekim3@usf.edu

S.-H. Lee et al. (eds.), *Perspectives in Performing Arts Medicine Practice*,
https://doi.org/10.1007/978-3-030-37480-8_8

hours, and neglect good health practice. Clearly, as the singer's instrument is the body, caring for it must be the priority. One of the main areas affected by the negligence of good health practice is the adoption of inefficient breathing habits. As singers focus their time on memorization, pitches, and color of voice, the practice of healthy breathing techniques is often left behind.

The ability to use the larynx efficiently is vital to the training of the healthy singer. The premise is that correct posture and proper breathing reduce tension in the vocal tract and improve vocal resonance. It has been commonly believed that the two most commonly neglected areas in voice students are posture and breathing. Posture is often hindered by mental and physical stress, bad habits, and emotional turmoil. Proper breathing is often neglected due to technical misconceptions and lack of body awareness. The purpose of this study was to examine if the *Fit-to-Play* course, *an integrated mind-body program*, had an effect on improving singers' posture, tension, and efficacy and specifically on increasing singers' breathing capacity.

Singers' Apparatus

Posture

Posture is critical for efficient function of the vocal tract. Good posture allows for freedom and flexibility of the respiratory muscles used in singing, such as the thoracic and the abdominal muscles. Postural deviations are known to produce obvious changes in respiratory function. Bad posture is often developed by slouching in front of the television, hunching over the computer, or carrying heavy bags. These habits force our bodies to adopt unnatural solutions that can cause tension in the shoulders, neck, jaw, and tongue, affecting the ability to sing freely. The singers' ultimate goal is to provide a relaxed environment for *inspiratory*, *expiratory*, and *pharyngeal* muscles to work efficiently. When the spine is in alignment, it reduces the tension on most muscles by distributing the weight over the heel bone (*calcaneus*) rather than over the balls of your feet (*metatarsal*), which balances the configuration of the *abdominal* and back muscles [1]. Like a straw when the *trachea* is bent, the air pressure is inefficiently distributed within the respiratory system, and tension is formed [2]. Students are often unaware of their posture as they strive to create a larger sound, developing more tension in the neck and torso.

Respiration

Respiration is activated as a basic motor function; however, singers must learn to control and coordinate both the *inspiratory* and *expiratory* muscles for efficient breathing. During *inspiration*, oxygen enters the nose and mouth and travels through the *pharynx* and *larynx* to the *cartilaginous* structure called the *trachea*. For singers, this process should be quiet as it indicates that the vocal *oscillator* is relaxed and open. The *trachea* then *bifurcates* into the *bronchi*, two branch-like structures, and further separates into *bronchioles*. These *bronchioles* lead to air sacs (or *alveoli*), where the carbon dioxide to oxygen exchange occurs. While oxygen is traveling through these *cartilaginous* structures to the *alveoli*, the *inspiratory* muscles and *diaphragm* work to expand the rib cage, which creates a negative pressure in the lungs, via expansion, and causes air to rush in. Shallow breathing may only involve movement of the rib cage to enlargen the lungs, while deep breathing engages diaphragmatic and abdominal movements. As such, the rib cage is able to move in three dimensions, vertically, horizontally, and anteriorally-posteriorally, to change the size of the thoracic cavity and adjust lung volume to meet the respiratory needs of the singer [3].

Exhalation begins when the lungs are optimally expanded. During normal exhalation, air is released due to the elastic recoil associated with the contraction of the *diaphragm* and other *inspiratory* muscles as these muscles return to their original position. This process increases the pressure with the lungs and forces the air out of the lungs. Singers must learn how to control the expiratory process by slowing down the descent of the rib cage and controlling the flow of air through the vocal tract. The necessary resistance to the volume of air flow is provided by the *external intercostals* and careful training of the *internal intercostals*, *rectus abdominis*, *external abdominal oblique*, *internal abdominal oblique*, and *transversus abdominis* (i.e., the *abdominal* muscles). With training, singers learn to control the rate at which the rib cage returns to its resting position. The purpose of this controlled exhalation is to create and maintain a constant power source that will provide the vocal *oscillator* with a steady controlled stream of air [3].

Phonation

Control of lung volume and efficiency is crucial for the regulation of *phonation*. Sound is produced because the vocal folds come together to build up *subglottal air pressure*. When subglottal pressure is great enough, the vocal folds are blown apart, initiating *vocal fold* vibration. By controlling *subglottal* pressure, one can modify airflow, *glottal* area, pitch, and overall volume [3]. Hence, the *vocal folds* are the *oscillator* of the human voice, much like the lips/mouthpiece of a horn or woodwind instrument. This is where the sound is created. Once the sound wave is generated, it is transferred to the *pharynx* and *oral cavity* where *resonance*, *tone*, and vocal color are shaped. If the airflow and pressure are not sufficient, the vocalist will usually compensate with excessive tension at the *oscillator* and other locations in the head and neck [4]. Further, voice production outside of the optimal range puts stress on the laryngeal muscles and can negatively impact vocal quality.

Resonance *and Tension in the Jaw*

The most important benefit of improved posture and respiratory functions for the singer is the increased *resonance* of the voice and overall *auditory* quality. The *resonators* that shape the sound of the voice are the jaw, tongue, lips, *palate*, pharynx, nasal cavity, and sinus shape [1]. Mastering the adjustments of these parts of the *vocal tract* is fundamental to vocal training. It enables the singer to be aware of how different methods of shaping the *vocal tract* can significantly improve vocal color, *resonance,* and *text declamation* [5]. If a coordinated diaphragmatic-abdominal breath is used to create a steady stream of air for the *vocal folds*, then tensions within the jaw, neck, and other *resonators* will hypothetically be released. This will improve overall movement of the jaw and allow for greater *resonance* and amplitude of the voice. Singers have the most control over the jaw and lips as *resonators* that enhance the color, *tone*, and volume of the singer's voice. As such, vocal training often includes rigorous exercises geared toward shaping these areas for optimal sound performance. This type of training can cause unnecessary tension within the facial muscles, unless the exercises are carefully monitored.

Methods

The fitness program is comprised of musician-tailored yoga, physical therapy exercises, and mental and free improvisation exercises. Pre-post measurements were conducted by (1) physical examinations including forward-retraction neck, deep flexor strength, *pectoral minor length*, and an endurance test; (2) a psychometric instrument containing a *health-pain-injury inventory* (HPI), *physical and mental efficacy* (PME), and *mental fitness and improvisation* (MFI) indicators; and (3) motion capture analyses showing range of motion for jaw movement and estimated breathing volume in four quadrants of the torso. Eleven voice performance students comprised of seven graduates and four undergraduates, eight females and three males, who were enrolled in *Fit to Play: Mind-Body Integration for Musicians* course in fall semesters between 2013 and 2017, participated in the study. The study was approved by the Institutional Review Board (Pro00014865).

Yoga

The concept of developing breath management and focusing the mind on coordinating *respiration* with movement has been active for thousands of years. One of the most commonly referred-to methods is yoga, which originated in ancient India. Yoga has been known to develop *cardiovascular* endurance and calm mind during moments of anxiety or panic. This practice could be extremely beneficial to the vocalist who wishes to improve their respiratory function and control their performance anxiety. It was believed in ancient India that each person was given a "predetermined number of breaths per lifetime" [6] (p.46). As a result, the primary form of breathing in yoga, *pranayama,* was developed with the purpose of extending each individual breath. *Pranayama* breathing is consciously coordinated and was believed to "enhance the ability to fully oxygenate your body" (p.44). Coincidentally, this method is exactly the same as that of diaphragmatic-abdominal breathing. Studies within yoga practitioners have found that *pranayama* breathing, or diaphragmatic-abdominal breathing, has been known to slow the heart rate, reduce oxygen consumption, and lower stress levels [7]. Specifically, the practice of the *Bhastrika* or *bellows* is described as a slow, deep *abdominal* breath, originating from the *diaphragm*. This type of breathing increases oxygen flow efficiency subsequently increasing overall blood flow [8].

The class included four 1-hour yoga sessions conducted by a certified yoga master which were followed by a 20-minute daily home practice. The yoga instruction included several forms of *pranayama* breathing focusing on the diaphragmatic-abdominal method of breathing, as well as coordinating muscle movement with the breath and developing body awareness.

Physical Therapy

A physical exercise program was adopted by a physical therapy and rehabilitation sciences clinical professor to improve posture, flexibility, muscular strength, and endurance in the upper body. After the initial testing, each student was given an individually prescribed set of exercises specifically addressing deficiencies, and he/she was required to execute these exercises for 20 minutes a day, recording this activity in a daily log. Flexibility/posture, muscular strength/endurance, and cardio endurance were measured by six parameters which were evaluated in a physical examination: forward head posture, *pectoral minor length*, *cervical range of motion*, *upper extremity/scapular strength* test, *deep neck flexor* endurance test, and endurance-aerobic test using YMCA step submaximal testing. Four intermittent instructional classes were provided to monitor the musicians to check if they were performing the exercises correctly.

Measurement

Physical Examination

Postural abnormality of the cervical spine was measured by the *craniovertebral* (CV) angle of forward head posture. When postural deviation persists, the muscular system adapts by either shortening or lengthening muscles causing weakness of muscles and limited range of motion. Physical examination included three major components and six measurements.

Flexibility/Posture

- Forward Head Posture (*craniovertebral* angle) – *Craniovertebral* (CV) angle is the angle formed by a horizontal line through the spinous process of C7 (seventh cervical spinal disc) and a line from the spinous process of C7 thru the tragus of the ear.
- *Pectoral Minor Length* – It is measured by placing the subject in a *supine* position and measuring the distance by which the shoulder sits above the table.
- *Cervical Range of Motion* – Active ROM was measured using a goniometer.

Muscular Strength/Endurance

- Upper Extremity/Scapular Strength Testing – Performed by *isometric* manual testing until movement was noted in specific muscles
- *Deep Neck Flexor* Endurance Testing – Measured as the length of time the *deep neck flexors* were held in proper positioning (lifted from the floor)

Endurance (Aerobic) Testing

- YMCA Submaximal Step Testing – Musicians performed 12-inch steps for 3 minutes, keeping pace with a metronome set at 60 beats per minute. Participant's pulse was taken immediately after completion of the task to determine submaximal aerobic capacity [9].

Psychometrics: Survey Questionnaire

The pre-post psychometric survey questionnaire included four parts: *health-pain-injury inventory* (*HPI*) asked questions about general health, health habits, drug/alcohol/caffeine/substance use, work hours, frequency of music-related pain and injury, pain locations, practice habits (daily practice hours, warm-up, and cool-down), and comfort with instrument and repertoire. *Physical and musical efficacy* (*PME*) included *physical awareness* and *comfort* levels on *posture*, *tension*, and *movement flexibility*, as well as *musical awareness* and *comfort on technique*, *tone*, and *flow/fluency*. The *mental fitness and improvisation* (*MFI*) measure provided information in terms of how long it took for *calming the mind*, *achieving imagery*, *mental practice*, and *mental recall*. Improvisation experiences were to indicate the degree of *comfort*, *in-the-moment experience*, and *satisfaction of their own sound*, *colleagues' sound*, and the *environment* during improvised performance. All variables were measured on a *Likert*-type numerical scale of 1–5. *Content validity* of the survey instrument was determined by a comprehensive analysis of the research literature and was tested in a previous pilot study [10]. All indicators were reliability tested with a larger sample dataset of collegiate voice and instrumental musicians in our previous published study [11].

Statistical Analysis

Nonparametric Wilcoxon paired samples signed rank tests were run to check for statistical significance in changes between pre- and post-measures for physical examination, PME, and MFI scores. A *nonparametric* test was appropriate with our small sample datasets because it does not assume *normality* and *pairing* takes data dependency into account [11, 12].

Motion Capture

An eight-camera *Vicon optical motion analysis* system (*Vicon*, Oxford, UK) was used to measure *kinematic* changes in the vocalists' *thoracic* and *abdominal* volume at the USF's Center for Assistive Rehabilitation and Robotics Technologies (USF CARRT). Prior to each data collection session, the instrumentation was calibrated following the manufacturer's guidelines. Passive, reflective spherical markers were placed on the torso, jaw, and head in order to track subjects' movements during singing trials. Each singer performed three trials of a scale and a song, which were averaged for the measurement.

Torso Volume

Breathing volume was estimated by calculating the change in torso volume in four regions as the subjects sang. Figure 8.1 shows the marker set up used to track the four torso regions on a digitized stick figure (from the *Vicon* Motion Capture System), inferior *abdominal* (IA), inferior *thorax* (IT), superior *abdominal* (SA), and superior *thorax* (ST), from one subject.

Breath volume of each region was estimated tracking the displacements of the markers outlining each region [9]. Each of the 4 torso regions was bounded by a total of 12 markers with 6 markers at the superior boundary and 6 makers at the inferior boundary as seen in Fig. 8.1.

The volume of each region was estimated using the following equation:

$$V = \frac{\left|(A-D)\ \left((B-D)\times(C-D)\right)\right|}{6} \tag{8.1}$$

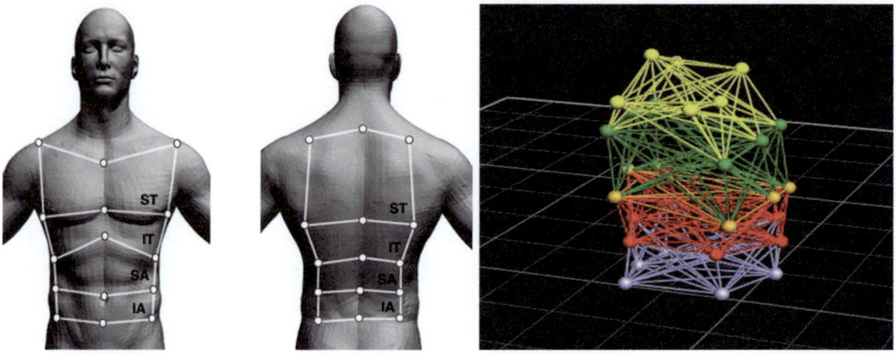

Fig. 8.1 Marker setup for vocalist and *VICON* capture shots of the four regions. Key Abbreviations in Figure: IA inferior *abdominal* (cyan color region), SA superior *abdominal* (red color region), IT inferior *thorax* (green color region), ST superior *thorax* (yellow color region)

$$V = \frac{|(A - D) \cdot (B - D) \times (C - D))|}{6}$$

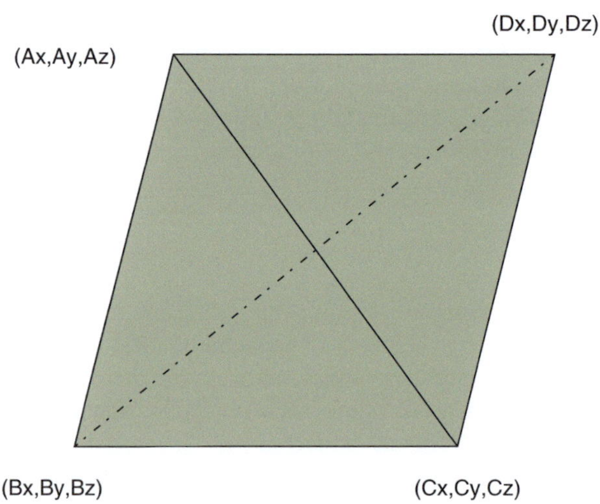

A MATLAB program was written to calculate the change in volume (measured in liters) in each region as the singer breathed or contracted the *diaphragm* (larger liter magnitude) or in (smaller liter magnitude) through the motion of the song.

Jaw Movement

In order to measure jaw movement, a new procedure was implemented. A head landmark was created as the midpoint between the two temple markers. A jaw land-

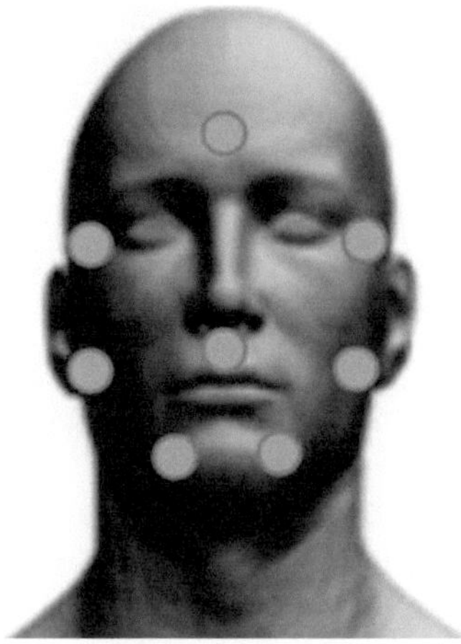

Fig. 8.2 Jaw marker placement

mark was created as the midpoint between the two lower jaw markers. The total distance the jaw moved relative to the head was calculated using the following equation (Fig. 8.2).

$$\text{Distance} = \sqrt{(\text{Hx} - \text{Jx})^2 + (\text{Hz} - \text{Jz})^2}$$

$$\text{Displacement} = \text{Distance}(i+1) - \text{Distance}(i) \tag{8.2}$$

Results

Physical Examination Results

Results of the *Wilcoxon* Signed Ranks Test show significant improvement in the strength/endurance of the *deep neck flexors*. This group of muscles is responsible for the movement of the head. Poor posture, including hunched shoulders, forces the head to move forward and weakens the deep flexor muscles over time. Table 8.1 shows the significant change in deep flexor adjustment ($p = 0.008$).

Psychometrics: Survey Questionnaire Results

The results in Table 8.2 show significant improvement in two areas of PME testing: "composite body awareness" (posture, tension, and movement flexibility) ($p = 0.046$) and "comfort in music technique" ($p = 0.038$).

Table 8.1 Physical examination: pre-post changes in singers ($N = 11$)

	Singers	Sig
Forward head (degrees)	–1.136	0.256
Forward head retract (degrees)	–1.315	0.189
Pectoral minor length R (cm)	–0.816	0.414
Pectoral minor length L (cm)	–0.343	0.732
Deep flexor (degrees)	2.668	**0.008**
Step (heart beats per min)	–0.534	0.594

Wilcoxon Signed Ranks Test based on negative ranks
Significant changes are in red boldface

Table 8.2 PME: pre-post changes in singers ($N = 11$)

	Singers	Sig
Body awareness		
Posture	–0.18	0.070
Tension	–1.000	0.317
Movement	–1.387	0.165
Compositie body aware	–1.99	**0.046**
Body comfort		
Posture	–1.811	0.070
Tension	–1.414	0.157
Movement	–1.350	0.177
Composite body comfort	–1.787	0.074
Music awareness		
Technique	–1.134	0.257
Tone	–0.816	0.414
Fluency	0.000	1.000
Composite music aware	–0.679	0.497
Music comfort		
Technique	–2.070	**0.038**
Tone	–1.823	0.07
Fluency	–1.190	0.234
Composite music comfort	–1.680	0.093

Wilcoxon Signed Ranks Test based on negative ranks
Significant changes are in red boldface

Table 8.3 shows singers' significant changes in MFI with "time taken to calm mind" ($p = 0.026$), "imagery of favorite music" ($p = 0.046$), and "satisfaction with the environment while improvising" ($p = 0.038$). Singers showed strong mental recall and calmness during the recall process: "recall first phrase" ($p = 0.038$), "recall whole recital" ($p = 009$), and "composite mental recall" ($p = 0.012$).

Table 8.3 MFI: pre-post changes in singers ($N = 11$)

	Singers	Sig
Calm mind (time took)		
Breathing	−1.403	0.161
Emptying mind	−2.220	**0.026**
Compositing calm mind	−1.550	0.121
Imagery		
Favority place	−1.342	0.180
Favorite music	−2.000	**0.046**
Composite imagery	−1.127	0.260
Mental practice		
Walking on stage	−0.552	0.581
First phrase	0.000	1.000
Whole recital	−1.342	0.180
Composite mental practice	−1.524	0.128
Mental recall recital		
Mental recall walk stage	−1.890	0.059
Mental recall first phrase	−2.070	**0.038**
Mental recall whole recital	−2.598	**0.009**
Composite mental recall recital	−2.527	**0.012**
Mental calmness walk stage	−1.611	0.107
Mental calmness first phrase	−1.730	0.084
Mental calmness whole recital	−1.933	0.053
Composite mental calmness recital	−1.969	**0.049**
Improvisation		
Comfort with my sound	−0.426	0.670
Comfort with collaborative sound	−1.625	0.104
Comfort with environment	−1.222	0.222
Composite comfort improvisation	−1.479	0.139
In the moment with my sound	−0.552	0.581
In the moment collaboration	−0.962	0.336
In the moment environment	−0.333	0.739
Composite in the moment	−0.931	0.352
Satisfaction with my sound	−1.518	0.129
Satisfaction collaboration	−1.725	0.084
Satisfaction environment	−2.070	**0.038**
Satisfaction composite	−1.548	0.122

Wilcoxon Signed Ranks Test based on negative ranks
Significant changes are in red boldface

In HPI, we observed a reduction in the frequency of pain report in three facial areas, i.e., cheek (3 to 1), lips (3 to 1), and jaw (5 to 3). This is interesting because other areas, specifically neck (4 and 4), shoulder (3 to 4), and headache (3 to 4), showed the same or higher frequency of occurrence. While statistically insignificant, we considered the reduction in the three facial areas as those areas may correlate with jaw *motion capture* analysis.

Motion Capture *Results*

The *motion capture* data displayed graphically in Figs. 8.3 and 8.4 showed that the singers have shifted their breathing pattern from chest breathing residing predominantly in the thorax (IT, ST) to the diaphragmatic-abdominal (IA, SA) breathing post-treatment. This finding is the result of expansion in the abdominal area.

This change in quadrant displacement also resulted in an increase in tidal volume by over a liter as shown in Fig. 8.5.

Our jaw movement data, and the analysis, were incomplete. More substantive data collection is necessary to validate our hypothesis.

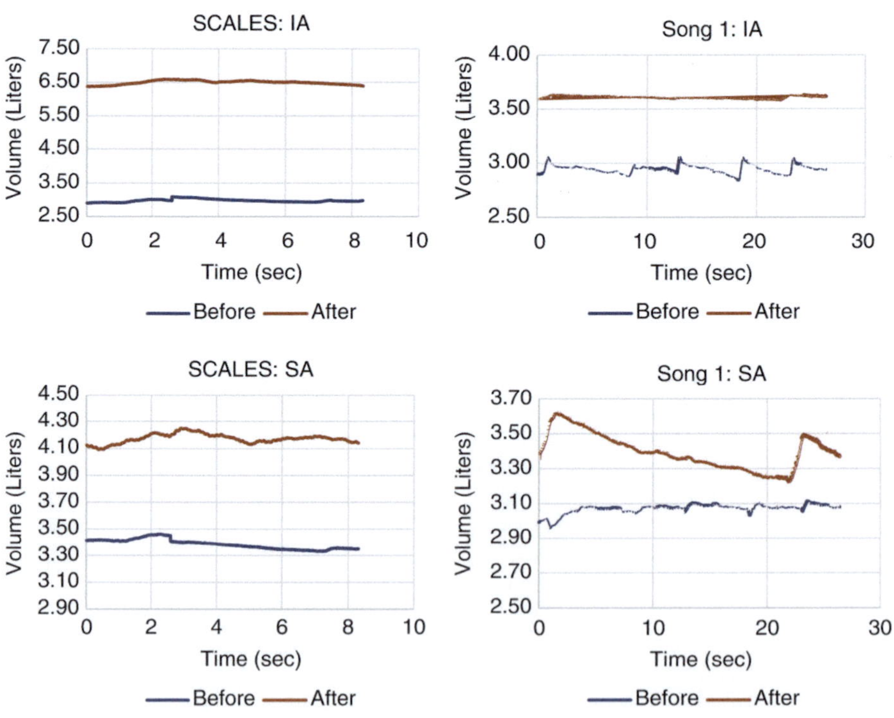

Fig. 8.3 IA, SA. Singer's breathing in *abdominal* quadrant in singing scales and song

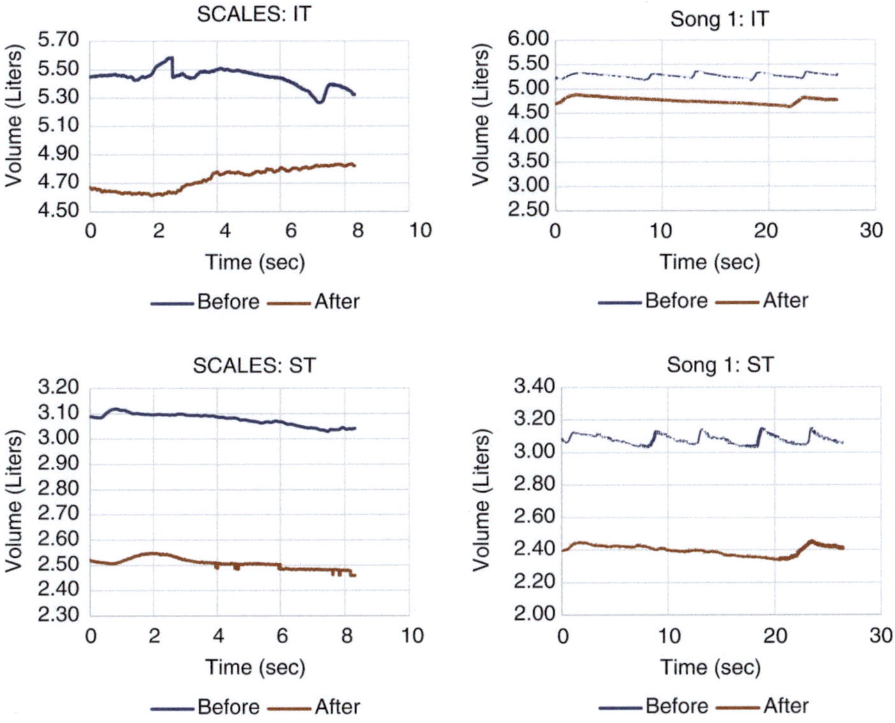

Fig. 8.4 IT. ST. Singer's breathing in thoracic quadrant in singing scales and song

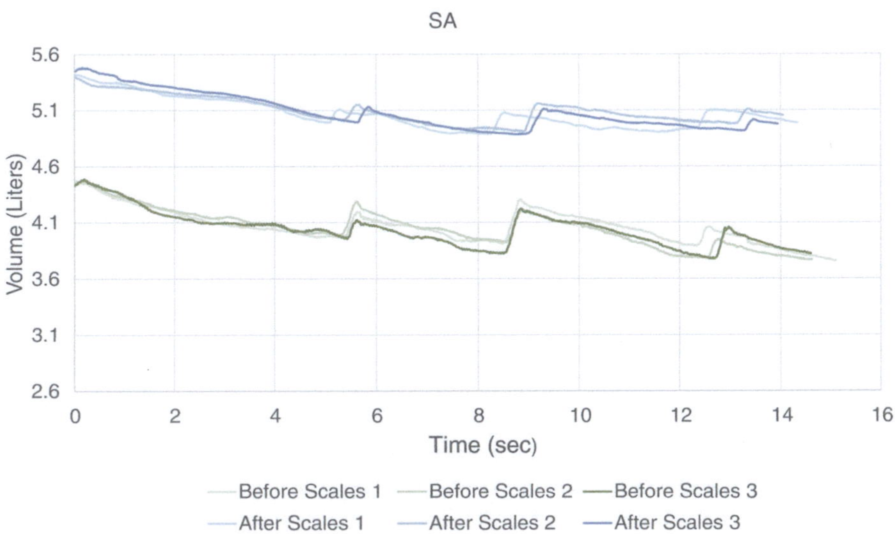

Fig. 8.5 SA. *Abdominal tidal volume* change

Discussion

Of the six pre-post physical measurements, only deep flexor endurance showed significant changes. The minimal improvement in posture, muscular strength and flexibility, and cardio endurance noted in this sample may be the result of two things: (1) it may be that the 20-minute daily exercises were not rigorous enough to demonstrate progress in the collegiate musicians whose musical demands may take priority and (2) a 16-week program may not be long enough to change postural habits and to build muscular strength and cardio endurance. Even so, singers felt positive about their progress in physical awareness and musical comfort. However, singers may already have greater bodily awareness since vocal training heavily relies on bodily awareness in the production of the sound. Students commented that the readings and discussions about memorization skills, performance anxiety, and peak performance were very useful. In a future study, the program's effects on music performance and anxiety can be added. We believe there were indications of relationships between jaw movement, tension, and pain. We plan to investigate the relationships between increased jaw movement, decreased tension, and decreased pain in the temporomandibular joint in a future study.

In conclusion, we posit this novel *Fit-to-Play* mind-body integrated program has a positive influence on collegiate singers' overall perception with demonstrated improvement on their breathing technique with the observed shift from *thoracic* to diaphragmatic-abdominal quadrants and the increased *tidal volume*. Increased tidal volume could potentially improve overall resonance in the voice as the singer learns to adjust the vocal tract. We can hypothesize a correlation between jaw movement and temporomandibular joint pain and tension in a future study.

Acknowledgments We appreciate the contribution of Tina Tidwell Bedore, Yoga E-RYT and CEO, Amour Movement Company of Tampa with her expert yoga instruction.

Conflict of Interest There are no known conflicts of interest associated with this publication, and there has been no significant financial support for this work that could have influenced its outcome.

References

1. Sataloff RT, Brandfonbrener AG, Lederman RJ, editors. Performing arts medicine. Chapter seven. Narberth: Science & Medicine; 1998. p. 137–88.
2. Webb JL. Promoting vocal health in the choral rehearsal. Music Educ J. 2007;93(5):26–31. https://doi.org/10.1177/002743210709300513.
3. Sapienza C, Ruddy BH, editors. Voice disorders. 3rd ed. San Diego: Plural Publishing; 2018.
4. Sataloff RT, Brandfonbrener AG, Lederman RJ, editors. Performing arts medicine. Chapter eight. Narberth: Science & Medicine; 1998. p. 139–203.

5. Hinds S. Argument for the investigation and use of overtone singing. J Sing. 2005;62(1):33–40. https://doi.org/10.1186/isrctn89892069.
6. Newman AT, Lee C. Breathing, alignment, and body awareness benefit many. Dance Mag. 2002;76(11):43–7.
7. Yeager S. Use less air through yoga: with some tips from ancient discipline, the eagle could replace your octopus. 2003 Mar. Retrieved from http://www.fwmedia.com/.
8. Chopra D, Simon D, editors. AARP the seven spiritual laws of yoga: a practical guide to healing body. 2nd ed. Hoboken: Wiley; 2012.
9. Hardwick D, Carey S, Lazinski M, Lee SH. Measuring the performer and performance. In: Lee S, editor. Scholarly research for musicians. New York, London: Routledge; 2017. p. 136–47.
10. Lee SH, Carey S, Dubey R, Matz R. Intervention program in college instrumental musicians, with kinematics analysis of cello and flute playing: a combined intervention program of yogic breathing and muscle strengthening and flexibility exercises. Med Probl Perform Art. 2012;27(2):85–94.
11. Lee SH, Carey S, Lazinksi M, Kim ES. Integrative intervention program for college musicians and kinematics in cello playing. Eur J Integr Med. 2019;25:34–40. ISSN 1876-3820. https://doi.org/10.1016/j.eujim.2018.10.014.
12. Ware WB, Ferron JM, Miller BM, editors. Introductory statistics: a conceptual approach using R. New York, London: Routledge; 2013.

Suggested Reading

Kearney K, Fults A, Lopez E, Carey S, Lee SH. Kinematic analysis of college vocalists participating in a mind-body integration program. Third USF-PAMA conference: life cycle of performing the artist. June 1–3 2018. Tampa, Florida.

Chapter 9
Health Benefits of Culturally Oriented Dance

Kyaien O. Conner, Juanita Patterson-Price, and Niche Faulkner

Introduction

Historically, African Americans have experienced barriers and disparities on the road toward becoming professional dancers in traditional classic forms. The lack of racial diversity in ballet and other dance forms has become one of the most discussed issues in the dance field of today. In an examination of the top international dance companies in 2015, few rosters included dancers of non-European descent [1]. In the United States, despite growth in the right direction, there remains an absence of African Americans and other dancers of color in the country's premier ballet companies [1]. More recently in the United States, a growing acceptance of different body types and a greater appreciation of diversity of dancers on stage have led to a rise in dancers of color on the concert stage. However, there remains a disconnect between dance on the professional stage and dance in university dance programs [2].

Disparities are persistent in higher education dance programs. Research suggests that in the academy, dance is both taught and practiced primarily by whites. A study which examined data on overall ethnicity in undergraduate dance programs indicated that African Americans represented only 10% of dance program

K. O. Conner (✉)
Department of Mental Health Law and Policy, College of Behavioral and Community Sciences, The Florida Mental Health Institute, University of South Florida, Tampa, FL, USA
e-mail: koconner@usf.edu

J. Patterson-Price
Department of Mental Health Law and Policy, College of Behavioral and Community Sciences, University of South Florida, Tampa, FL, USA
e-mail: juanitap@mail.usf.edu

N. Faulkner
Department of Dance, College of Arts and Architecture, University of North Carolina-Charlotte, Charlotte, NC, USA
e-mail: nfaulkn3@uncc.edu

S.-H. Lee et al. (eds.), *Perspectives in Performing Arts Medicine Practice*,
https://doi.org/10.1007/978-3-030-37480-8_9

participation, compared to white participation at 72% [3]. Additionally, studies have found that dance faculty in higher education are also primarily white (approximately 85% white, non-Hispanic) with less representation from racial and ethnic minorities [4]. Kerr-Berry [2] suggests that this imbalance of faculty representation is reflected in the number of students of color in higher education dance programs. The current dance curricula are largely based on a Eurocentric paradigm failing to integrate important cultural aspects of dance which impacts the dance student's educational experience in the classroom, in the studio, and ultimately on stage [2]. One potential strategy for engaging more students and faculty of color into higher education dance programs is to add courses and curricula related to culturally oriented forms of dance.

Culturally oriented dance is defined as a dance within a community or group that serves one or more purposes related to traditional practices, cultural transmission, social acceptance, or connectedness [5]. Examples of culturally oriented dance include West African, Afro-Brazilian, Flamenco, folk dance, and Haka dance. It is not modern dance, ballet, or jazz. It typically includes having a cultural or regional influence and is choreographed to cultural music. Culturally oriented dance can capture the imagination of individuals in ways that other forms of physical activity cannot due to its symbolic qualities [6]. Another important characteristic of culturally oriented dance is that it is often tailored to fit the needs of a specific population. It can be altered to match the age and health status of individuals without reducing the psychological and physiological health benefits. Alternations can take the form of modified intensity, variations in music choice, and movement selection tailored to participants. Little equipment is needed for cultural dance and practice space is often flexible [7].

Another characteristic of cultural dance is its link to culture. Culturally oriented dance may also be more accepted as a form of dance among ethnic minority groups due to reinforcement of their social norms. Cultural code of dress and behavior may be reinforced during cultural social dances and may be seen as more accepted from a community standpoint [8]. As such, the norms of the minority group are enforced and celebrated. Cultural dance may serve as an enjoyable group activity that strengthens ties with others while serving as a reminder of one's ancestral origins [9]. Culturally oriented dance can therefore help enhance cultural awareness, racial identity, and pride in addition to increasing physical activity and alleviating stress [10]. Research suggests that groups may be more likely to participate consistently in activities that are tailored to their specific cultural backgrounds. Several studies have demonstrated high retention rates when physical activities were tied to the specific cultural heritage of the targeted group [11–13].

West African Dance as a Culturally Oriented Dance Form

Traditional West African dance is the dance of the ancestors, coming from countries including Guinea, Senegal, Ghana, Mali, and the Ivory Coast. A dance may be hundreds of years old, preserved, and passed down from generation to generation. Its steps and movements, for the most part, represent everyday lifestyle. In the West

African worldview, dance is a conduit of individual and community healing. African conceptualizations of health integrate social, spiritual, physical, and mental realms [14]. The underlying belief is that in the community, mind and body must be incorporated through dance to facilitate healing, as well as transform and empower the individual and the group. Ultimately, West African dance plays an integral role in socialization, expression, and communication in West African countries. While each country and ethnic group has unique dances, dance is seen as a way to bring communities together involving all genders, age groups, and even outsiders (except during specific rituals that are closed to certain groups). It helps to build and maintain a healthy sense of self-esteem and offers an alternative cathartic experience for not only individuals but for the community as a whole [14].

Dance plays an important role for African Americans in the United States as a means of emotional expression, is symbolic of traditional African heritage, and is a means of interaction, support, and cohesion [15]. The significance of dance in the African American culture reflects an intrinsic cultural orientation toward physical expression and creativity [15]. Traditional West African dance can improve the physical dimensions of health through engagement in a variety of movements and step patterns that can be vigorous or mild for lower-intensity workouts. It can improve mental dimensions of health by relieving stress and anxiety [16]. It can further enhance social and mental health through addressing gender inequality [17]. It can improve the intellectual dimensions of health by providing new movement information to be analyzed and can improve the spiritual dimension of health by providing, through movement, a relationship with nature, the environment, and one's culture of origin [18]. Therefore, culturally oriented dance, and specifically traditional West African dance, has the potential to generate significant health benefits for African Americans but is seldom scientifically studied.

Descriptive reports and experimental studies document that culturally oriented dance has strong ties to health benefits and stress reduction for participants of varying ages and backgrounds. Cultural dance has shown promise in reducing problematic weight gain, stress management, increasing interest in physical activity, and increasing life satisfaction. For example, studies of culturally oriented dance interventions reveal decreased trait anxiety in American Indian women [19], increased bone density in older Viennese women [20], and decreased falling risk in elderly Japanese women [21]. Studies of traditional African dance demonstrated reduced BMI and improved fitness among African American women [22], lower stress and higher positive affect among college undergraduates [16], and reduced symptoms of depression and anxiety among African adolescents who had experienced trauma [23]. However, current research studies on culturally oriented dance tend to be largely descriptive in nature focused on the nature of recruitment efforts, observations, personal opinions about cultural dance, and methods for instruction, as opposed to using rigorous scientific and experimental designs.

Therefore, despite the available research demonstrating the strong benefits of culturally oriented dance, there is still insufficient empirical evidence to encourage funding support and, subsequently, implementation of cultural dance programs suffers.

To begin to address this gap in the literature, the authors utilized semi-structured interviews to examine the psychological and physical health benefits of traditional West African dance from the perspectives of pre-professional and professional dancers who participated in a West African dance conference. The goal of this investigation was to attain an in-depth understanding of the reasons for engaging in traditional African dance, the barriers or challenges to consistent participation, and the self-perceived benefits of such participation.

Methods

A written survey form and semi-structured interviews were conducted with 26 pre-professional and professional dancers who attended a West African Dance and Drum conference in South Florida. For the purpose of this investigation, pre-professional dancers are identified as dance majors in higher education dance programs, and professional dancers are operationalized as individuals who self-identify as such and are being paid to perform on a consistent basis. This venue was selected to engage a diverse group of participants who had a particular interest in cultural dance so that we could attain an in-depth understanding of the benefits and challenges of participating in such an activity from the perspective of a diverse group. This conference was a weekend-long event, which involved West African Dance and Drum classes led by master teachers from various West African countries for all ages and skill levels. All individuals who attended the conference were informed that they could participate in this research study, and they received a free dance class (worth $20) for participating. Of the 40 people who attended the conference, 26 individuals chose to participate (65% participation rate). Those who chose not to participate identified that they did not want to miss out on a dance class to participate in the interview as the primary reason for non-participation. Interviews were conducted on-site by a trained doctoral student in a back room to ensure confidentiality of response. Interviews lasted between 25 minutes and 45 minutes. In addition, participants provided demographic characteristics as well as answers to open-ended questions focused on the contributors and barriers to participating in cultural dance in a written survey. This study was approved by the University of South Florida's Institutional Review Board, and all study methods were conducted in compliance with this proposal including informed consent procedures (PRO 00033033).

Data Analysis

Qualitative techniques for thematic inquiry were utilized to ensure systematic and rigorous analysis of the semi-structured interviews. All interviews were audio-recorded, transcribed, and checked for accuracy. The thematic analysis process involved: (1) producing a comprehensive inventory of important ideas, expressions, terms, and phrases that reflected the language of participants, (2) generating categories under which identified ideas were placed, and (3) clustering the categories to identify broader themes and patterns that emerged from the data. Transcript data were first analyzed using in vivo (line-by-line) coding to categorize responses. Codes were subsequently clustered to generate emergent themes. Research team members (two) each independently coded all the transcripts and subsequently met to discuss any differences in the codes assigned to the text and to attain agreement about the final codebook. The final version of the codebook was utilized to re-code all the qualitative data. Categories of data were combined to create overarching themes, and matrices were utilized to identify broader patterns and recurring themes across the 26 interviews. Data saturation was reached after 23 interviews; however, we completed data analysis on all 26 interviews to ensure we captured the voices of all study participants.

Results

Participants

Participants were largely middle-aged, single African American women, who were well-educated and working either full time or part time. Of the 26 total participants, 10 identified themselves as pre-professional dancers and 16 as professional dancers. All participants identified having received some training in ballet or contemporary/modern dance. Having few opportunities for West African dance in their institutions of higher education, they all identified having to go into the community to study this cultural dance form. Having an opportunity to study West African dance to a greater degree was identified as the primary reason why the participants attended this conference (Table 9.1).

Qualitative analysis of 26 semi-structured interviews revealed a number of important themes. The first broad theme was overarching health benefits of African dance. Within this theme the primary sub-themes included (1) stress and anxiety relief, (2) improvement in mood, and (3) health promotion and disease prevention. The second overarching theme was challenges and barriers to participation in physical activity. Within this theme the primary sub-themes included (1) lack of time, (2) lack of finances, and (3) lack of motivation to participate in traditional forms of exercise. The third and final broad theme was connection, with sub-themes including (1) connection to culture, (2) connection to ancestors, and (3) connection to community. In the following paragraphs, we provide an in-depth explanation of these themes highlighted by participant quotes pulled directly from semi-structured interviews. Pseudonyms are used to protect the anonymity of study participants.

Table 9.1 Demographics of the participants

Gender	(*N* = 26)
Male	2
Female	24
Age	
Range	18–66 years
Mean age	36 SD = 3.56
Race	
White	5
African	16
Hispanic	1
Other	4
Marital status	
Single	15
Currently widowed	6
Divorced	3
Living with partner	2
Level of education	
Post-college	9
Bachelor's degree	6
Some college	6
High school graduate/GED	1
Associate degree/vocational graduate	3
Chose not to answer	1
Employment	
Full time	12
Part time	8
Unemployed	5
Retired	1
Self-identified professional dance status	
Pre-professional	10
Professional	16
Primary language spoken at home	
English	23
Spanish	1
French	2
Immigration status	
Legal immigrant	4
American citizen	21
Chose not to answer	1
Currently taking medications	
Yes	5
No	21
Diagnosed health condition	
Yes	6
No	18
Chose not to answer	2

Overarching Health Benefits of African Dance

Study participants were able to identify a number of health benefits associated with participation in African dance. Some of these benefits were aspects likely to be attained through participation in any form of dance. Participants stated that dance enhances one's ability to concentrate and enhances individual memory. Multiple participants suggested that having to learn new steps in a dance class on the spot translates in enhancing ability to remember things in real life. For example, Denise stated "[Dance] keeps my mind active. You know if I put a pencil here, I have to really walk away and come back and go 'what did I do with that pencil?'. So dance helps me to remember things. 1,2,3,4 this step after this step." Jennifer stated that "Dance gives you a different perspective on the world. It also helps meet new people, it can be a very social environment." However, there were a number of health benefits that participants identified as unique to African dance. These benefits included stress and anxiety relief, improvement in mood, and health promotion and disease prevention.

Stress and Anxiety Relief

Of the 26 participants interviewed, 20 identified stress and anxiety relief as a key psychological benefit of participation in a cultural dance form like African dance. Erika stated: "African dancing for me helps me to relax. Like, when I'm feeling stressed from school or with like things going on in my life like, when I do African dance I don't like, think about those stuff. So it just makes me feel relaxed and calm." Many participants identified being in an African dance class as a release. Alaina explained: "African dance is a release. It's, a… reliever! From daily life, from stress. It's healing, it's fundamental… um, it's a sanctuary for some and others…yeah you relieve just relieve and… freeness."

A specific aspect of African dance that led to this feeling of release was the involvement of live drumming. Theresa acknowledged: "African dance is a huge stress reliever for me, to really be at one with the drums." Natalie further echoed:

> It's like a release. Like you just let go, you just let the drums and the music move you, you don't really think about what movements you're doing you just do whatever your body feels like doing basically. So it's like a freeing experience, you don't have to think when you're dancing African dance, you just… do it!

Some participants actually expounded on the different form of release you are able to experience when participating in traditional African dance. Participants recognized that dancing in general can be a release but that African dance in particular provides a unique release due to the music and the connection to culture. Laura explained:

> I think it's just like, different types of release that are different from our culture. So you can dance in a way that is just different from everything you do in your own culture, which is nice. So you're kind of embracing this other side, and it's, it's just a stress reliever. And the

> energy you put out in African dance it's so invigorating. Even in dances like ballet, it has a different kind of release. I still feel like it's a form of stress relief but I feel like I take on a different personality and it's just, really fun.

Improvement in Mood

In addition to stress relief, participants overwhelming identified an improvement in mood as a benefit of African dance. Of the 26 participants interviewed, all 26 identified feeling happy when participating in African dance, and 20 identified that they *love* African dance. Participants referred to African dance as their *therapy* and as their *medicine*. Trina stated: "African dance for me is like my medicine. If someone does something bad to me, when I dance I… I'm just happy. It's like medicine." Lisa went on to explain: "I dance [African dance] because it's a passion of mine. My first passion actually. African dance is my therapy, it's a way of life for me, it's a way of expressing myself… it's the way I communicate myself to the world, basically without speaking. And it's something that I could not live without. Literally."

Health Promotion and Disease Prevention

Participants identified participation in African dance as a means for staying young and staying healthy. Kisha stated: "I love African dance. It keeps you healthy!" Lisa further explained: "I'm 25 years young, and I've been dancing professionally with West African since I was 13. And um, it has done… very well for my body! Everyone who's literally my age you know they're always asking me how do I stay in shape, how do I keep my physique and it's literally, cultural dance." This was consistently mentioned by study participants but seemed to be particularly salient for older study participants.

Participants were able to explain what they believe are the mechanisms behind why African dance is particularly helpful toward staying healthy. For some participants, it was the focus on the body, mind, and spirit that creates positive health outcomes. Kisha stated: "African dance actually is very therapeutic. It focuses on all aspects of your body so it can really keep you healthy and heal you. Mentally, physically and spiritually. It can heal you." Theresa explained:

> I think that African dance is interestingly more helpful athletically than a lot of other kinds of dance, because you do these very serious spurts of energy and then you rest and then spurts of energy and you rest and now they're starting to show that that's possibly the best thing that can happen on a mitochondrial level. (laughs) So, I think we're getting more benefit from It than I realized when I was younger. And I'm starting to realize why that the people who do it their whole lives don't look very old.

Participants discussed specific illness that they felt participating in African dance helped them to prevent. Marie explains that African dance is preventative for future heart disease. She stated: "African dance has cardiovascular benefits.

Like my endurance is top notch, it's the best it's ever been, like I don't get winded as easily. Especially going to class, I walk up like… stairs. Like three flights every morning and it's crazy, but, honestly it just works out really well 'cause I just feel so much better, I don't get fatigued as easily and I'm not always tired." Some participants identified having current health ailments that have been improved from participating in African dance. Fatima has scoliosis and had a hard time in traditional forms of exercise due to her back pain, but she found participating in African dance has significant health and healing benefits for her illness. Fatima said: "With my spine, like I was a couple of degrees away from getting a brace, needing surgery and within a couple of years it's, it's still a little curved but the pain is not like, anything it was before African dance. And so the physical benefits being able to like, be flexible and feel strong and do these grand movements is just a huge confidence boost, as well as feeling more energized."

Challenges and Barriers to Participation in Dance

The second overarching theme we identified is challenges and barriers to participation in dance. Although participants were able to easily identify the benefits of engaging in African dance, participants had a more difficult time identifying barriers and challenges. Often when asked about barriers or challenges to participation in African dance or other forms of dance, participants were confused by the question and required an additional prompt to understand. However, there were three sub-themes that consistently emerged: lack of time, lack of finances, and lack of motivation to participate in traditional forms of dance and exercise.

Lack of Time

Time was identified as a barrier by 23 out of 26 study participants. This was identified as a barrier to consistent participation in physical activity more generally and in African dance classes more specifically. Erika suggested: "I think time is a big factor. Like sometimes you get too busy with work and school, and stuff, so you don't like, find time to dance or do other stuff. So I think that's a big factor." When asked if there are any barriers to her participation in African dance classes, Aaliyah stated: "Time. I'm trying to figure out how I can live a regular life, you know go to work, come home and dance the dances that I want to dance." Tanya further elaborates: "Time is one [barrier], I don't really have time to like… if I didn't take this class I wouldn't be able to take another class because I'm like, so busy with my schedule and stuff. So… and I'm like always working, doing schoolwork, and I don't really have time to do anything else. So African dance is like, the only time I have to do something fun."

Lack of Finances

Another significant deterrent to consistent participation in dance was lack of finances. Other than a lack of time, money was the second more frequently cited reason for lack of consistent participation in dance generally and African dance specifically. Aaliyah stated: "[barriers are] Schedule and money. Finances. So sometimes the schedule but often it's the finances." Participants often stated that they would take many more African dance classes and would do so more consistently if they could afford to do so. Student participants noted that their dance education programs rarely offer West African dance courses, and if so it is often a single course. This requires them to have to go into the community and pay for classes separately, which comes with a significant financial cost. Lisa stated: "Some things are financially, you know you need finance to basically do them. But I was the type of person that, whenever I did not have the money I was just using whatever resources I can to study, or like, do it on my own, until I had resources. If I had unlimited resources, I would be in African dance class all the time."

Some participants identified that although finances could be a serious problem with being consistently engaged in physical activity, there were ways to get around that, which appear to be unique to the culture of attending African dance or other cultural dance classes. Justine explained:

> Honestly, I pretty much [African] dance regardless of the barriers, because at the end of the day this isn't for anyone else but for myself. And the thing is like, even if it cost money, there is a way to get to it. There are scholarships, people you can talk to, like, this African dance group that I dance with has provided such a great support system. Like you go to conferences, and if you can't foot the bill, they take donations from each other, in order to help you go. And I think that's really awesome because in a way dance brought us all together. Like a family!

Lack of Motivation to Participate in Traditional Forms of Dance

Although lack of time and lack of finances were identified as barriers to consistent participation in African dance classes, most participants identified African dance as a priority. It met so many of their needs (i.e., spiritual, psychological, emotional, and physical) that they were willing to sacrifice their limited time and resources to attend African dance classes. However, they were unwilling to make a similar sacrifice for traditional forms of dance (i.e., ballet, modern, jazz) or exercise (i.e., aerobics, weight lifting, going to the gym). When asked about participating in physical activity or going to the gym for exercise, Demetri stated: "The gym? Ummm no, I don't do anything else, I just dance. That's my life. I could do other things, I just don't want to." Participants consistently made comparisons between African dance and going to the gym. Participants did not identify themselves as "gym people." Empress stated, for example, "I'm more of a class person. I'm not a gym person. I'd rather go to a class. If it was African dance pump iron I'd be in there like yeah! Pumpin' weights." Denise mentions: "Gyms… seem a little sterile to me. If you put me on a treadmill, I get bored quickly. If you put me in a square box and say 'do this many of this' it's… it's bad. So… I know it's there but I mess with it."

Anna elaborated:

> African dance is fun and you don't really realize you're working out because you're so wrapped up in it being so fun, you know what I mean whereas at the gym you're just like 'how many reps I gotta do' 'oh my gosh I gotta add on this much weight', whereas [African] dance is fun and you just do like, lose yourself in it.

Some participants acknowledged that they felt uncomfortable or out of place in more traditional dance classes. These individuals candidly shared their experiences and suggested that African dance was a safe space to not feel judged or ashamed of the way they look or how American society expects them to look. Empress stated: "Psychologically, as a woman of size, I am able to… I'm not impacted by people's bias or fat shaming when I come and do African dance…Psychologically I am able to release tension, um, I'm able to release the words, descriptors that have been placed upon me as a woman of size and a woman of color, um from the Africana diaspora I'm able to release a lot of false perceptions that were never my own. That were put on to me just by being birthed in this (expletive) society."

Connection

Our third and final broad theme is connection. Participants consistently discussed the multiple connections they made when attending African dance classes. They identified a unique connection to their own culture or to a different culture that they wanted to learn more about. Some participants felt that African dance helped them to develop a connection to their ancestors, and others felt a strong connection to their community.

Connection to Culture

Participants consistently highlighted connection to culture as one of the many benefits of attending African dance classes. These were the added benefits not typically available in other types of dance classes. African American participants, and those from the African diaspora, frequently discussed how participating in African dance classes helped them to feel connected to their culture. Fatimah stated: "I know for me personally, it's my culture. I'm from Haiti. So, I basically feel like I'm at home, I'm in touch with my roots, so that's why, culturally, I love it [African dance]." Some participants discussed how participating in African dance classes helped them to feel pride in relation to who they are and to become more attached to their cultural identity. Brynn recalled: "Cultural dance energizes me and gives me a strong sense of pride." Erika further stated: "Cultural dance, it helps you to learn more and helps you to appreciate it more, and like, helps you learn where you came from. So you can understand like, who you are as a person."

Some participants took this opportunity to express their experiences of racism and oppression in the United States and how in some ways being a part of African dance helps to empower them to embrace their cultural identities and experiences. These were often occurrences individual participants experienced, but also experiences of African people more broadly, to whom participants felt connected. Jasmine stated: "African dance honestly helps me feel more in touch with my culture period, because the thing is like right now, nowadays it seems like everything is so… Americanized or… for lack of a better word whitewashed almost. And it seems like my culture just tends to fall to the wayside 'cause like, my history isn't what's taught in the history books. I mean it is, but you have to dig deep to find it and it's mentioned in like, 2 paragraphs on that page 196 of a textbook that's like maybe 722 pages."

Study participants who were not African American or did not identify with the African diaspora still saw a connection to culture and a benefit of learning about and connecting to a culture different from their own. Rose stated: "I think it's really important just, to engage the community. These are things that are fun and can engage the community in something that's different and it's like educational and putting out a different culture which is important. Like in the US we're all from so many different places and it's really cool to experience things from other cultures. Besides your own in like, this kind of setting." Jessica further stated: "I feel like it's just a way to immerse yourself in a different culture. You don't…I mean back home I didn't see a lot of conferences like this per se. But like, it's just a way to get outside of your own cultural bubble, especially like in a place like Tampa or Florida period where it's a melting pot just people celebrating different cultures is very special."

Connection to Ancestors

Beyond feeling connected to culture, African American participants and those from the African diaspora more broadly identified a connection to their ancestors through their participation in African dance. Brynn stated: "When I do African dance I feel that I am walking the path carved out by my ancestors while creating my own footsteps." Some participants felt that it was because of their ancestors that they are even able to dance. Aaliyah states: "It's because of my ancestors, God almighty, my ancestors and my DNA, and dance. If you don't dance you die." Some participants recognized the duality of connecting with ancestors as well as African teachers from the continent who come to teach them as being a uniquely rewarding experience, only available in an African dance class. Empress explained:

> Dancing African dance is absolutely reclamation of my identity. Absolutely, shared culture. As well, I to really look through the eyes of individuals who have just come here [from Africa] to share their culture. So not only am I connecting with my ancestors, I'm connecting with my contemporary folk. My contemporary ancestors to be so to speak. I believe that we're born, we die, we come back again, so I feel like we've all been together before and we're just coming back and meeting one another again, and we get to do it on this joyous journey through West African dance.

Connection to Community

More broadly, all 26 participants mentioned the benefit of connecting to community. Kisha states: "There is a certain sense of community that you get in different classes and in different cities and in different places. And when you have that sense of community that's really lovely." Community meant many different things for different people. For some it meant a community of dancers; for others it meant a community of people of shared culture; for others it simply meant a community of old friends and new friends. Kali stated: "Outside of the good workout, for me African dance is about really connection. Connecting with other people. The connection… which helps me spiritually, mentally… Connecting with people, feeling their energy. I'm big on energy! So it helps me, when I'm really feeling bad I'm like, I need to go to my African dance class and I feel liberated." Brynn states that African dance "Brings unity, to the people, together. I like that, because you get to see all different… races! Black, white, Persian, come together under one… having fun."

Discussion and Implications

The purpose of this study was to attain a deeper understanding of the benefits and challenges, of participating in African dance among pre-professional and professional dancers. Our analysis revealed a number of important themes including the overarching health benefit of African dance (e.g., stress and anxiety relief, improvement in mood, and health promotion and disease prevention), challenges and barriers to participation in physical activity (e.g., lack of time, lack of finances, and lack of motivation to participate in traditional forms of exercise), and connection (e.g., connection to culture, connection to ancestors, and connection to community). Our study suggests that African dance can yield multiple positive physical and mental health benefits for dancers. We also found that time and finances were a significant deterrent for individuals who want to participate in dance programs and African dance specifically. We found that for the racial and ethnic minority participants interviewed, African dance was strongly preferred over other forms of dance (i.e., ballet, modern/contemporary). Participants felt African dance met multiple needs at once and therefore was worth the extra time and finances needed to engage.

The results of this study should be viewed within the contexts of the study's limitations. This study used a convenience sample of participants who attended a West African dance conference in Tampa, FL. Therefore, the opinions and beliefs shared by these individuals may not be generalizable. However, we intentionally selected this group to attain an in-depth understanding of the benefits of participation in West African dance among pre-professional and professional dancers, something currently missing from the literature.

Despite the limitations, our findings add a unique contribution to the literature in this area and suggest multiple implications for future research and dance education.

Participants highlighted the significant health benefits, both psychologically and physiologically, of West African dance. West African dance is a high-intensity dance form which may have a greater impact on cardiovascular fitness than other dance forms. Therefore, it may be a beneficial supplemental or mainstream training activity in dance education programs. Further research is needed to examine this hypothesis. Future research should examine the psychological and physical health benefits of African dance and other culturally oriented dance forms as compared to other dance forms using rigorous research methods (i.e., randomized controlled trials) to have a better understanding of the unique benefits of adding more curriculum related to culturally oriented dance in dance education programs. Many participants started their dance training in traditional dance classes such as ballet; however, they identified feeling out of place or uncomfortable in those types of courses. This led to them not majoring in dance in their post-secondary education programs. Study participants also highlighted a lack of culturally oriented dance training offered in their institutions of higher education, leading them to go out into the community to further their training in this dance form. It is clear that dance training programs need to be more inclusive of different dance forms in order to promote sustained engagement and stronger motivation by racial/ethnic minorities in dance as an art form. It is very likely that including more culturally oriented dance curriculum in higher education could have a positive impact on the numbers of racial and ethnic minority dance students and dance faculty in the academy.

References

1. Hanson KM. Addressing racial diversity in ballet. 2015 January 18, 2019. Available from: https://www.britannica.com/topic/Addressing-Racial-Diversity-in-Ballet-2030912.
2. Kerr-Berry JA. Dance education in an era of racial backlash: moving forward as we step backwards. J Dance Educ. 2012;12(2):48–53.
3. Services HEAD. Dance annual summary 2002–2003. Reston: National Association of Schools of Dance; 2003.
4. Warburton E, Stanek M. The condition of dance faculty in higher education. In: Conference proceedings of the national dance education organization: Merging worlds: Dance, education, society and politics; 2004. p. 420–5.
5. Jain S, Brown DR. Cultural dance: an opportunity to encourage physical activity and health in communities. J Health Educ. 2001;32(4):216–22.
6. Conner M. Recreational folk dance: a multicultural exercise component in healthy aging. Aust Occup Ther J. 2000;47(2):69–76.
7. Ravelin T, Kylmä J, Korhonen T. Dance in mental health nursing: a hybrid concept analysis. Issues Ment Health Nurs. 2006;27(3):307–17.
8. Eyler AA, Vest JR, Sanderson B, Wilbur J, Matson-Koffman D, Evenson KR, et al. Environmental, policy, and cultural factors related to physical activity in a diverse sample of women: the women's Cardiovascular Health Network Project–introduction and methodology. Women Health. 2002;36(2):1–15.
9. Olvera AE. Cultural dance and health: a review of the literature. Am J Health Educ. 2008;39(6):353–9.

10. Murrock CJ, Gary FA. A culturally-specific dance intervention to increase functional capacity in African American women. J Cult Divers. 2008;15(4):168.
11. Whitehorse LE, Manzano R, Baezconde-Garbanati LA, Hahn G. Culturally tailoring a physical activity program for Hispanic women: recruitment successes of La Vida Buena's salsa aerobics. J Health Educ. 1999;30(sup2):S18–24.
12. Vahabi M, Damba C. A feasibility study of a culturally and gender-specific dance to promote physical activity for South Asian immigrant women in the greater Toronto area. Womens Health Issues. 2015;25(1):79–87.
13. Visram S, Crosland A, Unsworth J, Long S. Engaging women from South Asian communities in cardiac rehabilitation. Int J Ther Rehabil. 2008;15(7):298–305.
14. Monteiro NM, Wall DJ. African dance as healing modality throughout the diaspora: the use of ritual and movement to work through trauma. J Pan Afr Stud. 2011;4(6):234–52.
15. Farr M. The role of dance/movement therapy in treating at-risk African American adolescents. Arts Psychother. 1997;24(2):183–91.
16. West J, Otte C, Geher K, Johnson J, Mohr DC. Effects of Hatha yoga and African dance on perceived stress, affect, and salivary cortisol. Ann Behav Med. 2004;28(2):114–8.
17. Kerr-Berry JA. Using the power of West African dance to combat gender issues. J Phys Educ Recreat Dance. 1994;65(2):44–8.
18. Thompson D. The "Cronistas de Indias" revisited: historical reports, archeological evidence, and literary and artistic traces of indigenous music and dance in the Greater Antilles at the time of the "Conquista". Lat Am Music Rev. 1993;14(2):181–201.
19. Skye FD, Christensen OJ, England JT. A study of the effects of a culturally-based dance education model on identified stress factors in American Indian college women. J Am Indian Educ. 1989;29(1):26–31.
20. Kudlacek S, Pietschmann F, Bernecker P, Resch H, Willvonseder R. The impact of a senior dancing program on spinal and peripheral bone mass1. Am J Phys Med Rehabil. 1997;76(6):477–81.
21. Shigematsu R, Chang M, Yabushita N, Sakai T, Nakagaichi M, Nho H, et al. Dance-based aerobic exercise may improve indices of falling risk in older women. Age Ageing. 2002;31(4):261–6.
22. Engels H-J, Gretebeck RJ, Gretebeck KA, Jiménez L. Promoting healthful diets and exercise: efficacy of a 12-week after-school program in urban African Americans. J Am Diet Assoc. 2005;105(3):455–9.
23. Harris DA. Dance/movement therapy approaches to fostering resilience and recovery among African adolescent torture survivors. Torture. 2007;17(2):134–55.

Chapter 10
Analyzing the Use of the Fifth Position in Dance Training

Merry Lynn Morris, Paula Nunez, Andee Scott, and Stephanie L. Carey

Introduction

The fifth position closing action occurs repeatedly in ballet and contemporary dance classes, typically in *battement tendu*, *dégagé*,[1] and *grand battement* combinations, as well as in *rond de jambe*, *fondu*, *frappé*, *adagio*, *allegro*, *pirouette*, and traveling combinations. Dancers typically perform one hundred or more of the fifth position closing action with each leg during an hour-long class. The fifth position is a strenuous and anatomically difficult position to achieve because in its ideal iteration, the feet are fully crossed heel to toe and maximally outwardly rotated (Fig. 10.1) [1, 2]. Watkins et al. found that in fifth position the angle of deviation in the alignment of foot to knee was notably greater compared to the first position, placing the knee in a more vulnerable position [2]. Similarly, Negus, Hopper, and Briffa found greater compensated turnout in the fifth position when compared to the first position [3]. Compensated turnout is the difference between functional turnout angle and total (right and left) hip external rotation range of motion. Compensated turnout is typically achieved by employing additional mechanisms from the lower leg (e.g., knee external rotation, foot pronation) rather than from the hip [1, 3–10]. Dancers' prevalent use of compensated turnout is

[1] A *dégagé* movement is similar to a *tendu* in which the foot slides along the floor out to a pointed position (plantarflexed) except that the leg then is raised slightly off the floor. The closing action is similar to the tendu movement, except that the dancer is bringing the leg into the closing position on the floor from a raised position.

M. L. Morris (✉) · P. Nunez · A. Scott
School of Theatre and Dance, University of South Florida, Tampa, FL, USA
e-mail: mmorris3@usf.edu; paula3@usf.edu; andeescott@usf.edu

S. L. Carey
Department of Mechanical Engineering, Center for Assistive, Rehabilitation, & Robotics Technologies (CARRT), University of South Florida, Tampa, FL, USA
e-mail: scarey3@usf.edu

S.-H. Lee et al. (eds.), *Perspectives in Performing Arts Medicine Practice*,
https://doi.org/10.1007/978-3-030-37480-8_10

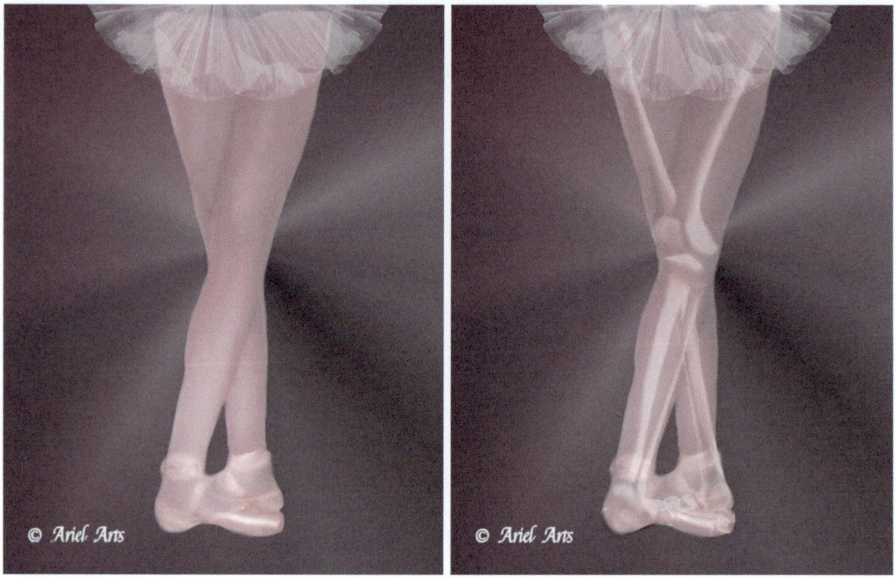

Figs. 10.1 and 10.2 Fifth position (180 degree) applied in classical ballet training

indicative of the anatomical difficulty of the fifth position. The dance-science literature suggests that these types of compensations can increase injury risk by placing torque on the knees and increasing the risk for meniscal, medial ligament, and patellofemoral injury [1, 2, 4, 8, 9, 11–15] (Figs. 10.1 and 10.2).

The seeds of this research grew from an initial teacher observation in which dancers in class were often seen bending and restraightening their legs (even if subtly) to accomplish the close to fifth position. This habit was particularly observed when the leg closed from the front and to a lesser extent in the side closing. Dancers often do this in order to recruit additional outward rotation from the knee joint, thereby achieving the correct look of the position [1, 8, 10]. When the knee is flexed, the collateral ligaments relax to enable further rotation [1, 8, 10]. Concern arose over how this might be damaging over time with respect to potential torque on the knee and its surrounding soft tissues, due to the frequent repetition of the movement. Additionally, if the goal of the exercise is to make sure dancers are developing stability and a strong, well-aligned, effective kinetic chain in the use of the leg, the pattern of constantly bending, twisting (externally rotating), and restraightening on a loaded knee joint may be antithetical to that training goal. This observed pattern of bending, twisting, and restraightening at the knee has negative implications for the whole kinetic chain of the spine, pelvis, hip, ankle, and foot.

The primary purpose of this study was to analyze the biomechanics of dancers' knee motions during a *tendu* closing from front in first, third, and fifth positions. The *tendu* movement was chosen because it is a standard, basic movement practiced in most dance training regimens. The foot slides out along the floor in a straight line to a pointed position and then returns back to its starting position. The leg should remain straight throughout. A secondary aim within the study was to better understand dancer's perceptions of the fifth position and what goals, images, associations, or prior knowledge undergird its performance. Quantitative motion analysis data were contextualized and combined with dancers' verbal reporting, instructor video analysis, and survey data to assess results.

Background

Lower body injuries in dance are common, with knee injuries and pain being frequent at anywhere between 15% and 39% [8, 13, 20–29]. Common types of knee injuries and conditions in dance include the following [8, 10, 11, 13, 15, 22, 23, 25–29]: chondromalacia patella, anterior knee pain, patellar malalignment, patellar femoral syndrome, patellar tendonitis, patellar dislocation or subluxation, plica syndrome, meniscus tear, medial collateral ligament tear, anterior cruciate ligament tear, and osteoarthritis. In a longitudinal cohort study of 1336 nonprofessional female dancers, Steinberg et al. found that knee injuries were the leading cause of complaints by adolescent dancers (14–16 years) [26]. Additionally, Sobrino and colleagues examined 486 injuries in professional dancers and learned that overuse injuries were the most frequent injuries and patellofemoral pain syndrome was the most prevalent overuse injury, followed by Achilles tendinopathy, patellar tendinopathy, and mechanical low back pain [25].

Dancer's "turnout" technique is probably one of the most important and frequent causes of the majority of knee pain and injury. Not surprisingly, efficient, healthful approaches to turnout use in dance are pervasive topics in the literature; yet effective assessment methods and practical training application for dancers remain challenging. Further, while knee rotation in movements such as *plié* and *grand plié* and in static positions [5, 6, 14, 30] have been studied, the *tendu* and *dégagé* movements have not yet been assessed, specifically in relation to their impacts in the repetitive torque at the knee during the closing action. Studies have also indicated that the biomechanically efficient means of achieving turnout/outward rotation is initially and predominantly from the hip joint, rather than from knee joint rotation (tibial external rotation) especially while the feet are weight-bearing [1–20].

Researchers and practitioners have observed that in order to accommodate certain repetitively practiced positions such as fifth position, a dancer often recruits the outward rotation available at the knee when bent and then restraightens into the appropriate position in order to achieve additional turnout [1–3, 8–11, 20, 27]. In fact, it is commonly observed that dancers adopt a variety of different types of compensatory strategies to achieve maximal turnout of the legs in various positions [1, 3–10]. Analysis of these practices may lead dancers and dance educators toward better strategies for implementing efficient pedagogy. This study combines precise motion analysis imaging technique with intentional observational analysis by dance movement experts and dancer response to evaluate the strategies dancers employ when closing the leg, with specific attention to the knee joint. Few studies incorporate dancers' descriptions of how they experience the movement in their bodies, as this study does. Listening to what dancers say about the movement experience is important for gleaning a more complete understanding of movement compensations and injury risks. The outcomes of this study will add further insight to the current understanding of dancers' approaches and strategies in closing actions of the leg to fifth position.

Methods

In this study, multiple methods of data collection were used to glean an understanding of the biomechanics of closing to fifth position, as evidenced by motion analysis data, video analysis by dance instructors, and dancers' descriptions after performing the movement in verbal reports. Additionally, to better understand dancers' perceptions of the position and the goals, images, associations, or prior knowledge that undergird its performance, a survey was distributed to dancers.

Participants

Twenty-three undergraduate dance majors from a large urban research university were recruited to participate in the study under an approved Institutional Review Board (IRB #00008440) protocol. Ten of the twenty-three participants took part in the quantitative motion analysis, ten took part in the studio analysis portion, and all participants provided verbal explanations of their closing strategies. The same ten participants who completed the studio analysis portion also completed the survey portion. Twenty-one students were female and two were male, with age range between 18 and 23 and comprised of intermediate and advanced dancers having at least 10 years of prior dance training. The participant pool was a cross section of sophomores, juniors, and seniors. Participant data was not collected on race or ethnicity.

Motion Capture

The motion capture session took place at the University of South Florida's Center for Assistive, Rehabilitation and Robotics Technologies (CARRT) motion analysis lab. The participant had measurements such as height, weight, hip width, knee width, and ankle width taken and recorded for the purposes of accurate motion analysis. The participant wore tight fitting shorts and a short-sleeved shirt or leotard. Twenty-seven small (approximately 0.5 inch in diameter) spherical reflective markers were attached to the participant on the following boney landmarks: shoulders, clavicle, sternum, C7, T10 vertebrae, back, anterior and posterior iliac spines, thighs, knees (medial, lateral), tibias, ankles, and first and fifth toes, using a combination of neoprene with Velcro straps and double-sided tape.

The participant performed the following dance movements: *tendu* front and side closing into first, third, and fifth positions and closing with the foot flat on the ground with straight legs. Three trials for each action were performed on both right and left legs. The principal investigator (PI) on the study, also a dance professor, provided instructions verbally and physically to the participant. No music was used; the principal investigator rhythmically cued dancers for timing.

The participant was videotaped while completing these trials. Total time for each participant for this portion was approximately 2 hours.

The dancers' *tendu* movements were tracked using an 8-camera optical motion analysis system (Vicon Motion Systems, Denver, CO), and knee angles were calculated in each position: first, third, and fifth. To ensure reliability, composite measurements of three trials were used.

Video Analysis by Dance Movement Experts

At the University dance studio, participants performed *tendu* and *dégagé* front and side closing into first, third, and fifth positions and closing with the foot flat on the ground with straight legs. Three trials for each action were performed on both right and left legs at the barre. The PI provided instructions verbally and physically to the participant. The dance movement sequences were performed in exactly the same way as in the motion analysis lab with verbal cueing by the principal investigator and the same pace maintained without music. A second sequence of *tendus* was performed with ballet music to mimic the conditions of a regular ballet class. The same music was used for each participant. The participant wore traditional dancewear with ballet shoes. Total time for this portion was approximately 20 minutes.

All three trials of dance movements were videotaped. Three dance movement experts from the University's Dance Faculty watched and evaluated the video recordings of all three trials on both right and left legs. The assessment focused on the movement mechanics of the dancer's lower body, with specific attention to what occurred at the knee. The dance movement experts were each given four questions to answer with regard to the analysis of the action after reviewing the videos. The questions were as follows:

- *Question 1*: Do you see any changes or differences in the basic mechanics of the action when the dancer closes to the first position, then third, and then fifth?
- *Question 2*: If the answer to the above question is yes, please describe the main changes or differences you observe.
- *Question 3*: What, if anything, do you perceive occurring at the knee joint when the dancer closes first, then third, and then fifth?
- *Question 4*: Please describe any other important details you notice in how the dancer appears to be accomplishing the *tendu* and *dégagé* actions.

One of the faculty members regularly teaches ballet; another regularly teaches modern dance and choreography; and the third regularly teaches dance improvisation, Laban movement analysis, and kinesiology. All three of the instructors are experienced dancers and choreographers with at least 20 years of dance teaching experience. Two of the instructors possessed expertise in anatomy and kinesiology.

Verbal Reports by Dancers

The participants verbally reported their strategies and kinesthetic sensations after completing the movement series. These comments were recorded on paper and then transferred to an electronic document. These verbal reports occurred in both the motion capture session and the studio portions of the study, directly after the participant had finished completing the entire movement series. First, the participant was asked to describe how they accomplished the closing action to first, third, and fifth positions and to describe any differences in their strategies among the positions. The participant was then asked to describe any feelings/sensations elicited during the closings to first, third, and fifth positions.

Survey

Ten of the twenty-three participants filled out a short 8-question survey of their perceptions of the fifth position. The questions were related to how dancers understood the position and what associations they ascribed to it. For example, in some of the questions, dancers viewed images of 180-degree turnout positions and less turned out images of the feet/legs and were asked to use adjectives to describe how they view those positions. Another question asked dancers to agree or disagree with the following question: "I view 180-degree turnout as the 'ideal' to work towards." And, dancers were asked to reply yes or no to this question: "I find the 5th position, flat, 180 degree turnout, with the feet fully crossed a *more beautiful* position than a 5th which is less turned out, such as the ones pictured below." Questions were designed with simplicity in mind, using terms with which dancers would be familiar. Many questions were close-ended questions such as yes/no or agree/disagree. The goal was to elicit easily quantifiable results contextualized with qualitative responses targeting the research goal. Completing the survey took approximately 15 minutes.

Results

Motion Capture Portion

Results showed the average range of motion (ROM) of knee flexion and rotation increased incrementally from first to third to fifth positions in both right and left legs.

Table 10.1 Average knee angles in degrees with standard deviation (STD) during tendu closing

Position	Side	Knee flexion ROM degrees (STD)	Knee abduction/adduction ROM degrees (STD)	Knee rotation ROM degrees (STD)
First	Right	6.9 (2.2)	2.3 (0.8)	5.3 (2.4)
	Left	6.1 (2.3)	2.2 (0.7)	4.9 (1.9)
Third	Right	10.3 (2.7)	1.6 (0.4)	5.8 (2.8)
	Left	9.2 (3.0)	1.7 (0.4)	5.8 (2.3)
Fifth	Right	12.0 (3.0)	1.9 (0.5)	6.5 (2.7)
	Left	10.3 (4.1)	1.8 (0.6)	6.3 (2.2)

The average ROM figures in Table 10.1 reflect all dance participants (10/10) exhibiting the flexion, rotation, and restraightening pattern at the knee, during the closing action of the *tendu*. The ROM reflected the highest degree of knee flexion and knee rotation in the fifth position closing. For the right leg, there was a 5.1-degree difference between the flexion in first versus fifth, and there was a 1.2-degree difference between rotations in first versus fifth. For the left leg, there was a 4.2-degree difference between the flexion in first versus fifth, and there was a 1.4-degree difference between rotations in first versus fifth. Abduction angles for each closing position were also calculated. As would be expected, abduction decreased incrementally from first to fifth positions. This finding is logical and is due to the fact that the dancers were gradually adducting the legs in each of the three positions. Although abduction angles were calculated, they were not of target concern in the study as they do not present the same type of injury risk flexion accompanied with rotation at the knee is likely to cause.

Video Analysis by Dance Movement Experts

Three dance faculty evaluated the videos and answered four questions about what they observed. A summation of the answers to those questions follows:

- *Question 1*: Do you see any changes or differences in the basic mechanics of the action when the dancer closes to the first position, then third, and then fifth?

All three instructors answered yes to this question for 100% of participants.

- *Question 2*: If the answer to the above question is yes, please describe the main changes or differences you observe.

The key theme noted by all three instructors is as follows: More compensatory adjustments in the foot, ankle, knee, and pelvis were observed during the third and fifth closings, rather than the first position closing. Compensatory adjustments usually referred to winging or pronation of the foot, bending and rotating the knee, and tilting the pelvis (anterior and/or posterior) as well as pulling the hip/pelvis back, often on one side more than another.

- *Question 3*: What, if anything, do you perceive occurring at the knee joint when the dancer closes first, then third, and then fifth?

For 100% of participants, instructors observed bending (flexion) and outward rotation at the knee during the third position closing and usually to a greater degree in the fifth position closing, but not in the first position closing. One instructor sometimes noted the adjustment at the knee as more of a "softening" than a flexion action. This pattern was noted by all three instructors as occurring most obviously in the front closing, but the same pattern could also be seen in the side closing (particularly the side *tendu* or *dégagé* closing in front of the supporting leg). This pattern usually occurred at about the half-way point of the closing action, and it was followed by a restraightening of the knee once the feet reached their final position. For example, one instructor commented:

> The tendu in 1st or 3rd has less impact and it is easier for the dancer to maintain the natural rotation during the closing. When the dancer closes in 5th position I see a small misalignment and pronation that increases the strain on the knee joint. The dancer is using her quadriceps, kneecap, and hip muscles correctly, but slightly forcing the turnout from the knee down when she closes her foot in 5th position.

Instructors perceived variations among dancers in terms of the extent of flexion and rotation observed, and there were variations between right and left legs, in terms of how the closing was accomplished. At times, dancers employed significant winging of the foot (pronation) in conjunction with the flexion and rotation at the knee, while others moved the pelvis back (anterior tilt) in addition to the flexion and rotation at the knee, in order to accommodate the closing action. Further, instructors noted that for some dancers, the muscles around the knee cap (quadriceps) appeared to remain engaged throughout the movement trajectory, while other dancers seemed to noticeably release the muscles around the knee cap and then re-engage as they completed the closing. Instructors noted that dancers often used the friction of the floor to help maintain the end position and desired turnout. Dancers who utilized a more modified turnout generally exhibited less flexion and rotation of the knee joint during the third and fifth closings.

- *Question 4*: Please describe any other important details you notice in how the dancer appears to be accomplishing the *tendu* and *dégagé* actions.

Within this question, instructors often commented about the correctness of the dancer's approach in terms of body mechanics and the quality of the movement. They noted when dancers appeared to be working "within their range" rather than forcing their turnout or improperly using their body mechanics (e.g., employing excessive pelvic and spinal adjustment). They noted when dancers appeared to be "grounded" and when they were appropriately engaging their leg muscles in a "spiraling action" and "using resistance." Instructors also made general postural alignment observations regarding the visual correctness of the dancers' beginning postures. In some cases, dancers' weight placement appeared too far forward or back and in other cases, dancers appeared to have an anterior pelvic tilt or lordosis. Instructors generally viewed neutral pelvic alignment, effective use of turnout initiation from the top of the leg (hip), and an active core engagement/abdominal lift as "correct." When students deviated from these notions, the movement was viewed as less efficient and less correct. Commentary also included an observation about leg contour/shaping and how the shaping of the leg impacted the dancers' ease or difficulty with the movement. In some cases, dancers' leg shapings as well as hip width seemed to better accommodate the fifth position closing (e.g., hyperextended dancers and dancers with larger thigh mass appeared to have more difficulty in the closing). Overall, there was an acknowledgement of the varied and subtle differences among dancers' postural and movement strategies and a concern for the biomechanical compensations taking place.

Verbal Reports by Dancers

Dancers reported more difficulty and greater physical adjustment in the pelvis, hips, and knees during the third and, particularly, fifth position closing than in the first position.

When dancers were asked how they accomplished the *tendu* closing from the front, the majority described initiating the movement by "pulling the toes back" and then "lifting/pulling up" (in the pelvis), as they drew the leg into the closing position. For example, "When I close from devant [front], I think of lifting my hips up and pulling back the big toe."

Most dancers noted that their focus was on keeping the leg "turned out" (outwardly rotated) during the entire action. Several dancers specifically mentioned the use of the inner thighs "wrapping outward" as the leg closed, and others mentioned that they engaged the outer thigh or back of the thigh during the action. A few dancers described feeling the engagement of their "gluts" (gluteal muscles) during the action. Other dancers mentioned "tucking the pelvis" or "bringing the pelvis under" as the leg drew in as well. The majority of dancers focused upon what the gesture leg was doing (the leg performing the *tendu*), but some described the need to pull up, shift their weight, and maintain turnout on the supporting leg as well.

When dancers were asked if the method of closing differed between first, third, and fifth, dancers reported that the basic strategy was the same for all: pulling toes back, maintaining turnout, and lifting, but that more work and additional strategies had to be adopted in the fifth closing such as further tilt of pelvis, bending of the knee, and additional winging of the foot.

For the purposes of this study, we were most interested in how dancers described knee adjustments or sensations. Here are representative samples of the variety of responses dancers' reported:

> For first, it is a little bit easier to execute – easier to keep my hips up – it feels like a more stable position. third feels relatively easy as well. But fifth is most difficult, especially closing into the front, because my knee has to bend in order to actually close the foot into the position. It is so difficult to create space in this position. It is so difficult to go from the

feeling of length in the outward movement of the tendu and then it feels like I have to foreshorten that length. It is hard to create space. When I bend the knee, it allows me pull my toes back. I feel like it doesn't come naturally from my thigh at all. My calves get in the way and my thighs get in the way. In plié, I can find a beautiful fifth.

For all the positions, I tried to close with a gradual articulation of the foot: toes, metatarsal, heel. Third was similar to first. In fifth, it was harder to get the toes back; I had to focus more on that. I tried to keep the hip and knee turned out in the whole movement. Moving the leg in fifth feels like the hip has to pull back more to close the leg (note: dancer demonstrated an anterior tilt of pelvis when she made this statement).

I feel the turnout coming from my inner thighs wrapping outwards and I feel it in the calf a little. I try to keep my knee straight. I am hyperextended so I have to bend the knee to close it in all positions. I pull up my knee to close as well. I need to wing the foot to close it in.

For all of the positions, the heel leads out and the toes pull back to close. I try to maintain turnout in both legs. I try to keep my knees straight especially in fifth because it feels like it wants to relax or bend. Keeping the knees straight is most challenging in the fifth position. Half-way in it feels like the knee wants to bend. I think it bends because of the turnout.

In the fifth, I had to think more about the toes leading. In both third and fifth, I had to pull up the lower abs and gluts a lot more – more in fifth than the other positions. I had to pull up more on the standing leg to make room for the leg to close. I also felt my shoulders go down as I pulled up. I also have to bend the knee in order to close fifth – when it is about an inch away from the fifth position. Bending the knee helps to accomplish the visual look of turn-out. I also have to tilt my pelvis (anterior pelvic tilt) and re-correct it to close fifth.

Lastly, dancers were asked to describe any *feelings/sensations* associated with accomplishing the closing action in first, third, and fifth. There were sometimes repeat comments made from the previous questions when answering this question. The goal of this question was to have dancers reflect upon not just the strategies they used to accomplish the action but how the action felt in their bodies (e.g., difficult, easeful, fluid, natural, painful, etc.).

Examples of participants' responses are as follows:

In first, it feels like it just happens naturally. The third is odd – partly because we don't use it that often, but it feels better than fifth. Fifth is like...I am constantly finding new things to fix. I feel antsy, like there is no point of stillness, just constant fixing.

First feels more grounded because you can stand easier on both legs. In fifth, I kind of almost feel like my knee is twisting outwards. I feel relatively grounded in third. I feel like I have to fight against the outward twisting – my body/pelvis wants to go with it.

I feel like I can't straighten the knee all the way and close the leg. It feels like their isn't space [in fifth]. With the first position I feel more centered and it feels more natural. Third and fifth, I feel like I have to shift my weight more onto one leg – to the ball of the foot. I feel more pulled up in first; I feel like I can hold my core better. In third and fifth I am concentrating on closing the legs so much that I can't focus as much on my upper body.

Third and fifth particularly awkward feeling, especially side closing.

first position very easy. Typically adjusting is in fifth – knee and hips both feel as if they have to shift side to side/rotation to get to the crossed closing. Almost feels like patella is moving/rotating. In third, I felt pretty stable, first felt most stable, fifth felt least stable.

I feel more torqued in the front mostly in the fifth because of how I have to pull my toes back to close. Inside of my knee, I feel that it is pulling in a way that shouldn't be. I feel that torque about half way into the closing.

Also, feel that a little in the third position. And, in the side closing to the front.

As a goal – the "true fifth" is still in my head – as the standard.

In third and fifth positions it was harder to turn-out because the leg is not coming back at all the way underneath you. I plant the heel in fifth and then continue turning out the foot to get the final fifth closing –the aesthetic. It is hard to bring the leg back to the original starting position.

Survey Results

Question 1: My responses to viewing the foot/leg positions below are (circle all that apply):

Dancers were shown images of 180-degree fifth positions front and side views.

As can be seen by the graph in Fig. 10.3, 90% of participants marked *ideal*, 60% marked *contorted*, and 60% marked *beautiful*. The responses of *uncomfortable*, *awesome*, and *injurious* came in at 40% followed by *other* at 30%, *ouch* at 20%, and *odd* and *perfect* at 10%.

The responses in the category of *other* were "aesthetically pleasing as a trained dancer," "unique," "symmetrical," and "wish my turnout looked like that."

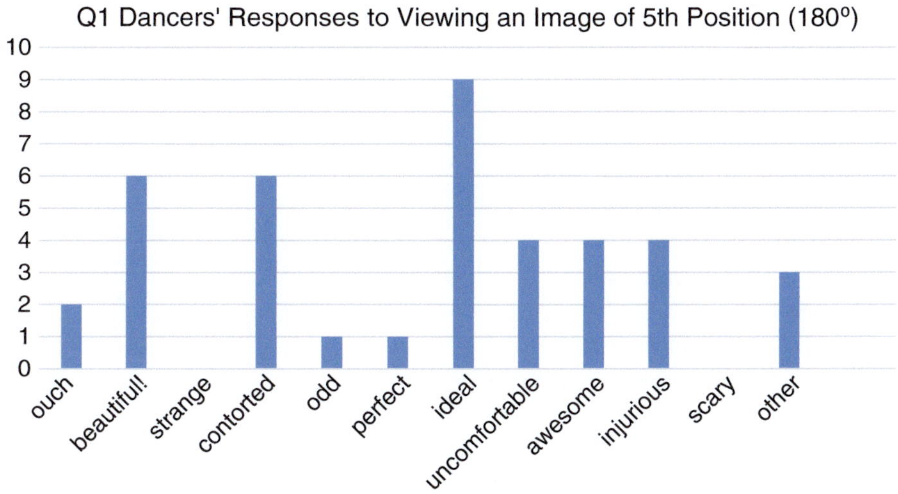

Fig. 10.3 Question 1

Question 2: Explain your response to the pictures.

This question asked dancers to explain their answers to question 1. In this question, dancers acknowledged that although they found the 180-degree position "more pleasing to the eye," it was "worse for the body." In addition, it is worth noting that many of them described that this is how they were *taught* to see. The statements below effectively capture the key ideas expressed in the responses:

> I know it's the ideal, but all I can think about is the pain in the knees. That's probably because I've never been able to have perfect turnout without my knees hurting.
>
> I believe the pictures are ideal because they all have a correct toe to heel position. They do look contorted because it does not look like a normal bodily position.
>
> 5th position does not look uncomfortable, but it does appear contorted and injurious. The "X" shape of the legs and the alignment of the toes and heels is unique, pleasing to the eye and beautiful. To me, the position only becomes uncomfortable when performed.
>
> That is what I feel we have been taught to strive for in our 5th positions.

Question 3: When I compare the two foot positions below my reaction is that Image A is (circle all that apply for you):

For this question, dancers viewed Image A – a 180-degree version of the fifth position – and Image B, a fifth position with modified turnout (less than 180 degrees). The images dancers were shown are similar to those pictured in Fig. 10.5.

As can be seen in the graph in Fig. 10.4, 90% of participants marked *more aesthetically pleasing*, followed by 70% marking *more beautiful* and *more ideal*, 60% marking *more perfect*, 50% marking *more correct*, and 20% marking *other*.

Only 10%, one participant, marked *less perfect* or *less beautiful.*

Question 4: When I work in the fifth position in class, I work within my turnout range, but, ideally, if my body enabled it, I would like to have "perfect" turnout.

100% agreed (10/10).

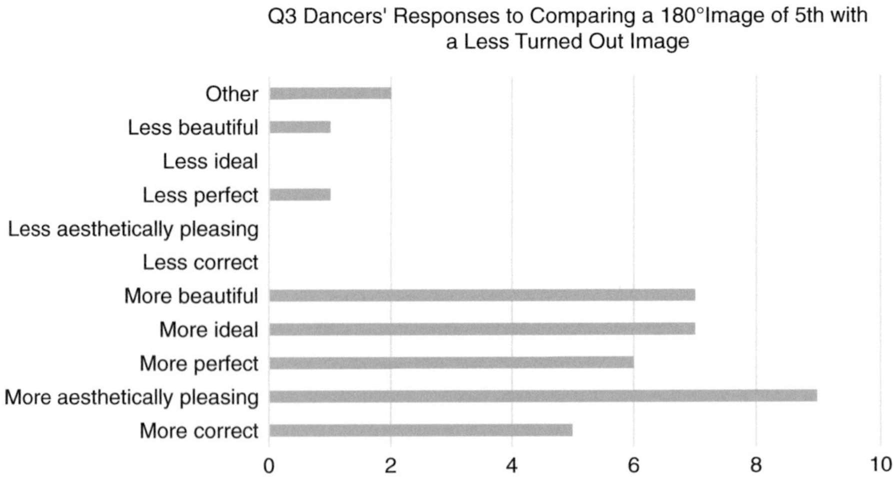

Fig. 10.4 Question 3

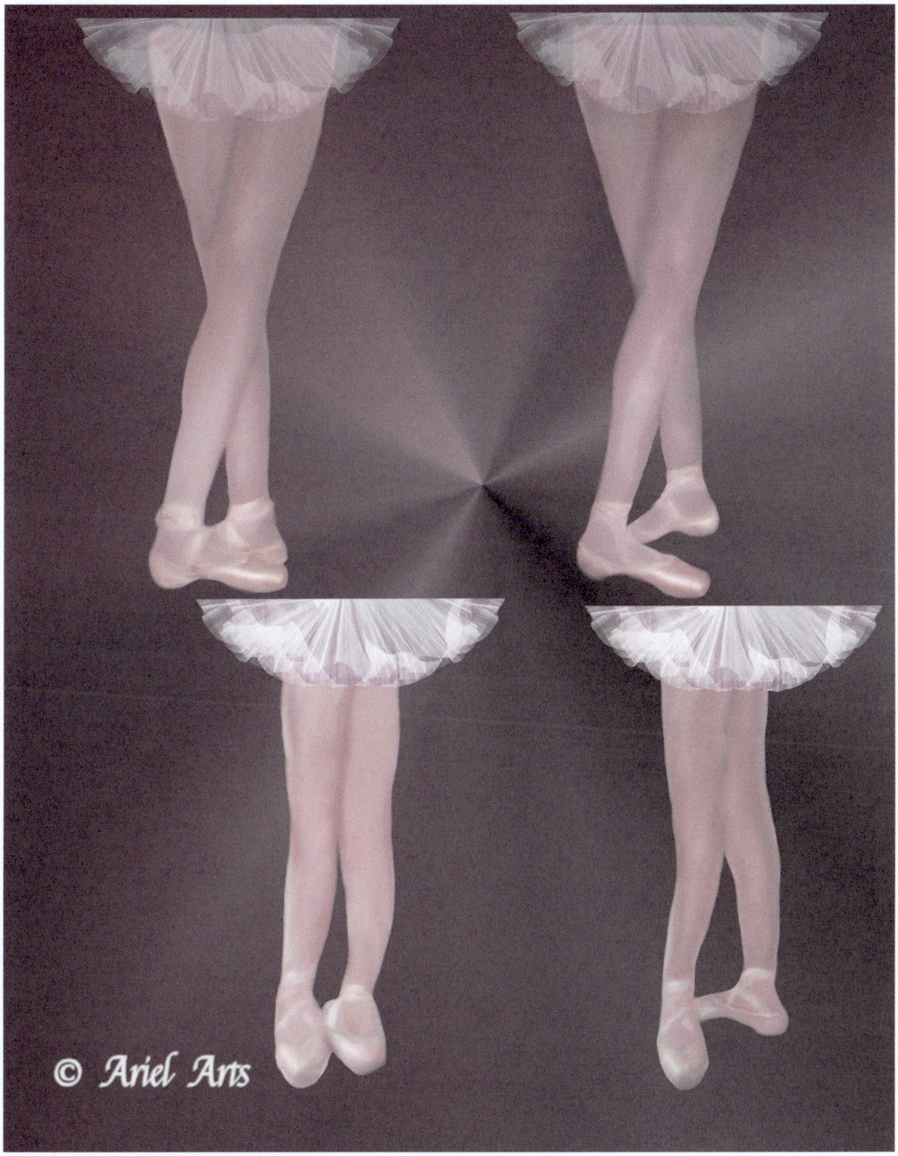

Fig. 10.5 Images of fifth position: 180-degree and modified turnout versions

Question 5: I view 180-degree turnout as the "ideal" to work toward.

70% agreed (7/10) and 30% disagreed (3/10).

As can be seen by the graph in Fig. 10.6 for question 6, 100% of participants marked *hard work*, 70% marked *generally uncomfortable*, 60% marked *awkward*, 30% marked *other*, and 20% marked *annoying* and *painful*.

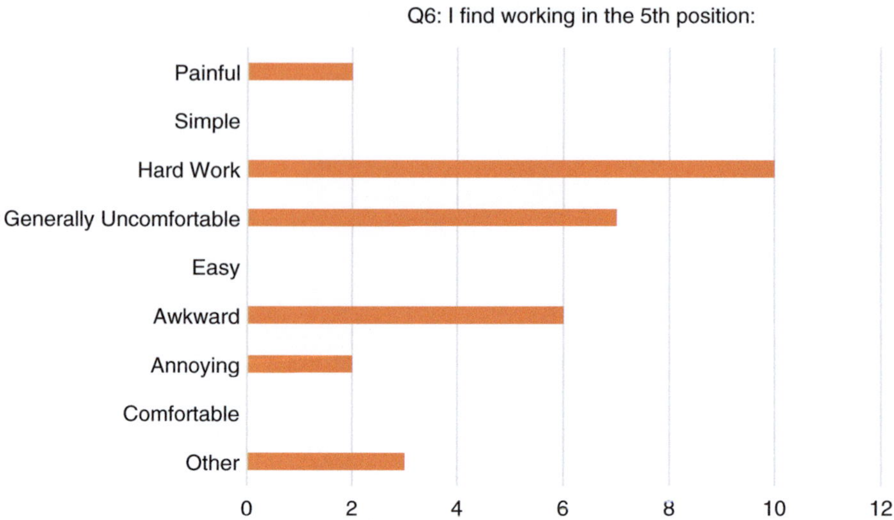

Fig. 10.6 Question 6

Answers for *other* were "movement hindering," "normal because we learn this position is significant in the beginnings of training," and "complicated."

Question 7: I was taught that the fifth position ideally is a flat 180-degree position, with the feet fully crossed toe to heel.

Yes = 80% (8/10)
No = 10% (1/10)
Yes and no = 10% (1/10)

The participant who marked "yes and no" explained, "I have had different teachers with different approaches toward working in the fifth position." The participant who marked no explained, "I was taught to always work on turnout not the idea that my fifth position had to be perfectly 180."

Question 8: I find the fifth position, flat 180-degree turnout with the feet fully crossed a *more beautiful* position than a fifth which is less turned out, such as the one pictured below.

Yes = 80%, (8/10)
No = 20%, (2/10)
Comments for this question included:

I think the body can naturally look beautiful in any position

I like the look of straight lines, that is what I find beautiful

A better image is produced when the legs are fully crossed and are almost 2-D

Although still correct, this type of 5th has essentially been taught to me as less technically correct.

Limitations, Reliability, and Validity

Limitations of this research include not having all twenty-three participants engage in each aspect of the study. Time and resource restrictions meant that only ten participants took part in the quantitative motion analysis data collection. However, within this cohort of participants, a clear biomechanical pattern could be seen. Participants in other portions of the study evidenced a pattern consistent with the motion analysis data, as revealed through visual observation. This study also focused only upon collegiate dance students, limiting the generalizability of the results. Future research should analyze different age groups and dance training contexts to determine if the observed pattern is similar across varying groups. The relatively small sample size for this study is also a limitation, and a larger sample size would bring additional validity to the study.

Reliability of the study was addressed through the multiple trials dancers performed in both the motion analysis lab and the dance studio; the analysis performed consistently by three dance instructors, all yielding similar observations (high inter-rater agreement); and the consistency of the research procedures. The survey instrument developed for the study involved input by several dance experts and was designed with multiple factors in mind, including language use, alignment with the research goal, question sequencing and style, and internal consistency [31].

Validity of the study is evidenced through the study being reviewed by an ethics board – the Institutional Review Board (IRB) – as well as the use of triangulation in the study. Multiple data sources were used to identify and understand the movement mechanics of the action: quantitative motion analysis data, analysis by three dance movement experts, dance participants' self-reports, and dance participants' survey data. These four data sources produced convergent results.

Discussion and Summary

The primary goal of this research was to determine if dancers frequently employ flexion and rotation at the knee joint to accommodate the closing action of the leg to fifth position, in such common training movements as *tendu* and *dégagé*. In order to have a basis of comparison, data were collected on first, third, and fifth position closings. The leg gradually crosses (adducts) further over the midline from first to third to fifth, while maintaining turnout (outward rotation); thus, it was helpful to see what changes might occur as the leg crossing became greater with outward rotation maintained. The study focused upon the front closing due to an initial observation suggesting that this closing required the most adjustment and accommodation at the knee joint. The high level of repetition of this movement within technique training, specifically, ballet, makes analyzing this potentially injurious action relevant.

Quantitative data analysis demonstrated that the first position closing exhibited the least amount of knee flexion and rotation indicating that the dancer was able to more effectively perform the closing movement of the leg in this position, maintaining a straight, well-aligned leg throughout the movement trajectory. Study results show a gradual increase of degrees of flexion and rotation at the knee from first to third to fifth. This finding coincides with dancers' verbal descriptions, and it further coincides with video observations of the dancers performing the movement, showing greater biomechanical accommodation during the third and particularly, the fifth closing.

The results of this study prompt two key questions for dance educators:

1. What is the purpose of the movement?
2. Is the purpose of the movement being achieved effectively if dancers are repetitively bending, rotating, and restraightening their knees with each closing?

The researchers in this study suggest that the purpose of the movement needs to be examined carefully to align intention with outcome. If the goal is to train dancers' muscle strength and neuromuscular patterning in terms of building a strong, well-aligned, stable leg, with effective use of outward rotation, it is questionable as to whether the constant compensatory actions at the knee are facilitating that goal. Existing research suggests that employing excessive rotation from the knee joint presents significant injury risk [1, 2, 4, 8, 9, 11–15]. If the goal is purely an aesthetic one, how much value should be placed upon a foot position in relationship to the dancer's overall artistic development and training goals? Can other methods be employed yet retain similar aesthetic ideals? Dance training practices should be called into question, especially in light of the dance-science research now available. Some choices have simply become traditional, habitual practices, passed down over time but not thoroughly examined from multiple perspectives [32]. Is this physical training practice doing what it is intended to do with regard to producing highly proficient dancers who can sustain their involvement in dance?

Of additional importance is listening to how dancers describe their sensations of the movement as they close into the fifth position. Whereas closing into the first position was most often described with words such as "grounded," "natural," "centered," "stable," and "comfortable," closing into the fifth position was most often described with words like "awkward," "difficult," "bound," "torqued," and "uncomfortable." One dancer stated: "Fifth is like....I am constantly finding new things to fix. I feel antsy, like there is no point of stillness, just constant fixing." Other dancers stated:

> First position very easy. Typically adjusting is in fifth – knee and hips both feel as if they have to shift side to side/rotation to get to the crossed closing. Almost feels like patella is moving/rotating. In third felt pretty stable, first felt most stable, fifth felt least stable.

> I feel more torqued in the front mostly in the fifth because of how I have to pull my toes back to close. Inside of my knee, I feel that it is pulling in a way that shouldn't be. I feel that torque about half way into the closing.
>
> Also, feel that a little in the third position. And, in the side closing to the front.

Only one dancer (1/23) reported that the fifth position closing felt "stable," and she attributed this to the fact that she has to pay more attention to squeezing and pulling up. Her sensation may be more linked to the act of employing more conscious muscular engagement and control in her body rather than the "stability" of the position itself. This dancer also described that she had to "force" her turnout at the end in fifth. When dancers are training, what bodily sensations do we, as dance educators, want to instill in the dancer as "healthy"? If it is important for dancers to have functionally healthy relationships to their bodies, physically and mentally, how do we, as dance educators, facilitate those relationships in how we teach?

The survey results distributed to dance participants indicate another important dimension regarding the study. According to the study data, the majority of dancers have been taught that 180-degree turnout (90 degree on each foot) is the *ideal* to which they should strive. They also view the position simultaneously as contorted, uncomfortable, awesome, and injurious. Although most of them acknowledge that 180-degree turnout is not achievable in a functionally healthy way, they have been taught that it is the aesthetic goal and that it is *more beautiful*, *more perfect*, *more ideal*, and *more correct* than a less turned out foot position. In fact, in many cases, dancers associate this extreme 180-degree foot position with the notion of being a good dancer, even though it is not a biomechanically safe or functionally efficient position and it, alone, does not equate to dancing proficiency [15]. However, this notion has been perpetuated over time, specifically in the classical ballet canon [33]. The mental image of the movement sets up an expectation. As one dancer stated: "As a goal – the 'true fifth' is still in my head – as the standard." Thus, regardless of whether they have an understanding of a healthy sense of turnout or working within their bodily range, the majority of dancers still work toward this extreme aesthetic image of the feet. The problem with this emphasis is that the dancers may be overemphasizing the visual look of the foot position instead of working toward the functional purpose of the movement action overall. The researchers suggest that dance educators consider how dancers are instructed as to the goals of their training regimens and how priorities are expressed (verbally and physically). How well do dancers understand the purposes of the movements they are doing in daily practice? Do these practices attend to the dancers' health and longevity in the art form? What images and ideas are perpetuated and why?

As this study as well as prior research indicates, the fifth position closing action (specifically from the front) is biomechanically highly complex and difficult for dancers. In order to do it as expected, they employ various compensatory strategies, which may be damaging over time. This particular movement is anatomically difficult due to the significant hip outward rotation and adduction which is maintained as the hip extends toward a very small, tight, closed base. Dancers describe feeling that there is "no space" for the leg to close, even when they try to pull up as much as possible. Few muscle groups perform the combination actions of hip adduction, outward rotation, and extension (lower gluteus maximus and lower three of six deep rotators); this means that there needs to be a refined and intensive selective recruitment of muscle groups and fibers. These muscle groups may not function optimally from a position of flexion when the leg is drawn into the fifth from the front. Additionally, the more powerful adductor muscles of the hip, which are necessary to recruit in the action, also perform flexion rather than extension actions, making the extension action potentially more difficult to access. Regardless of muscular complexity, there are anatomical limitations with regard to what degree of external rotation most hip joints can achieve. Dance science studies have shown that 90° hip rotation (180-degree bilaterally) is not common or feasible for individuals; rather, the research indicates that "a range of 60° to 70° is contributed by the hip, while the distal aspects of the lower extremity contribute approximately 10° to 35°" [18]. When the dancer compensates and attempts to bend at the knee to achieve greater outward rotation and close the foot into the desired fifth position, another muscular challenge presents. The biceps femoris would likely be the prime mover in this action, as it flexes and outwardly rotates the knee, but it is also an abductor, which is not helpful to the adduction goal of the movement. This issue likely adds to the need for constant "adjusting" as dancers in this study reported and demonstrated.

Although the reported values for the degrees of flexion and rotation are relatively small and visual observation indicates that this movement compensation pattern can be quite subtle, we suggest that this type of repetitive torque over time to the soft tissues of the knee joint can compromise the joint stability and may lead to patellar misalignment or more severe knee injuries. Additionally, we question how this neuromuscular pattern of bending, rotating, and restraightening may be contradictory to the actual technique goal in terms of training a straight, strong, stable, well-aligned leg.

The data from this study prompt multiple possible avenues of additional inquiry.

Further studies should analyze the other compensatory actions occurring throughout the kinetic chain during the closing action of the leg including pelvis, spine, ankle (subtalar joint), and foot motion. Additionally, a suggested intervention and follow-up study is to examine alternative third/fifth closings to reduce the need for potential injurious torque and strengthen the kinetic chain. Closing into a *plié* in fifth position (without restraightening) or closing up to a *relevé* (or *sous-sus*) fifth could be alternative methods for the closing. The *plié* closing could create the necessary space for the leg, while working on the dancer's sense of grounding and stability. Knee-foot alignment would still need to be attended to as in any *plié* movement. The *relevé* (or *sous-sus*) closing, in which the dancer rises onto the demi-pointe (ball of the foot/metatarsal heads), would also create space for the leg, while effectively working the crossing action of the leg and tight fifth closing in preparation for movements such as a *soutenu* turn. An additional option would be to have the dancer modify their outward rotation to reduce the bending and rotation at the knee, but this would require an adjustment to traditional aesthetic expectations of the position (Fig. 10.7).

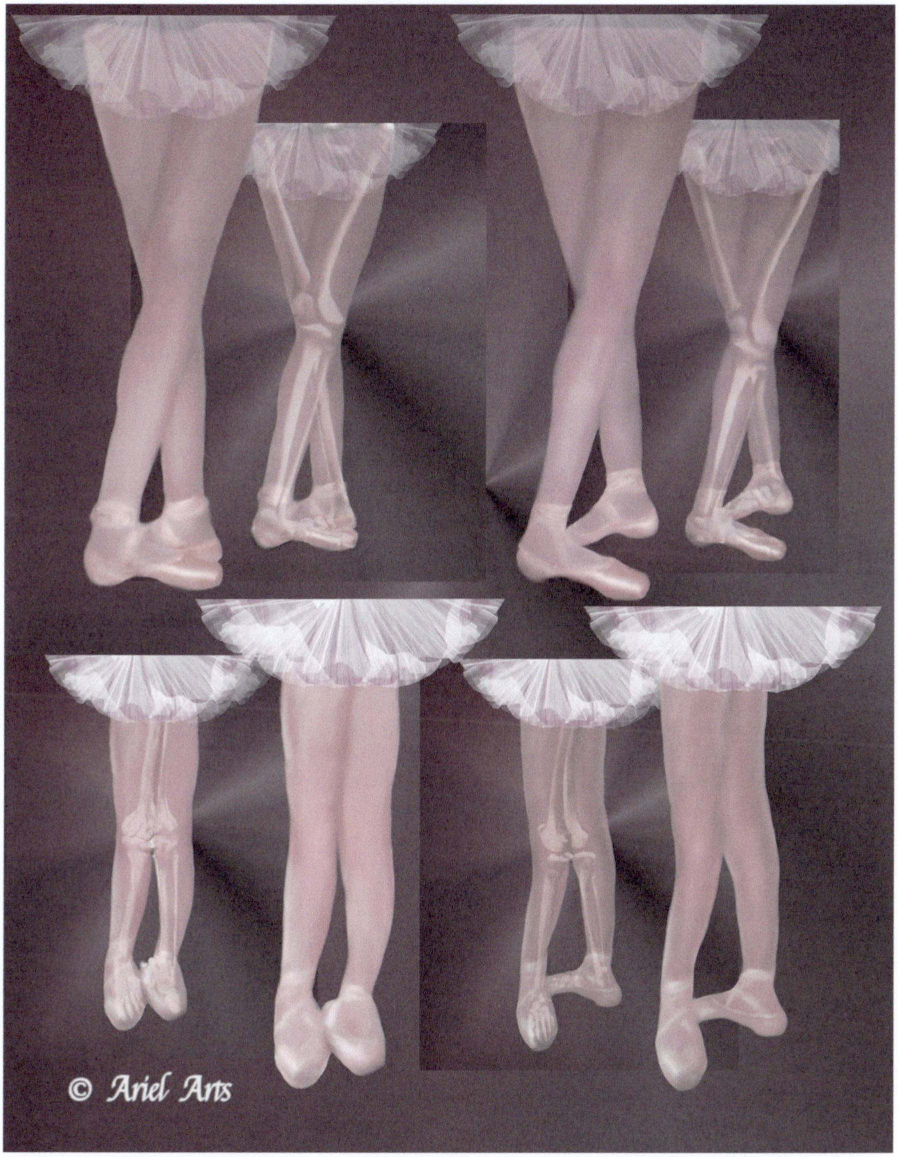

Fig. 10.7 Images of fifth position: 180-degree and modified turnout, front and side views (Author has received full permissions to use original artwork by Ariel Arts© for this manuscript)

Acknowledgments The authors gratefully acknowledge the dance participants who served as research participants for this study and Nyssa Masters' contribution. Special appreciation is expressed to Ariel Arts for providing original artwork for this publication.

References

1. Wilmerding V, Krasnow D. Turnout for dancers: hip anatomy and factors affecting turnout International Association for Dance Medicine and Science 2011:1–7. https://www.iadms.org/page/323. Accessed 20 Dec 2018.
2. Watkins A, Woodhull-McNeal AP, Clarkson P, Ebbeling C. Lower extremity alignment and injury in young, preprofessional, college, and professional ballet dancers. Med Probl Perform Art. 1989;4:148–53.
3. Negus V, Hopper D, Briffa NK. Associations between turnout and lower extremity injuries in classical ballet dancers. J Orthop Sports Phys Ther. 2005;35(5):307–18.
4. Deighan MA. Flexibility in dance. J Dance Med Sci. 2005;9(1):13–7.
5. Carter SL, Duncan R, Weidemann AL, Hopper LS. Lower leg and foot contributions to turnout in female pre-professional dancers: a 3D kinematic analysis. J Sports Sci. 2018;3:1–9.
6. Quanbeck AE, Russell JA, Handley SC, Quanbeck DS. Kinematic analysis of hip and knee rotation and other contributors to ballet turnout. J Sports Sci. 2017;35(4):331–8.
7. Grossman G. Measuring dancer's active and passive turnout. J Dance Med Sci. 2003;7(2):49–55.
8. Motta-Valencia K. Dance-related injury. Phys Med Rehabil Clin N Am. 2006;17(3):697–723.
9. van Merkensteijn GG, Quin E. Assessment of compensated turnout characteristics and their relationship to injuries in university level modern dancers. J Dance Med Sci. 2015;19(2):57–62.
10. Clippinger KS. Dance anatomy and kinesiology. Champaign: Human Kinetics; 2007.
11. Scioscia TN, Giffin JR, Fu FH. Knee ligament and meniscal injuries in dancers. J Dance Med Sci. 2001;5(1):11–5.
12. Grossman G, Krasnow D, Welsh TM. Effective use of turnout: biomechanical, neuromuscular, and behavioral considerations. J Dance Educ. 2005;5(1):15–27.
13. Solomon R, Minton S, Solomon J, editors. Preventing dance injuries. 2nd ed. Champaign: Human Kinetics; 2005.
14. Faria F, Atalaia T, Carles ML, Coutinho I. Knee angular displacement analysis in amateur ballet dancers: a pilot study. Eur J Phys. 2013;15(4):215–20.
15. Fitt SS. Dance kinesiology. 2nd ed. New York: Schirmer Books; 1996.
16. Welsh TM, Rodriguez M, Beare LW, Barton B, Judge T. Assessing turnout in university dancers. J Dance Med Sci. 2008;12(4):136–41.
17. Pata D, Welsh T, Bailey J, Range V. Improving turnout in university dancers. J Dance Med Sci. 2014;18(4):169–77.
18. Champion LM, Chatfield SJ. Measurement of turnout in dance research–a critical review. J Dance Med Sci. 2008;12(4):121–35.
19. Liederbach M, Hagins M, Gamboa JM, Welsh TM. Assessing and reporting dancer capacities, risk factors, and injuries: recommendations from the IADMS standard measures consensus initiative. J Dance Med Sci. 2012;16(4):139–53.
20. Coplan JA. Ballet dancer's turnout and its relationship to self-reported injury. J Orthop Sports Phys Ther. 2002;32(11):579–84.
21. Gamboa J, Roberts L, Maring J, Fergus A. Injury patterns in elite preprofessional ballet dancers and the utility of screening programs to identify risk characteristics. J Orthop Sports Phys Ther. 2008;38(3):126–36.
22. Ekegren CL, Quested R, Brodrick A. Injuries in pre-professional ballet dancers: incidence, characteristics and consequences. J Sci Med Sport. 2014;17(3):271–5.
23. Arendt YD, Kerschbaumer F. Injury and overuse pattern in professional ballet dancers. Z Orthop Ihre Grenzgeb. 2003;141(3):349–56.
24. Hincapie CA, Morton EJ, Cassidy JD. Musculoskeletal injuries and pain in dancers: a systematic review. Arch Phys Med Rehabil. 2008;89(9):1819–29.
25. Sobrino FJ, de la Cuadra C, Guillén P. Overuse injuries in professional ballet: injury-based differences among ballet disciplines. Orthop J Sports Med. 2015;3(6). https://doi.org/10.1177/2325967115590114.

26. Steinberg N, Siev-Ner I, Peleg S, et al. Injury patterns in young, non-professional dancers. J Sports Sci. 2011;29(1):47–54.
27. Stretanski MF, Weber GJ. Medical and rehabilitation issues in classical ballet. Am J Phys Med Rehabil. 2002;81(5):383–91.
28. Jenkinson DM, Bolin DJ. Knee overuse injuries in dance. J Dance Med Sci. 2001;5(1):16–20.
29. Winslow J, Yoder E. Patellofemoral pain in female ballet dancers: correlation with iliotibial band tightness and tibial external rotation. J Orthop Sports Phys Ther. 1995;22(1):18–21.
30. Barnes M, Krasnow D, Tupling S, Thomas M. Knee rotation in classical dancers during the grand plié. Med Probl Perform Art. 2000;15(4):140–7.
31. Cozby PC. Methods in behavioral research. New York: McGraw-Hill; 2007.
32. Wilmerding V, Krasnow D. Dance pedagogy: myth versus reality. Proc Int Symp Perform Sci. 2011;201(1):283–9.
33. Morris ML. Re-thinking ballet pedagogy: approaching a historiography of fifth position. Res Dance Edu. 2015;16(3):245.

Chapter 11
A Case Report: Using Multimodalities to Examine a Professional Pianist with Focal Dystonia

Sang-Hie Lee, Juan Sanchez-Ramos, Ryan Murtagh, Tuan Vu, Dustin Hardwick, and Stephanie L. Carey

Introduction

Dystonia is a neurological condition in which muscles contract or extend involuntarily, causing repetitive, twisting movements and abnormal posturing. The condition can affect one part of the body (focal dystonia), two or more adjacent parts (segmental dystonia), or multiple segments of the body (general dystonia). The muscle contraction can be mild to severe and can interfere with performance of daily tasks. Task-specific dystonia is a subtype of focal dystonia that is triggered by specific repetitive or over-practiced motor activity. Writer's cramp and musician's dystonia are two of the most common forms of task-specific focal dystonia, though

Electronic Supplementary Material The online version of this chapter https://doi.org/10.1007/978-3-030-37480-8_11 contains supplementary material, which is available to authorized users.

S.-H. Lee (✉)
School of Music, College of the Arts, University of South Florida, Tampa, FL, USA
e-mail: slee@usf.edu

J. Sanchez-Ramos · R. Murtagh · T. Vu
Department of Neurology, Morsani College of Medicine, University of South Florida, Tampa, FL, USA
e-mail: jsramos@usf.edu; rmurtagh@usf.edu; tvu6@usf.edu

D. Hardwick
School of Physical Therapy & Rehabilitation Sciences, Morsani College of Medicine, University of South Florida, Tampa, FL, USA
e-mail: dustinhardwick@usf.edu

S. L. Carey
Department of Mechanical Engineering, Center for Assistive, Rehabilitation & Robotics Technologies (CARRT), University of South Florida, Tampa, FL, USA
e-mail: scarey3@usf.edu

S.-H. Lee et al. (eds.), *Perspectives in Performing Arts Medicine Practice*,
https://doi.org/10.1007/978-3-030-37480-8_11

it can occur in any movement with extensive practice. It is estimated that 1–2% of all professional musicians will develop focal dystonia at some point in their career, which is often career ending [1].

Functionally, dystonic posturing in focal dystonia is thought to occur due to impaired balance of inhibition and excitation [2]. Electromyographic studies have demonstrated coactivation of antagonist muscles, prolonged agonist activation, and abnormal firing of proximal musculature during skilled tasks [3–5] all of which suggest impaired inhibition. Studies using transcranial magnetic stimulation (TMS) have confirmed the presence of impaired cortical and surround inhibition [6, 7], while other studies have demonstrated impaired cortical gamma-aminobutyric acidergic (GABA) neurotransmitter system, and important inhibitory neurotransmitter levels [8, 9]. These disruptions in inhibition and excitation are thought to occur primarily due to changes in the neural structures of the basal ganglia, which are responsible for controlling inhibition and excitation during planned movement [10, 11]. Structural changes in the sensorimotor cortex and cerebellum are also involved, either directly or through their projections to the basal ganglia [12]. These structural and functional changes are known to be a result of maladaptive neuroplasticity to prolonged, intense, repetitive movement [13–15]. While we have learned a great deal in the last decade about the contributing factors and neuropathology of focal dystonia, we have yet to develop a universally effective treatment.

In a longitudinal study of skilled pianists' hand biomechanics, we encountered *three* pianists who demonstrated focal dystonic symptoms (10% of $n = 31$). We examined the anomalous behavior of one pianist using multimodality and explored restoration of the impaired piano playing. The purpose of this case analysis was to learn about the etiology of pianist's focal dystonia and gain insights into a holistic rehabilitation strategy including development of a vibrotactile motor-integration device.

Patient Information

The subject is a 53-year-old male professional pianist, a successful college music professor and administrator, who developed focal dystonia in the left hand. He had led a tightly organized life to meet the demands of a multiple-career role as a performer, teacher, and administrator with family responsibilities for many years. The first sign of dystonic symptoms appeared while he was working on a computer keyboard for many uninterrupted hours. The initial examinations occurred during 2011 and the retraining program was conducted in fall of 2016.

Our pianist had had serious pain and injury during his college years (some 30 years ago), caused by over practicing difficult octave and heavy consecutive chord passages with tightened muscles and without periodic rests. The pianist had sought chiropractic treatment, acupuncture, deep muscle-tissue massage therapy, and neurology induction velocity test, of which, deep muscle massage was the most helpful in relieving pain and allowing him to resume playing [16].

The onset of dystonic symptoms took place in 2008 when he was working on a computer keyboard for many uninterrupted hours preparing an institutional self-

Table 11.1 Timeline

1984–1985	Background	Right-hand injury playing Chopin's Octave Etude for 11 hours the day before college music school final examination. Sought chiropractic, acupuncture, deep-tissue massage therapy, and neurology induction velocity tests
1987		Reinjured the same hand playing Bartok's Sonata with heavy chords
2005		Coauthored a published article, "Pianists' rehabilitation: Three cases" in collaboration with the current researcher [15]
2008	Onset of focal dystonia	Left third digit involuntary extension. Uneven touch control
2011	First visits and examinations	Interview with the researcher: Discuss lifestyle, time commitment, and workload. Mindfulness meditation sessions. Examination by a hand surgeon. Hand measurement. MIDI recording of 16 musical examples
2016 (September–November)	Intervention and retraining	Use C3 vibrotactile feedback. Retraining with *slow-finger-walk technique*

study document. When he became a part of our piano study in 2011, we examined the subject's lifestyle factors such as career roles, work load, work schedule, practice habit, family responsibilities, and recreational activity. As a division chair and faculty at a community college, he also taught several other music courses beside piano. Having a reputation as one of the premier piano teachers in the city, he taught many students at his home studio, extending his work hours to evening. Thus, for decades, the subject led a tightly organized life from early morning to evening. Maintaining an active performing life meant that he practiced in between duties, grabbing moments, likely in a psychologically and physiologically heightened state with little respite or escape in between (Table 11.1).

Physical Examination

Our hand surgeon's examination revealed that the subject's hand was exceptionally large, with the span reaching an octave and a half (10.5″, as compared to the normal octave 7.5″) and all hand and finger joints were hypermobile. Hypermobility in the musician's hand has both positive and negative effects: it allows flexibility and range while at the same time weakens joint strengths and stability (Fig. 11.1).

We measured the pianist's hand length, hand width, and composite measurements of finger length and finger span between each two of all five digits of the hand. Adopting Wagner's hand studies [17], we added active ulnar deviation and the ratio of hand and arm weights. Hand and arm weights were measured after complete deadweight relaxation training at wrist and elbow joints. Multiple measurements were done to ensure reliability. In measuring hand biometrics, we excluded radial deviation at the wrist and handgrip strengths which are not germane in skilled piano technique [18]. The pianist's hand measurement affirmed the hand surgeon's exami-

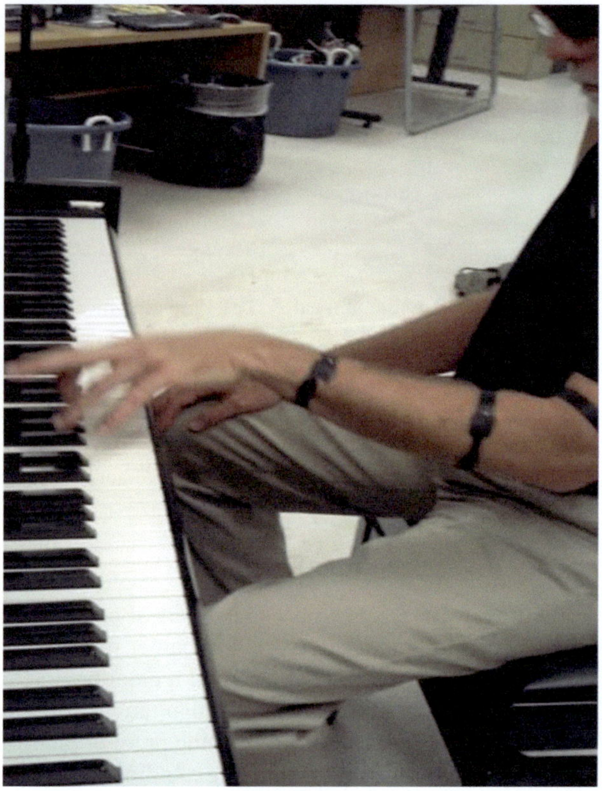

Fig. 11.1 Pianist with focal dystonia in the left third digit

nation, showing larger than the average male hand with wide span and wrist agility, indicative of favorable hand attributes for skilled piano performance [17, 18].

Diagnostic Assessment

Musical Instrument Digital Interface (MIDI)

The pianist played 16 prototype skilled piano technical exercises on a hybrid MIDI piano (Exercises #11 & 12 irrelevant-skipped). Yamaha AvantGrand, N3 version, is a state-of-the-art instrument that combines the traditional key hammer action and electronic Musical Instrument Digital Interface (MIDI), a digitized computer language that describes musical note names, key press and release times, and the speed of key press (key velocity). The MIDI data helps to obtain an electronic signature of the piano performance [19]. Each exercise was played several times to collect enough playing information. Key velocity evenness was measured by standard deviation (SD) calculated from the quantitative MIDI units (0–127). Temporal evenness was measured by SD of note duration in milliseconds. MIDI data showed uneven touch control in key velocity (sound volume) and key duration (tone articulation). Overall, evenness control in the left hand was more problematic than the right hand. We also saw the non-dystonic right hand showing lack of evenness control in playing polyphonic exercises (pressing down more than one key at the exact same time in exercises #7, 8, 13, and 14 – velocity – and #7 and 8, duration). We attribute this lack of evenness control in the right hand possibly to the past injury [16] (Figs. 11.2 and 11.3).

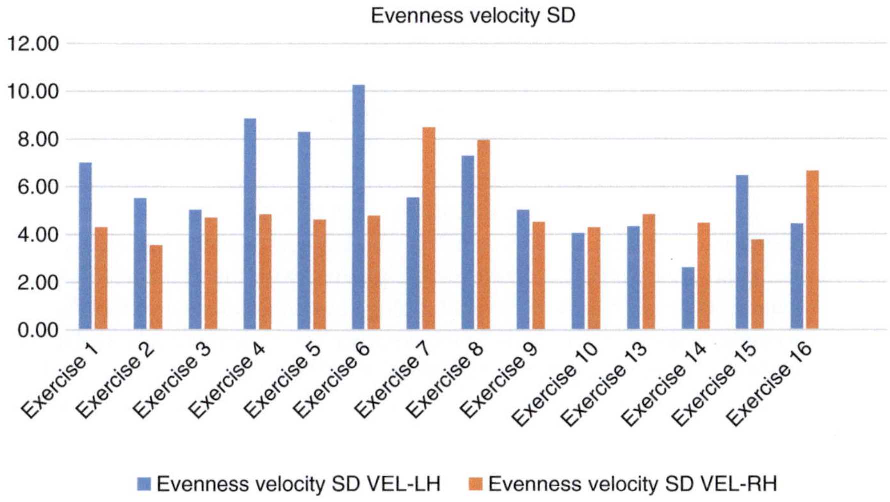

Fig. 11.2 MIDI key velocity evenness (both hands)

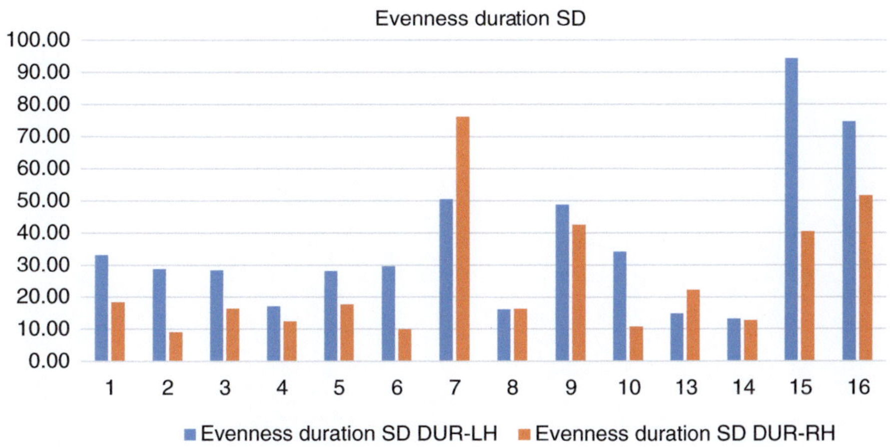

Fig. 11.3 MIDI key duration evenness (both hands)

Functional Magnetic Resonance Imagining (fMRI)

MRI was performed using GE HDXT 3.0T MRI (Milwaukee, WI). The patient was placed in the scanner and provided with an MRI-compatible keyboard. fMRI was performed using blood oxygen level–dependent (BOLD) technique with imaging acquired during alternating periods of rest and movement (simulated playing of the keyboard). After acquisition, images were transferred to the Invivo Dynasuite® (Gainesville, FL) workstation for post-processing. The subject played three sets: first, simple tapping on a flat board on his chest with the afflicted left hand; second, a five-finger scale with the left hand; and third a five-finger scale with the right hand. In all three playing sets, the subject felt as if he was really playing the keys. During the first and second playing with the afflicted left hand, the subject's middle finger involuntarily flew away from the normal flexed position. We tested the right hand playing the scale to discern the difference in the brain image.

fMRI images showed greatly enhanced activity in contralateral (right) primary sensorimotor cortex, supplementary motor area, and parietal-occipital regions during simulated playing with the left hand. Ipsilateral sensorimotor area (left) and parietal-occipital area were also active, while playing with the affected left hand, but less than the contralateral side. Finger tapping showed less sensory motor activities. Conversely, simulated playing with the non-dystonic right hand revealed markedly diminished activation of the contralateral (left) sensorimotor cortex and no activation of the ipsilateral (right) sensorimotor and parietal-occipital cortices (Figs. 11.4, 11.5, and 11.6).

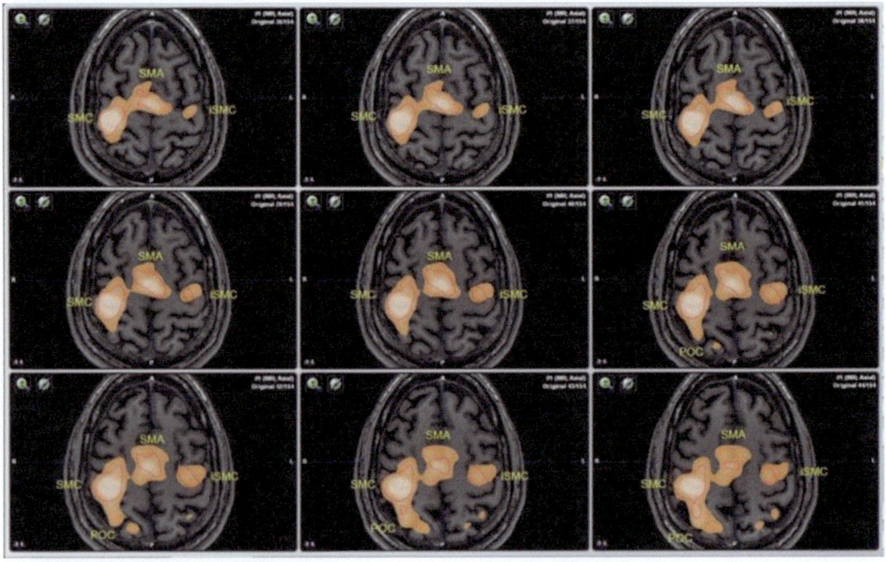

Fig. 11.4 fMRI affected hand (L) playing

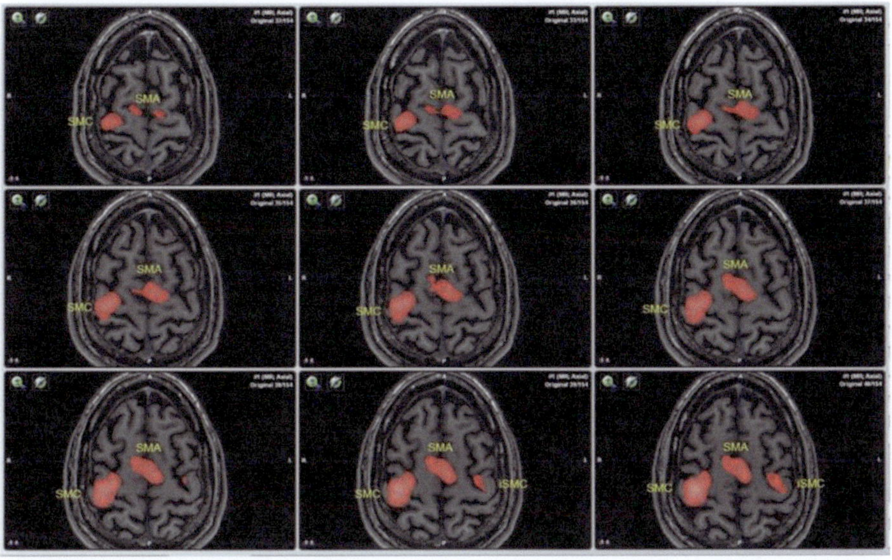

Fig. 11.5 fMRI affected hand (L) tapping

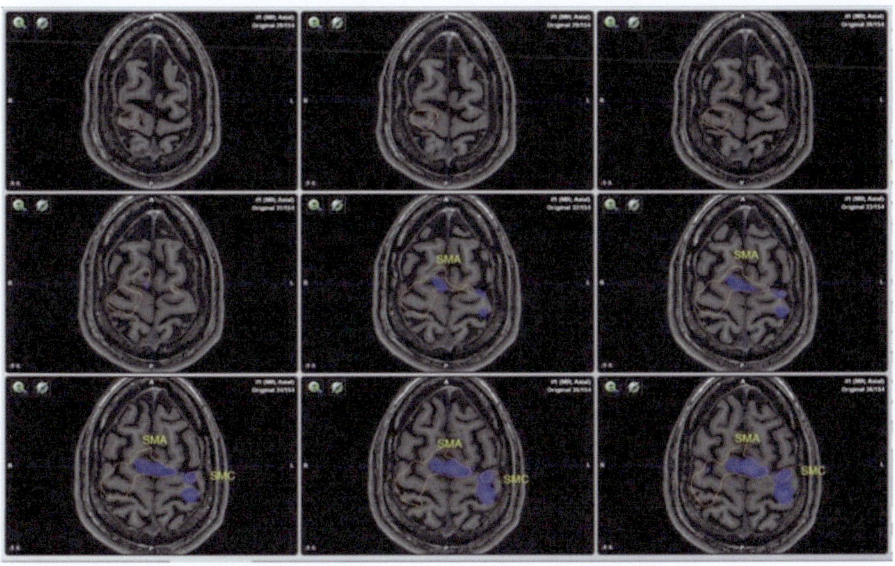

Fig. 11.6 fMRI unaffected hand (R) playing

Electromyographic Analysis

Since the subject has dystonic extension of the left middle finger when playing the piano, the muscle responsible for this dystonia is presumably the left EDC. For this study, a 37 mm concentric needle was inserted into the EDC and secured in place. The signals were analyzed using an EMG machine (Nicolet/Viasys), with filter settings of 20–10 kHz, time base of 100 ms/div, and gain of 100 μV/div.

No EMG signal was detected at rest when no dystonia was seen. Low amplitude EMG signals, indicative of muscle activity, was seen when the subject's left hand was extending forward even though no dystonia was observed (these signals were presumably from activities of distant muscles involved in supporting the posture). Oscillating EMG signals were seen when the subject moved his left fingers in simulated playing the piano. After he ceased playing, distinct and periodic signals were detected when the subject was exhibiting dystonic posturing of the middle finger. For comparison, EMG of the left EIP, not clinically observed to be affected in the subject's dystonia, showed no specific EMG signals (Figs. 11.7 and 11.8).

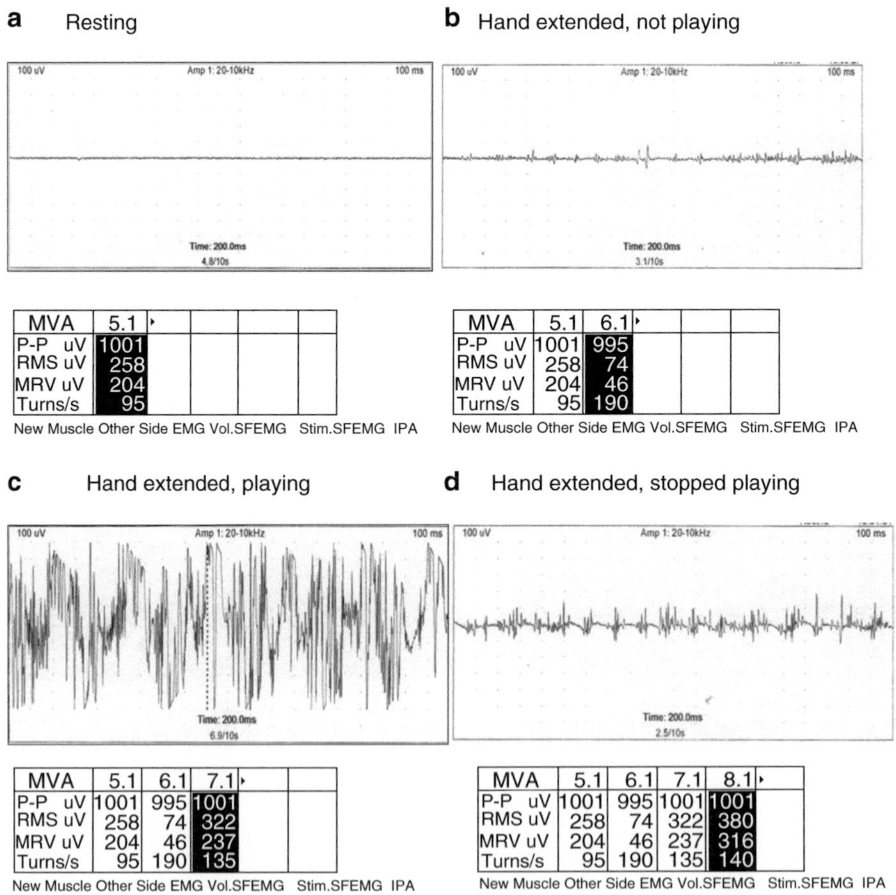

Fig. 11.7 nEMG EDC (L fingers 3–5) affected finger muscle

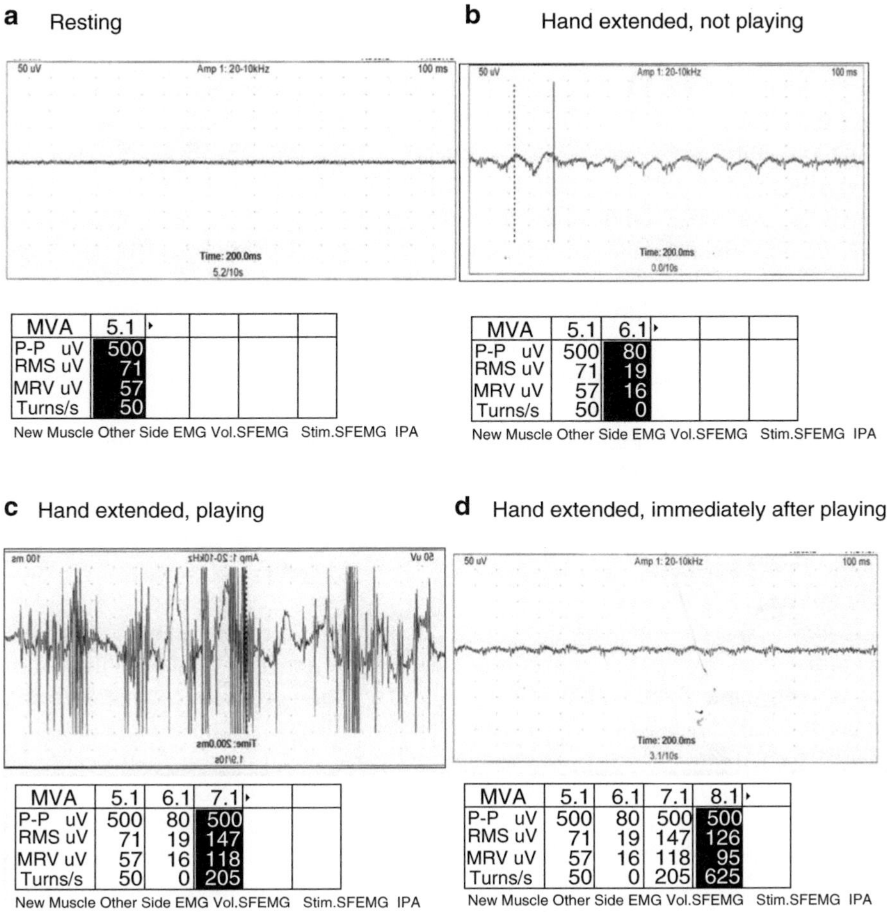

Fig. 11.8 nEMG EIP (L index finger) unaffected finger muscle

Intervention

Vibrotactile Feedback

Vibrotactile feedback has been applied to interfere with the abnormal integration within the basal ganglia in a posturing of co-contraction of the agonist and antagonist muscles and ameliorate the dystonic posturing allowing for motor relearning with proper sensory integration [20]. We placed C3 vibrotactile sensors (Engineering Acoustics Inc.), approximately 1 inch in diameter, over the muscle bellies of the flexor digitorum profundus and superficialis and extensor digitorum muscles associated with the dystonic posture during piano performance. The vibration was tuned in amplitude and frequency using the supplied software until a perceptible buzz was felt by the participant and was activated during the performance on the piano.

Retraining

Four 1-hour retraining sessions were conducted biweekly between September and November of 2016 under the pianist–researcher–pedagogue's guidance. Using C3 vibrotactile sensors, we applied the slow-finger-walk pedagogy (one finger lifting at the MC joint and transferring the finger weight to the consecutive finger with the minimum tension as in easy-pace walk). This encourages awareness of the most efficient motion with a firm MCP–PIP arch and tension-free finger–hand–forearm coordination [18]. *Slow-finger-walk technique* is a method adopted from the traditional finger technique school that emphasizes moving each finger up and down to press the key with the minimum tension and efficient motion. Sound volume is controlled by applying the necessary key speed without excessive force, using gravity as in a steady walk with no stomping or attacking. The subject was assigned to practice the 16 prototype exercises 20 minutes daily with the frame of mindfulness meditation previously introduced in 2011. The video shows the initial playing recorded in March 2011 followed by four progressive retraining sessions conducted in September–October 2016. https://drive.google.com/file/d/0B8G4WyMEWdOFcWQ5WkhvU29jVjQ/view?ts=57e89cb2 (Video 11.1)

Figure 11.9 shows changes in the key velocity and duration evenness control at the initial meeting (2011) and during intervention sessions (2016). Vibrotactor seems to have interfered with both velocity and duration evenness control, showing higher standard deviation "with stimulator (vibrotactor)" than "no stimulator" in all measurements. Key velocity evenness showed improvement showing with decreased SD (3-1-2011, 9-9-2016, and 9-16-2016), with slightly higher SD on September 23 and again lower SD in the last session on October 14. Neither duration (showing even articulation of tones) nor timing evenness (note down to note down, denoting playing time) showed a pattern of improvement throughout the retraining period. Accordingly playing tempo remained the same as shown in the video.

Modifying Lifestyle

We suggested modifying lifestyle and allotting some downtime and recreational time to allow caring for self.

Follow-Up Outcomes

After the fall of 2016, the pianist reported continuing to practice *slow-finger-walk technique* but found it difficult to adhere to this technique while working on regular repertoire, chamber, and church music when his old technical habits dominate playing. However, he finds this new technique useful and effective in teaching (Table 11.2).

Scale (Exercise 5)	Velocity (MIDI unit 127) SD	Duration (ms) SD	Timing (ms) SD
3-1-2011 no stim	8.30	28.21	28.04
9-9-16 no stim	8.51	30.37	24.07
9-9-16 w stim	6.73	39.29	24.95
9-16-16 no stim	5.21	38.32	37.68
9-16-16 w stim	4.32	49.97	42.21
9-23-16 no stim	8.01	29.14	22.95
9-23-16 w stim	7.78	32.05	31.57
10-14-16 no stim	6.62	28.37	23.88
10-14-16 w stim	5.14	36.80	39.57

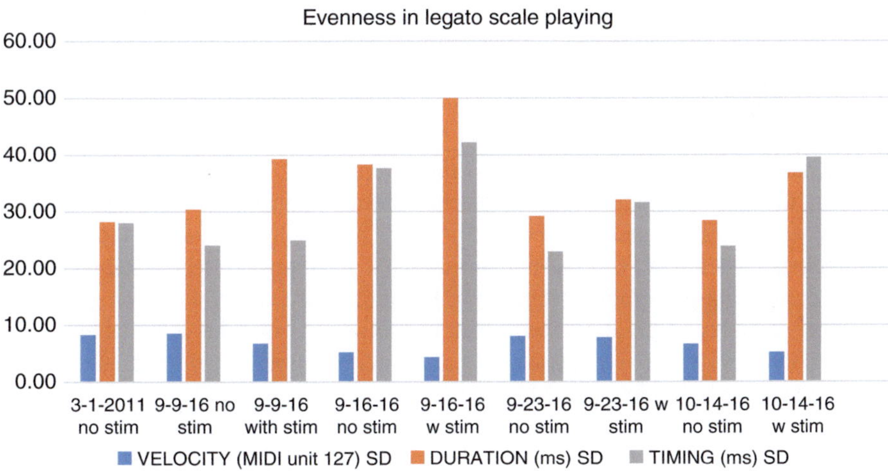

Fig. 11.9 Evenness changes

Table 11.2 Pianist's lifestyle and retraining

Life before modification	*Life after modification*
Tight schedule	Meditation
Multiple roles:	Increased recreation
Teacher	Motorcycle riding
Administrator	Reading for fun not just work
Performer	Weight loss
Accompanist	Lightened administrative duties
Father	More time with friends
Husband	Positive personal outlook on life at 50
Neglect care for self	Family vacation to Russia
	Actively involved in teenage son's music and daughter's dance performances
Playing before retraining	*Playing after retraining*
Involuntary middle finger flying	More even touch control each session
Uneven touch and tone control	Using *finger-walk technique* in teaching
	Continue to play the old way

Discussion

This case report described intensive multimodal examination and individualized intervention. MIDI data showed some evidence of progress in evenness key depression (sound volume) but not in hold-note duration (articulation) or timing (tempo). The audio and video recordings showed clear progress up to the third session and somewhat declining or plateauing thereafter. The fourth session recorded no improvement over the third, when the pianist came in somewhat disarrayed and confessed not having practiced.

The underlying maladapted neurophysiology in focal dystonia presents a major challenge to developing long-lasting treatments. The most common forms of treatment include sensorimotor retraining, botulinum toxin, trihexyphenidyl, ergonomic changes, physical therapy, and pedagogical retraining. Literature reveals that treatments show improvements in symptoms in only 50% of cases [21–25]. Furthermore, treatment effects are not durable in long-term follow-up, and as result, many treatments are abandoned because improvements in symptoms are insufficient to lead to meaningful performance improvements [23, 24, 26]. Without changing the underlying physiology, the symptoms will re-emerge once treatment is stopped. Long-lasting treatment effects will only occur when motor retraining is combined with treatments that change the underlying neurophysiology.

Even though the *finger-walk-meditation* strategy rehabilitation program was effective to a certain degree, staying in this mode of playing outside the lab sessions is unrealistic. Therefore, we continue our search to develop an effective biofeedback device paralleling pedagogical retraining. From this case study, we can hope that a complete recovery of pianist's focal dystonic symptoms may be achievable with a biofeedback device applied consistently along with deliberate and exclusive practice of retraining technique (Fig. 11.10).

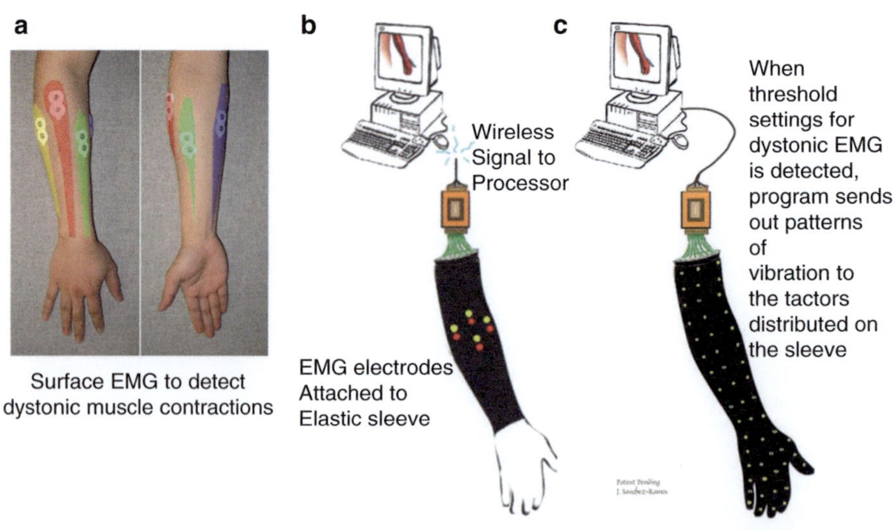

Fig. 11.10 Computerized peripheral sensorimotor integrator

An implication of this case study is to acknowledge that the *gradual* development of all-inclusive piano technique, that is, finger technique, arm and its weight, coordinated upper body movement, whole body engagement, and the mind–body integration, is imperative to sustain healthy playing at all ages. Importantly for our case, during the 6-year span, our subject modified his lifestyle by cutting down administrative work, enjoying non-work-related reading, riding motor cycle, losing weight, in general accepting the decline of his piano playing capabilities, and continuing to enjoy occasional ensemble performance and keeping his regular church music playing.

There are many limitations of the study. While we have examined several physical aspects of this pianist, we did not include psychological examination that might have shed lights to the lifestyle examination. As one reviewer observed, for a lifetime career pianist, losing the dexterity of a part of one hand would have caused depression and other psychological issues. The lifestyle of this pianist is not unusual for career musicians; their financial and social life depends on managing hectic and multiple roles as a musician/teacher/family person. This study provides us with a glimpse into the nature of a musical career as well as the perseverance of the musician's fortitude to sustain and manage a reasonable and artistically satisfying life.

Informed Consent Below is his communication granting permission of the use of video rehab sessions.

Monday, March 26, 2018 at 8:11 AM

Hi Sang-Hie,

Thanks for the message… Of course I have no issue with the use of any video in which I appeared, and don't mind if anybody recognizes my voice, etc. I don't keep the reason for my inability to play anymore a secret…

My best always,

Acknowledgments We appreciate USF Neuroscience Collaborative Seed Grant (2010–2012) and USF Office of Research and Innovation Early Career Researcher Grant (2015) that enabled this study and 30 other pianists' hand studies.

We appreciate our subject pianist's cooperation in this experiment.

We are thankful to Dr. Robert Belsole for his careful examination of our pianist' hand.

We thank Jeff Chodil for his assistance with data management.

Additional Information Financial disclosure/conflict of interest concerning the research related to the manuscript: There is no conflict of interest.

References

1. Altenmüller E. Focal dystonia: advances in brain imaging and understanding of fine motor in musicians. Hand Clin. 2003;19(3):523–38, xi.
2. Lin PT, Hallett M. The pathophysiology of focal hand dystonia. J Hand Ther. 2009;22(2):109–13.
3. Cohen LG, Hallett M. Hand cramps: clinical features and electromyographic patterns in a focal dystonia. Neurology. 1988;38(7):1005–12.
4. Hughes M, Mclellan DL. Increased co-activation of the upper limb muscles in writer's cramp. J Neurol Neurosurg Psychiatry. 1985;48(8):782–7.

5. Farmer SF, Sheean GL, Mayston MJ, et al. Abnormal motor unit synchronization of antagonist muscles underlies pathological co-contraction in upper limb dystonia. Brain. 1998;121(Pt 5):801–14.
6. Chen R, Wassermann EM, Caños M, Hallett M. Impaired inhibition in writer's cramp during voluntary muscle activation. Neurology. 1997;49(4):1054–9.
7. Beck S, Richardson SP, Shamim EA, Dang N, Schubert M, Hallett M. Short intracortical and surround inhibition are selectively reduced during movement initiation in focal hand dystonia. J Neurosci. 2008;28(41):10363–9.
8. Levy LM, Hallett M. Impaired brain GABA in focal dystonia. Ann Neurol. 2002;51(1):93–101.
9. Marjańska M, Lehéricy S, Valabrègue R, et al. Brain dynamic neurochemical changes in dystonic patients: a magnetic resonance spectroscopy study. Mov Disord. 2013;28(2):201–9.
10. Peller M, Zeuner KE, Munchau A, et al. The basal ganglia are hyperactive during the discrimination of tactile stimuli in writer's cramp. Brain. 2006;129(Pt 10):2697–708.
11. Zeuner KE, Knutzen A, Granert O, et al. Increased volume and impaired function: the role of the basal ganglia in writer's cramp. Brain Behav. 2014;5:e00301.
12. Delmaire C, Vidailhet M, Elbaz A, et al. Structural abnormalities in the cerebellum and sensorimotor circuit in writer's cramp. Neurology. 2007;69(4):376–80.
13. Quartarone A, Bagnato S, Rizzo V, et al. Abnormal associative plasticity of the human motor cortex in writer's cramp. Brain. 2003;126(Pt 12):2586–96.
14. Quartarone A, Rizzo V, Bagnato S, et al. Homeostatic-like plasticity of the primary motor hand area is impaired in focal hand dystonia. Brain. 2005;128(Pt 8):1943–50.
15. Weise D, Schramm A, Stefan K, et al. The two sides of associative plasticity in writer's cramp. Brain. 2006;129(Pt 10):2709–21.
16. Lee SH, Hanks K, Schwartz J. Pianist's rehabilitation: three cases. Med Probl Perform Art. 2005;20(2):35–9.
17. Wagner C. The pianist's hand: anthropometry and biomechanics. Ergonomics. 1988;31(1):97–131.
18. Lee SH. Pianists' hand ergonomics and touch control. Med Probl Perform Art. 1990;5(2):72–8.
19. Neninger CR, Sun Y, Lee SH, Chodil J. A complete motion and music capture system to study hand injuries among musicians. *ANS ERRSD* – 13th robotics & remote systems for hazardous environments. 11th emergency preparedness & response. Knoxville, TN, August 7–10, 2011 on CD–ROM[1], American Nuclear Society, LaGrange Park, IL.
20. Huang K, Starner T, Do E, Weinberg G, Kohlsdorf D, Ahlrichs C, Leibrandt R. Mobile music touch: mobile tactile stimulation for passive learning. CHI 2010; tactile interaction April 10–15, 2010, Atlanta, GA, USA.
21. Jabusch HC, Zschucke D, Schmidt A, Schuele S, Altenmüller E. Focal dystonia in musicians: treatment strategies and long-term outcome in 144 patients. Mov Disord. 2005;20(12):1623–6.
22. Zeuner KE, Bara-jimenez W, Noguchi PS, Goldstein SR, Dambrosia JM, Hallett M. Sensory training for patients with focal hand dystonia. Ann Neurol. 2002;51(5):593–8.
23. Zeuner KE, Shill HA, Sohn YH, et al. Motor training as treatment in focal hand dystonia. Mov Disord. 2005;20(3):335–41.
24. Schuele S, Jabusch HC, Lederman RJ, Altenmüller E. Botulinum toxin injections in the treatment of musician's dystonia. Neurology. 2005;64(2):341–3.
25. Van Vugt FT, Boullet L, Jabusch HC, Altenmüller E. Musician's dystonia in pianists: long-term evaluation of retraining and other therapies. Parkinsonism Relat Disord. 2014;20(1):8–12.
26. Sheean G. Restoring balance in focal limb dystonia with botulinum toxin. Disabil Rehabil. 2007;29(23):1778–88.

Chapter 12
Discrepancies in Pianists' Experiences in Playing Acoustic and Digital Pianos

Pablo Arencibia

Discrepancies in Pianists' Experiences in Playing Acoustic and Digital Pianos

Digital piano technology has evolved significantly over the last few decades. Nowadays, digital pianos are replacing acoustic pianos in many applications including practicing, teaching, amateur playing, and professional playing with the main reasons being cost, portability, and flexibility.

Digital pianos' weighted-action mechanisms have significantly improved over the last few decades to simulate acoustic pianos. The sound of most digital pianos is based on sampling technology by reproducing recorded sounds of acoustic pianos. Supported by these developments, manufacturers claim that the experience of playing their digital pianos is now very close to playing real acoustic pianos. However, it is a common perception among professional pianists that there are significant differences in the experience of playing the acoustic and digital pianos. Some people claim the sound is different, some think there are problems with the keyboard feel, some say they do not react naturally, and others refer to differences in the touch and tone. This article aims to provide an objective perspective on the virtues and drawbacks of digital pianos to illuminate some of the pianists' frustration when playing them.

This information may help the modern digital piano manufacturers to develop better replacements for acoustic pianos. Digital pianos may never be able to fulfill the demands of skilled pianists completely, and acoustic pianos are likely to remain preferred; however, with improved digital pianos, pianists may feel more comfortable and satisfied whenever they are in a position to use them. It is also beneficial to understand the impact of digital piano in music education because digital piano

P. Arencibia (✉)
University of South Florida, Tampa, FL, USA
e-mail: pablo6@mail.usf.edu

S.-H. Lee et al. (eds.), *Perspectives in Performing Arts Medicine Practice*,
https://doi.org/10.1007/978-3-030-37480-8_12

usage is increasingly common in the field. A better understanding of the differences between acoustic and digital pianos and how they are played by skilled pianists can help us to understand physical and aesthetic consequences in learning to play the piano using digital instruments.

There is limited scholarly literature on and about digital pianos. Therefore, the documentation issued by manufacturers is a key source to understand their features. Digital music instruments work largely using the Music Instrument Digital Interface (MIDI) standard [1], which includes the parameters used to define the characteristics of the notes being played when the keys are depressed and released and the depressing key velocity. It may include other parameters such as modulation, balance, pan, and portamento; however, they are generally considered not relevant in the acoustic piano sounds. In this chapter, some detailed analysis of different touch and tone mechanisms between digital and acoustic pianos is discussed to inform the overall knowledge in playing digital pianos. This knowledge may help pianists' approach to digital piano playing with less tension and efficient use of the body.

Sound and Haptic Feedback

Satisfaction of skilled pianists with their piano-playing experience on a digital piano may be related to all elements that they perceive from the instrument, including even the visual and olfactory aesthetic sense of the instrument. However, the two most important elements in the relationship of the musician with the piano are the *audio feedback* and the *haptic feedback* [2, 3]. *Audio feedback* is defined as the pianist perception of the sound produced by the piano in response to pianist inputs to the keys and pedals. *Haptic feedback* is the pianist experience of texture, movement, pressure, and any other feeling perceived by the haptic sense coming from the piano keys and pedals. (Extended piano techniques, e.g., *inside piano*, are not considered in this study because most digital pianos are not intended to be played in these ways.)

Pianists playing the piano are aiming to obtain a certain resulting sound using their playing technique and actions. It is not only a matter of the sound quality itself but how this sound is related to all the different subtle nuances in the pianist way of playing the piano [3]. Usually, pianists refer to the response of the piano as the capacity of the instrument to react properly with its sound to the different ways it is played.

The haptic feedback is the sensorial perception that occurs when the pianist makes contact with a piano key or depresses the different pedals, including a wide variety of elements such as the resistance that the keys offer to be depressed, the length of the keys' movement until they reach the key-bed, the deceleration of the keys when they reach the key-bed, the differences in resistance through the key travel, the texture of the keys' surface, and others [4]. Based on his/her previous playing experience and training, the performer uses both audio and haptic information to adjust the way of playing the instrument, consciously or unconsciously, to obtain the desired sound result.

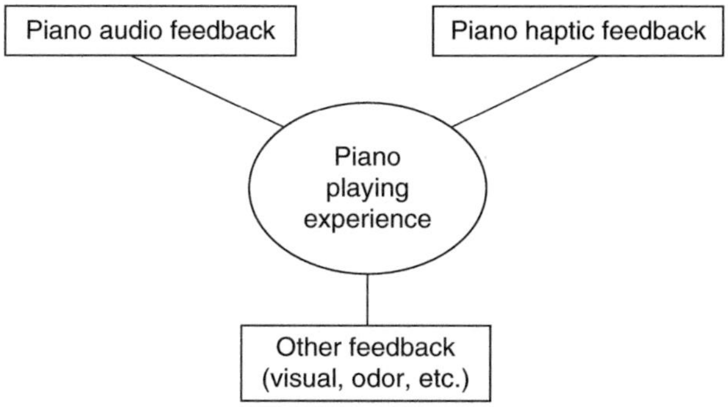

Fig. 12.1 Piano-playing experience breakdown. Elements constituting pianist experience

The importance of the haptic feedback perception was illustrated by Galembo [5] in his experiment in which a number of skilled pianists were blindfolded and asked to play three different acoustic pianos built by different manufacturers. All of them were able to recognize the different pianos, even when they had headphones on their ears playing white noise that did not allow them to hear the piano. However, when a blind listening experiment was conducted in a way they could only hear a few piano notes being played by other pianists, they were not able to properly distinguish one piano from another.

This high-level breakdown of the piano-playing experience from the pianist's feedback elements can be illustrated as in Fig. 12.1.

Piano Audio Feedback: The Sound Pianists Hear and How They Control It

The pianist's capacity to control the touch-sound in playing is considered to be one of the main elements of the art of piano interpretation [3]. These nuances constitute the personal *sound* of each pianist. Even when playing the same instrument, differences are perceived when different pianists play [6]. If the resulting sound of the piano is different with each pianist, it means that each pianist is playing the piano in a particular way that leads to these sound results. Therefore, skilled pianists playing a digital piano would expect it to respond in a consistent way to the subtle changes they are doing (consciously or unconsciously) in their playing. Touch is a word used to describe all these different aspects and nuances of body and hand posture, movement, speed, force, and pressure on piano keys and pedals that could have an impact in the resulting piano sound [3]. Not surprisingly, piano touch is one of the most discussed and controversial aspects of studying piano and creating the desired sound.

Bernays and Traube [7] conducted an experiment to identify objectively specific changes pianists make in their way of playing according to the timbre they try to produce. A number of adjectives were selected to name different subjective timbres (*dry*, *bright*, *round*, *velvety*, and *dark*). A computer-controlled piano was used, and several pianists were asked to play a few music pieces while aiming to obtain each of these timbres. The performances were recorded, and all the data captured by the piano computer system was extracted and analyzed. The output of this analysis was a list of playing parameters that the pianists had been altering whenever trying to obtain a specific timbre. The data were captured by the computer-controlled piano; therefore it is possible that there were additional parameters changed by pianists not captured by the computer system. This list provides at least a subset of parameters being modified by pianists as they look for different sound results. The parameters they found relevant to piano-playing changes are:

- Hammer velocity
- Key depression depth
- Attack duration (delay between initial key depression and hammer launch)
- Soft pedal depression
- Sustain pedal use
- Sustain pedal depression
- Release duration (time taken to complete key releasing)
- Right-hand chords overlap

In order to analyze how the piano may react to these and other changes in the pianist's subtle ways of playing and how these may differ in an acoustic piano compared to a digital piano, the large complexity of the elements involved in the piano playing and their influence over the audio feedback perceived by the pianist can be broken down into three areas: key action, pedal action, and unpredictability as shown in Fig. 12.2.

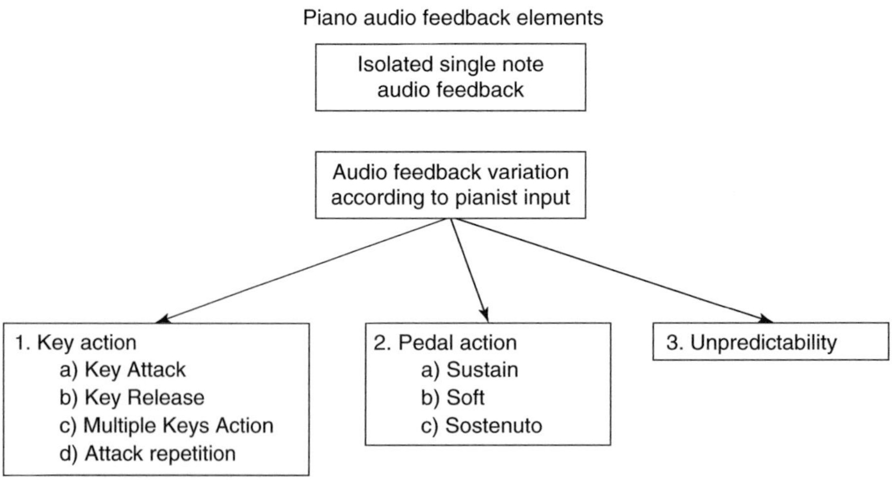

Fig. 12.2 Piano audio feedback elements. The audio perceived by pianists according to the way they are playing

Isolated *Single Note Audio Feedback*

Analyzing the sound of just one piano note without considering any other parameters is a very limited approach. However, this is an important starting point to understand the differences between an acoustic and a digital piano. Nowadays, the most widely used technology in digital pianos is sampling [8]. This technique consists of recording the sound of an acoustic piano and reproducing it (after certain processing) when the corresponding digital piano key is played. So, the obvious question is: Is there a relevant difference in the sound of a digital piano compared to an acoustic piano when a single note is played without taking into consideration other parameters? It might seem intuitive that if the sound is a recorded note of an acoustic piano, it should be almost indistinguishable due to the high fidelity of modern audio systems that can be enjoyed when listening to recorded music. However, the sound emitted by the piano through its soundboard (and the entire acoustic structure) is very complex. Each area of the soundboard emits different sounds as detailed by Ortmann [9]. Appropriately, some digital pianos aim to solve this complex acoustic property issue by incorporating multiple speakers to reproduce sampled sounds that are recorded from different microphone positions inside an acoustic piano [10].

Another consideration is that in order to save memory space and processing time, some digital pianos use short duration recordings of acoustic piano tones, capturing only the initial length of the sound. In this case, when a digital piano key is depressed for a longer time, the system uses a repeated sound sample (called loop) gradually reducing its intensity to extend the duration of the note, which may not match the acoustic piano tone quality.

Consequently, while the isolated digital piano key press produces high-quality sound close to the acoustic piano sound, the resultant tone quality may be degraded according to the quality of the audio system employed and the digital sample quality and length.

Key Action

The piano keys are the main interaction point between the pianist and the instrument. They offer a wide variety of possibilities to the pianist, not only in what notes and when they are played but also "how" they are played. As shown in Fig. 12.2, the actions and combinations over the piano keys can be broken down into key attack, key release, multiple key action, and attack repetition.

Key Attack: Hammer Velocity

The hammer velocity as a consequence of the key attack is one of the most important parameters to take into consideration. The hammer's speed when it hits the strings is probably the most influencing factor on the produced sound [9]. The hammer speed is determined by the way the key is played by the pianist. The hammer may hit the strings at any speed from 0 m/s up to 5 m/s or more [11]. This is a continuous range, so the number of different speeds at which the hammer can strike the strings is infinite.

The hammer speed determines the wave amplitude of the produced sound which defines the sound intensity, but it also determines the sound timbre. That is because at different speeds, the profile of the generated sound wave changes. Generally, at higher speeds, the higher partials (wave harmonics) increase their amplitude in relation to the resulting final wave, but this is something that changes for each piano and even for each note, so the possible variations are infinite again [9].

The pianist induces a hammer speed through the complex set of mechanical elements that are part of the piano action, converting the key movement into a resulting hammer movement. The way in which the force applied to the key translates into the hammer speed is also complex due to mechanical features such as the double escapement which can convert small finger movements into significant hammer displacements providing pianists with a wide range of control possibilities over this speed. The touch or the way in which the pianist depresses the key also influences the final hammer speed because it causes changes in the hammer acceleration during its traveling [11]. In fact, the level of control a pianist can have over the hammer speed is highly related to how the piano is regulated which depends on the piano design and manufacturing and also on the way it is serviced.

Hammer velocity in most digital pianos is enacted by the sensors to capture the key velocity which is mapped to a hammer speed or sound intensity [12]. Some digital pianos reproduce parts of the internal piano mechanism to have a more accurate reading of the speed at which a piano hammer would be hitting the string if it was impulsed by a real piano action [13]. A specific type of digital pianos called hybrid pianos have an acoustic-like piano mechanism with a hammer shank that moves as it would in an acoustic piano so that the speed reading can be as accurate as possible [10]. This speed is mapped into a recorded sound of a particular timbre that is reproduced with a variable intensity attempting to reproduce the resulting sound of an acoustic piano.

As previously mentioned, the sound produced by a modern digital piano is normally based on recorded samples from acoustic pianos. Clearly, digital piano manufacturers are finding it impossible to record all the infinite number of sounds that an acoustic piano produces in their infinite hammer-action velocities and the resultant variety of timbre combinations. So usually a few recordings are made at a certain discrete number of velocities that are considered to be “good enough” to capture the timbre variations of the piano [14]. These are called velocity layers.

The measured velocity at a digital piano is normally mapped to a 7-bit number as described in the MIDI specification [1] which means that the infinite speed range is represented by only 128 possible values. (Note: There are certain digital pianos that use a higher precision but it is still finite and limited.) This measured value is translated into one of the recorded sample sounds or a combination of them that is finally played through the digital piano speakers.

This is one of the most obvious areas to look into when analyzing digital piano's quality. The calculation of the piano hammer speed is based on the information the sensors capture from the digital piano key movement, and this is a complex mathematical challenge [11]. Van den Berghe, De Moor, and Minten further concluded that digital piano systems cannot accurately calculate the hammer velocity based on their readings [15]. Some modern digital pianos have up to three different sensors to improve this measurement [12], but it is unknown if this is enough to solve the mathematical challenge described by Askenfelt and Jansson [11]. This problem is partially resolved in hybrid pianos with an acoustic-like piano action to generate real movement from a physical hammer mechanism [10] instead of calculating it. But even in this case, once the hammer velocity is measured, it is a challenge to accurately map this speed into the right sound intensity and timbre combination. Furthermore, digital pianos use a limited number of sampling recordings (velocity layers) that may not be enough to emulate the nuances in touch that a professional pianist expects. Most digital piano manufacturers do not disclose the number of velocity layers they use in their products.

Key Attack: Timing

As alluded earlier, the piano action is made of a number of mechanical elements that transform the pianist touch into the hammer movement. As in any mechanical system, this transformation is not instantaneous. There are mechanical lag times involved, and also the hammer needs to travel a certain distance before it reaches the strings which also takes time. Depending on how the key is played by the pianist, the hammer hits the strings either before or after the moment when the piano key reaches the end of its movement in the key-bed [16]. In fact, the key might never reach the key-bed and the hammer may still hit the strings. The proper mapping of these time nuances (action timing) in digital pianos can affect the pianist perception of the instrument quality. This problem is solved in hybrid pianos for the reasons explained above, but it is a challenge to implement this feature in other regular digital pianos, and no evidence has been found that any manufacturers have taken it into account.

Key Attack: Additional Touch Considerations

As mentioned above, the overall sound of the piano varies from one pianist to another according to their way to play the instrument (their touch). For many years there has been controversy about how much the pianist can influence the timbre of a piano note by changing the way they attack the piano keys [17]. Nowadays, the majority of researchers and experts agrees that at the key attack time, the only sound production parameter that pianists can influence is the hammer velocity, and therefore any change in *timbre* would be associated with a change in intensity, both caused by the different *hammer velocities*. In other words, timbre changes cannot be produced independently of the intensity [6, 9, 18]. Nevertheless, Suzuki [19] found a slightly different result when completing an experiment on this subject. According to his results, in the high register notes of the piano, slight differences in tone could be produced using different touches without varying the intensity. However, he concludes that these differences are much less noticeable than what most pianists would expect.

This overarching evidence that control of tone depends solely on key velocity might seem to invalidate all the efforts from pianists through centuries who have been refining their technique to obtain the desired sound quality from the piano, differentiating from many different ways of playing in order to produce different results [20].

However, this is not true because this refined technique of playing affects many parameters in the piano mechanism and sound, including the hammer velocity, while closely associated to sound intensity, can have a very complex and rich impact on the produced timbre. Additionally, there are other audible elements that can change the *tone* of individual notes, that is, the additional noises produced by the piano mechanism and the pianist's body. Two distinguishable sounds have been identified: the finger key (FK) sound and the key bottom (KB) sound [21].

The finger key sound is the sound produced by the pianist finger and the key top when they get in touch. This sound can be heard only when the pianist finger reaches the key with a previous velocity and therefore knocking the key on its way down. If the pianist touches the keys very gently or if the fingers are in contact with the keys before pushing them, the FK sound is greatly reduced or completely eliminated. This is something the pianist can control (consciously or unconsciously) by using different touches or ways to attack the keys [21].

The key bottom sound is produced when the key reaches the end of its travel range and hits the key-bed of the piano. This sound can also be controlled by the pianist according to the technique being used, because depending on the force applied to the key during its travel range, it will reach the bottom at different speeds and under different pressures from the fingers. In fact, the piano can be played without the key even reaching the key-bed and therefore not producing this sound at all. This can be achieved by applying just the right amount of force in order to stimulate the hammer movement without pushing the key all the way to the bottom of its travel range [21].

Goebl, Bresin, and Fujinaga suggested that these sounds are perceptible and an educated audience can even identify how the keys were attacked and, therefore, what kind of touch was used regardless of the velocity of the hammer (intensity) [21]. This was observed only for extremely different touches (i.e., gently pressing the key vs. attacking the key with high initial speed in order to exacerbate FK and KB sounds); however, it may be possible that more subtle differences in touch are perceived in the sound. There is no evidence or documentation that any digital pianos have implemented any features to mimic these sounds. It is possible that the digital pianos with high-quality keys and key-beds generate similar sounds compared to acoustic pianos, but no documentation has been found in this regard. Furthermore, the original acoustic piano recordings that are used as part of the sampling technology do not have any distinction on the type of touch used, and therefore these noises may or may not be recorded as part of the sample and finally not corresponding with the expectation of the pianist playing the digital piano.

Key Release: Sound Dampening

When a piano key is released, a felt damper makes contact with the vibrating strings to stop the sound. It takes a certain amount of time (usually short) for the sound to completely stop, and, during this time, the sound timbre changes due to the friction of the damper felt into the keys [22]. The dampening sound varies according to the pitch of the note being dampened. Furthermore, lower notes in the piano use thicker strings that accumulate higher energy, while vibrating at a lower frequency, and therefore it takes a longer time for the damper to extinguish the sound than on higher pitch strings [23]. Not only does it take longer, but the dampening sound of these thicker strings is different because of their shape and material composition, as well as the difference in the damper shapes. In addition, by varying the speed at which the fingers release the keys, the pianist can alter the way the dampers touch the strings, modifying the time it takes to extinguish the sound and its timbre during the process [22].

The dampening length and sound together with the dampening time precision are very important for musical articulation. As seen by Repp [24], the overlap time between one note and the next one is a fundamental aspect of piano playing, and the subjective perception of different articulations varies according to a significant number of factors such as playing speed, pitch, etc. It is important that the pianist has fine control over the note dampening process in order to obtain the desired results in terms of articulation. On top of these considerations, the piano dampers could have additional influence over the sound. For example, the faint noise they make when they leave the strings right before the hammer hits them can be significant.

There is no evidence that any digital pianos incorporate functionality to map the speed of key release or other dampening effect elements. It is also not part of the MIDI standard [1]. Some digital pianos allow the player to choose different profiles of sound extinguishing (shorter or longer sound releases), but they are not related to the way the pianist releases the keys in real time [12]. This evidence suggests that the nuances in the sound dampening process are not mapped in digital pianos. Therefore, pianists may not perceive the same response in digital pianos compared to acoustic pianos in relationship to the sound extinguishing process which has a significant impact on their perception of musical articulation.

Multiple Key Action

Pianists seldom play one note at a time, but often notes are played together to form chords or polyphonic textures. All the above-described sound-producing elements come into play in complex sequences of notes being played and released. This situation combined with the pedal usage (addressed below) creates many interactions in the piano sound. Open strings that are not being stopped by dampers resonate by sympathy with compatible frequencies, and the piano's soundboard, bridge, and other elements resonate with a combination of notes instead of single ones. Due to the physical nature of these piano components, they react in many different ways to the vibration of the strings, sounding not as a sum of the individual sounds but producing new timbres based on the combination of multiple frequencies vibrating simultaneously [9]. Furthermore, all these vibrating elements of the piano can react not only to the string's sound but also to stimuli coming from outside the piano, amplifying and adding to sounds such as the natural sound reverberation of the room, sound from other musical instruments playing, etc.

Some modern digital pianos include string resonance features that aim to reproduce part of this sounding complexity by simulating the strings sympathetic vibrations [12]. Some of them also incorporate features to simulate the soundboard resonation [10]. However, no documentation has been found about the effectiveness of these functionalities, so it is unknown how much of these complex processes are covered. And there is definitively no functionality documented about the reaction of the piano vibrating elements to sounds occurring outside of the *instrument.*

Attack Repetition

Piano hammers can hit a string that is already vibrating and producing sound. This is possible by using the sustain pedal or by depressing a piano key that has not been totally released using the double escapement mechanism [6]. Since the string is already vibrating, the sound resulting from the new hammer strike is different than the one produced when the string is stimulated from a static situation. The resulting sound will be different depending on the hammer velocity but also depending on the string vibration amplitude and phase at the moment when the second strike occurs. No documentation of any features in digital pianos addressing these issues has been found, and there is nothing in the MIDI protocol to consider these situations separately [1].

Piano Pedals

The piano pedals constitute another critical interaction point between the pianist and the instrument. In most cases, pedals are not intended to produce sound by themselves, but they open a large set of possibilities for the pianist to alter the sound being produced by the instrument. The traditional piano has three pedals: sustain, soft, and sostenuto, each having its own sound *faculty*.

Sustain Pedal or Damper Pedal

The sustain pedal adds an enhanced layer of sound effect in performance. The movements of the pedal, which is intended to extend sound duration by opening all strings and soundboard vibrations without the dampening effect, can create sound by themselves. A quick release or closure of the piano dampers creates noises that can resonate in the strings and in the instrument body. Furthermore, the mechanical noise of the pedal reaching the limits of its travel range can be more or less noticeable depending on how the pianist is acting on the pedal and according to the piano construction and regulation.

Using the sustain pedal also modifies the note's timbre and intensity depending on when it is depressed (before, during, or after playing notes on the keyboard) [9]. These sound changes are mainly caused by the sympathetic resonance of other strings with the harmonic components (partials) of the already existing sound (see the Multiple Key Action section), including noises. It is easy to have a glimpse of this effect by depressing the sustain pedal of a grand piano without playing any keys and then producing sounds like clapping or talking close to the strings and soundboard. The strings and the rest of the instrument will resonate in many different ways to these stimuli.

During normal piano playing, all these complex resonances take place amplifying and modifying the sound being produced. The sustain pedal adds to the resonance at different depressing deepness. This means that when the dampers release the strings they may stay at different distances or even touching them slightly (a technique referred to as half-pedaling or even quarter-pedaling). This significantly affects the way the strings resonate [22].

Last but not least, each time the pedal is released, it dampens the sound of the piano similarly to the way it was previously described in the Key Release section, allowing the pianist to finely control how the sound is extinguished according to the speed variations of the pedal movement. In this case, it affects not only one single note but the entire set of piano strings multiplying the expressive possibilities of the dampening process for the pianist [22].

Digital pianos offer some advanced features for sustain pedals including half pedaling, release and catch (capturing resonance remnants by depressing the sustain pedal right after keys or pedal itself is released), and string resonance as in the case of multiple key actions [12]. At this point, there is no documentation about digital pianos featuring different pedal movement speeds and timing to affect the resulting sound, suggesting that this significant part of the acoustic piano sound behavior is not mapped.

Soft Pedal

Using the soft pedal while playing a grand piano modifies the sound tone and intensity by displacing the area of the hammer's surface that gets in touch with the strings and in some cases making the hammer to strike a lower number of strings each time (2 instead of 3 or 1 instead of 2) [22]. It also works differently in different registers of the piano due to the different number of strings per note and different materials and shapes. Similarly to the sustain pedal, the soft pedal can be used at any deepness level creating an infinite number of possibilities of tone and intensity variability to the sound produced by the piano.

There is no documentation about soft pedal functionality in digital pianos other than just creating an overall change of the sound intensity and timbre [13]. In fact, not all digital pianos feature a soft pedal.

Sostenuto Pedal

The sostenuto pedal is added in the late modern pianos to be used when the desired tone needs to be sustained while the other tones are dampened. This feature is used effectively in the piano literature by postromantic and contemporary composers. The mechanism of this pedal is relatively simple, and its operation does not offer any parameters that can be varied continuously in a wide range. Not all acoustic pianos, particularly older models, have incorporated sostenuto pedal.

Piano Sound *Unpredictability*

Acoustic pianos are purely mechanical machines. Piano action parts are made of materials like wood, felt, and metal, causing them to suffer changes due to temperature and humidity conditions as well as usage wear [16]. They are manually adjusted by a piano technician, and the piano is tuned by hand (with the help of computerized tools for tuning precision). Also, the piano strings vary in length, thickness, and even construction materials depending on the register. These physical and mechanical characteristics of the acoustic piano vary significantly in mechanical regulation and sound production. Further, the complexity of the interaction among the sound-producing elements offers infinite possible variations in playing the piano (hammer velocity, note dampening speed, pedal depressing, etc.). These mechanical and natural factors introduce uncertainty in the sound control for the pianist. Regardless of how skilled the pianist is, the unpredictability of the sound exists. Skilled pianists deal with this uncertainty by reacting to the variability and adjusting their playing to obtain the desired sound [25]. Thus, skilled piano playing involves constant fine adjustment of piano touch based on the sound that the pianist hears in the moment as he/she creates a coherent and satisfactory musical result. This uncertainty and variability is a source of inspiration as well. Hearing sounds slightly different than expected can boost pianists creativity, making them react to the resulting sound and look for new ways to generate expressive music that is coherent to the sound that has just been produced.

Digital pianos are computer-controlled instruments, and, in them, acoustic piano's infinite possibilities are reduced to a predefined set of parameters. The perception of the uncertainty existing in the acoustic piano by the performing pianist is eliminated or at least greatly reduced. For skilled pianists who have developed a very fine control of their fingers and foot movements in order to produce fine nuances of sound, it is likely that they will be able to perceive much less uncertainty in the sound produced by the digital piano compared to an acoustic piano. At the same time, they may find that predictability restricts spontaneity and creativity during stage performance.

Piano Haptic Feedback

The other main interaction element between a pianist and a piano is the tactile feedback. Every time the pianists make contact with a piano, they perceive textures, resistances, and many other inputs from the piano mechanism that they use to adapt their playing to produce the desired results. This haptic feedback is not always directly related to the sound that is produced, and not feeling it does not necessarily limit the expressive possibilities of the instrument. However, if it is different than expected, pianists would lack information about how the piano reacts and may feel uncomfortable to apply the same movements and force they would apply to an acoustic instrument. The two main haptic interaction elements between the pianist and the piano are the keys and the pedals.

Key and Pedal Movement and Resistance

The main interaction points between the pianist and the instrument are the keys. Keys offer resistance to be depressed caused by the weight and inertia of the moving piano action parts and internal friction [2]. It is necessary to apply a certain force to overcome this resistance and move the key in a way that it can also propel the corresponding hammer to eventually hit the string(s) and produce the expected sound.

This resistance, however, varies depending on the location of the key within its travel range. As the key moves down, different parts of the mechanism are moved, and the resistance of the key changes accordingly. Due to elements in the piano mechanism such as the double escapement system, this resistance also varies according to the velocity of the key movement [2]. Furthermore, if the sustain pedal is depressed, the key resistance is slightly reduced because the dampers' weight is already lifted by the pedal.

When the key reaches the bottom of its travel range, it touches the key-bed preventing further movement, and this is felt by the pianist. Depending on the materials of the mechanism, the deceleration of the key reaching the bottom is different, and this is also perceived [11].

When the key is released, it returns to its rest position. This movement involves certain acceleration and deceleration of the key that depends on the weight and friction of the piano mechanism components [4]. The pianist can perceive that the keys are *lighter* or *heavier* depending on how this movement happens while the keys still have some contact with the pianist's fingers. Last but not least, the key top is touched by the pianist's fingers when playing, and the key material texture, such as wood, ivory, and synthetic product, is perceived. Almost all these considerations apply to piano pedals as well. For instance, the sustain pedal has different resistances to the pianist's foot depending on where it is within its travel range.

Importantly, these haptic feedback sensations that the pianists perceive are closely related to sound production and dampening effects. A pianist would expect certain sound quality results according to what it is perceived through the keys and the pedals, which means that both areas are very closely related to each other [8] and to body control. Digital pianos do not resemble these characteristics effectively enough [4] to allow the pianist to train the haptic control efficiently.

Modern high-end digital piano keys are adjusted so that the overall resistance is the same as it is found in a grand piano action. Also, their key tops are often made of the same materials that would be found in acoustic pianos [13]. However, these features are not enough to provide a similar overall haptic experience to the pianist because of the other elements discussed above.

One solution that is already implemented by some digital piano brands is the production of the hybrid pianos [10]. Because of their physical mechanism, very similar to acoustic instruments, the keys generate haptic feedback that the pianist perceives as very similar to acoustic instruments. Also, the velocity sensors can measure the actual speed of the hammer shank which means that the relationship between the pianist actions and the hammer movement is preserved and tracked for sound generation. This approach solves many of the problems in this area for digital pianos. However, some important parts of the mechanism are still not included into the hybrid mechanism, such as dampers and pedals, and therefore some elements of the haptic feedback are not perceived by the pianist as in an acoustic instrument. In reality, the hybrid mechanism adds significant weight, cost, and complexity to the instruments taking away some of the advantages of the digital pianos.

Developing a computer-controlled mapping of the piano action is an alternative solution that has been proposed in academic environments. In this case, a computer makes the necessary calculations to determine the resulting hammer velocity and other parameters resembling the acoustic piano mechanism according to the key and pedal movements. An electromechanical system translates variable resistance forces to the keys in real time in order to provide haptic experience to the pianist. There is significant theoretical and experimental research on this topic [4, 15], but no evidence has been found of any commercial implementations, likely due to the technical and cost challenges involved in the development of a practical version of such system. There is also no information about the real potential of these mechanisms to provide a realistic haptic perception to the pianist.

Conclusions

The number of variable features involved in piano playing is very large, and complex interactions occur between the pianist and the instrument. There is an infinite number of possibilities in which pianists can influence these parameters as part of their playing, modifying the sound that is perceived (audio feedback). The pianists also use haptic perceptions (haptic feedback) in order to adjust their playing to obtain the desired sound. Digital pianos implement a number of features to mimic both the audio and haptic elements of acoustic pianos with different degrees of success. In many cases, these features are not enough to closely imitate the complexity of the acoustic pianos, and some acoustic piano features are not mapped at all.

Digital pianos' haptic feedback is not realistic in many areas because not all the nuances in piano mechanical response are simulated. Significant improvements have been made in some models, such as the hybrid pianos, to minimize this gap, but even in this case, there are elements of interaction that are not properly mapped.

Regardless of pianists and educators preferences, it is already a reality that digital pianos are replacing acoustic pianos in some applications, including performance and education situations. Understanding the real limitations of these instruments is important to support the usage of acoustic pianos whenever possible. On the other hand, improving digital instruments will benefit performers, teachers, and students in situations when acoustic pianos cannot be used. Trying to map all acoustic piano elements into a digital piano may be impractical and even impossible, but identifying the ones that have the highest impact in the pianist overall experience including the bodily efficient movement will be very useful to continue improving the quality of these instruments.

Acknowledgments I would like to express my deepest appreciation to Dr. Sang-Hie Lee for her invaluable guidance and support throughout the duration of this project.

References

1. The MIDI Manufacturers Association. The complete MIDI 1.0 detailed specification. 3rd ed. 2014. https://www.midi.org/specifications/item/the-midi-1-0-specification. Accessed 2 Nov 2017.
2. Gillespie B. The touchback keyboard. Paper presented at: Proceedings of the 1992 International computer music conference. San Francisco, CA; 1992.

3. MacRitchie J. The art and science behind piano touch: a review connecting multi-disciplinary literature. Music Sci. 2015;19(2):171–90. https://doi.org/10.1177/1029864915572813.
4. Oboe R. A multi-instrument, force-feedback keyboard. Comput Music J. 2006;30(3):38–52. https://doi.org/10.1162/comj.2006.30.3.38.
5. Galembo A. Perception of musical instrument by performer and listener (with application to the piano). Paper presented at: Human supervision and control in engineering and music international workshop. Kassel, Germany; 2001. p. 257–66.
6. Hart HC, Fuller MW, Lusby WS. A precision study of piano touch and tone. J Acoust Soc Am. 1934;6:80–94. https://doi.org/10.1121/1.1915706.
7. Bernays M, Traube, C. Expressive production of piano timbre: touch and playing techniques for timbre control in piano performance. Paper presented at: Proceedings of the 10th sound and music computing conference (SMC2013). Stockholm, Sweden; 2013. p. 341–46.
8. Horváth P, Töröcsik D. Magnetic issues of a haptic keyboard. Rz Elektrotech. 2013;02b/2013:61–3.
9. Ortmann O. The physical basis of piano touch and tone. London: K. Paul, Trench, Trubner & Co. Ltd; 1925. p. 186.
10. Yamaha Corporation. N3 AvantGrand Hybrid Piano Specs. n.d. https://usa.yamaha.com/products/musical_instruments/pianos/avantgrand/n3/specs.html#product-tabs. Accessed 2 Nov 2017.
11. Askenfelt A, Jansson EV. From touch to string vibrations. II: the motion of the key and hammer. J Acoust Soc Am. 1991;90(S1):2383–93. https://doi.org/10.1121/1.402043.
12. Clavia Digital Musical Instruments. Nord piano 3 specification. n.d. http://www.nordkeyboards.com/products/nord-piano-3/nord-piano-3-specification. Accessed 2 Nov 2017.
13. Kawai Musical Instruments Manufacturing. Kawai VPC1 virtual piano controller specifications. n.d. http://www.kawaivpc.com/en/specifications/. Accessed 2 Nov 2017.
14. Roland Corporation. What is SuperNATURAL technology? 2013. http://www.rolandus.com/blog/2013/06/04/what-is-supernatural/. Accessed 2 Nov 2017.
15. Van den Berghe G, De Moor B, Minten W. Modeling a grand piano key action. Comput Music J. 1995;19(2):15–22. https://doi.org/10.2307/3680597.
16. Askenfelt A, Jansson EV. From touch to string vibrations. I: timing in the grand piano action. J Acoust Soc Am. 1990;88(1):52–63. https://doi.org/10.1121/1.399933.
17. Goebl W, Bresin R, Galembo A. Once again: the perception of piano touch and tone. Can touch audibly change piano sound independently of intensity. Paper presented at: Proceedings of the international symposium on musical acoustics. Nara, Japan; 2004.
18. Haas M. Tone colours on the piano: acoustic predisposition or contextual illusion. Piano J Eur Piano Teach Assoc. 2017;112:18–22.
19. Suzuki H. Spectrum analysis and tone quality evaluation of piano sounds with hard and soft touches. Acoust Sci Technol. 2007;28(1):1–6.
20. Neuhaus H. The art of piano playing. New York: Praeger Publishers; 1973. p. 240.
21. Goebl W, Bresin R, Fujinaga I. Perception of touch quality in piano tones. J Acoust Soc Am. 2014;136(5):2839–50. https://doi.org/10.1121/1.4896461.
22. Taguti T, Ohtsuki K, Yamasaki T, Kuwano S, Namba S. Quality of piano tones under different tone stoppings. Acoust Sci Technol. 2002;23(5):244–51. https://doi.org/10.1250/ast.23.244.
23. Askenfelt A, Jansson EV. From touch to string vibrations. III: string motion and spectra. J Acoust Soc Am. 1993;93(4):2181–96. https://doi.org/10.1121/1.406680.
24. Repp BH. Acoustics, perception, and production of legato articulation on a digital piano. J Acoust Soc Am. 1995;97(6):3862–74. https://doi.org/10.1121/1.413065.
25. Goebl W, Bresin R. Measurement and reproduction accuracy of computer-controlled grand pianos. J Acoust Soc Am. 2003;114(4):2273–83. https://doi.org/10.1121/1.1605387.

Part III
Practice

Chapter 13
Musculoskeletal and Associated Conditions in the Instrumental Musician

Dusty Marie Narducci

Introduction

Musicians can be classified as instrumentalists and noninstrumentalists. The information in this manuscript is directed toward instrumental musicians and the clinicians providing medical care for musculoskeletal injuries among this population. The material presented in this chapter serves to provide an overview, evidence, and future directions of common playing-related musculoskeletal disorders (PRMDs). Methods for obtaining the content of this chapter include a comprehensive review of the literature as well as practitioner-based experience. Although acute injuries are possible, chronic injuries from overuse or misuse explain the majority of musculoskeletal complaints seen in musicians.

Focus will be placed on injuries associated with the following instrument categories: percussion (e.g., piano, drums, cymbals, triangle, chimes, tam-tam, glockenspiel, timpani, bells, and xylophone), woodwind (e.g., flute, piccolo, clarinet, recorder, bassoon, and oboe), upper and lower stringed (e.g., violin, viola, cello, bass, harp, and dulcimer), brass instruments (e.g., trumpet, trombone, tuba, French horn, cornet, saxophone and bugle), and electronic (e.g., keyboard). The following types of musculoskeletal pathologies will be reviewed: overuse injuries (e.g., tendinosis), nerve compressions (e.g., carpal tunnel), myofascial dysfunction, osteoarthrosis, neurological disease (e.g., dystonias), bursitis, and hypermobility syndrome. Musculoskeletal injuries in instrumental musicians most commonly affect the shoulder, wrist, spine/neck, elbow, and hand/fingers [1]. The chapter will assist the reader in recognizing, treating, and preventing common musculoskeletal conditions in the music-making population.

The relationship between fatigued state, adaptive patterns, injury, and poor technique is thought to determine the cumulative risk of musculoskeletal injury among

D. M. Narducci (✉)
Morsani College of Medicine, University of South Florida, Tampa, FL, USA
e-mail: dustynarducci@usf.edu

S.-H. Lee et al. (eds.), *Perspectives in Performing Arts Medicine Practice*,
https://doi.org/10.1007/978-3-030-37480-8_13

this population. Gender, anatomical proportions, age, lifestyle, comorbid medical conditions, substance use, and decreased muscle conditioning also contribute to the prediction of injury. Playing-related musculoskeletal injuries are described as any pain, weakness, tingling, or physical symptom that interferes with normal playing affecting up to 86% of professional musicians [1–4].

Association Between Musicians and Sports Athletes Regarding Musculoskeletal Conditions

Musculoskeletal injuries in musicians are thought to reflect instrument-specific and repetitive physical load placed on the body [5, 6]. This is a similar finding in athletes who have injuries based on specific movement required by their sport. Similar to athletes, musicians are also at risk of developing psychological symptoms/conditions [7]. Sports athletes often receive supplemental training to help prevent anticipated injuries associated with their specific sport, anatomical form, or training pattern [8, 9]. Lack of resources, deficits in education, and negative connotations are just a few of the reasons that musicians do not seek health care for PRMDs [10–12]. Unlike the wide variety of sports medicine and physical therapy professionals addressing musculoskeletal injuries, experts who specialize in optimizing anatomical function in the music-making population are limited [13]. The consequences of injury, if not addressed, can result in temporary and even permanent hazard in their careers.

Risk Factors for Playing-Related Musculoskeletal Disorders

It is imperative that health-care providers treating musicians obtain a good history of the patient in order to understand any existing or potential physical and psychological factors. Change in musical load or intensity of playing (practice, teacher, instrument), teacher, general and specific physical fitness (flexibility, injury, anatomical deformities), diet, psychological stress, exercise habits, and substance abuse may affect a musician's risk and recovery from PRMDs [14, 15]. Implementation of well-designed prospective studies is needed to identify more accurately causative relationships of the etiology and risk of PRMDs in instrumental musicians [16].

Repetitive highly complex movements are made on a daily basis for extended periods of time in the process of developing and maintaining appropriate neurological, sensory, and musculoskeletal abilities to become a skilled musician [17, 18]. As musicians gain experience, the need for practice is intensified inevitably placing them at higher risk for PRMDs [18, 19]. The hours a musician performs on a weekly (about 28–40 hours) and daily (about 2–6 hours) basis should be accounted for [20]. Time spent undergoing independent practice, rehearsal and performance conditions, frequency of rests during rehearsals and performances, and instructor factors should also be considered. Sustained high levels of playing or sudden increases in playing burden lead to overuse and overload of the musculoskeletal system placing undue strain on the body. These factors, paired with poor injury management, represent a strong risk for PRMDs. Following periods of decreased playing such as during vacation, musicians also do not consistently return to play in an appropriate step-wise manner. Educating musicians on how to implement a graduated return to activity can allow them to return to play without injury.

Although some physical risk factors are not modifiable, their potential burden should be noted. Playing conditions such as temperature, required travel, breaks, and length of rehearsals and performances may be unavoidable, but indirect efforts may limit these inconveniences. Demanding repertoires, although sometimes mandatory, may be better managed with mental practice rather than repetition. Individual size and proportions, elements of anthropometry, are generally inalterable, but adjustments to technique, instrument, and conditioning may help to prevent impending risk [19, 21]. Frequent and formal breaks would allow musicians to recover from the constant strain and load placed on muscles, tendons, and joints [8]. A general recommendation of 5-minute rest breaks for every 25 minutes of play may help to limit PRMD risk [9, 18]. The length of breaks and frequency may need to be increased for those musicians performing more complex repertoires. Rest periods of 3–7 days may optimize the recovery of tissues and protect their integrity following an acute musculoskeletal injury [18, 19, 21].

Gender and Age

The relationship of the development PRMDs in musicians with gender and/or age has been investigated. Kok et al. conducted a cross-sectional study evaluating reported PRMDs among amateur musician orchestra students and found a higher independent prevalence in younger, female musicians [22]. A similar cross-sectional study of 357 members of Dutch orchestra students assessed PRMDs using a questionnaire. An independent association of a higher prevalence of PRMDs with female gender, younger age, higher body mass index (BMI), and playing a string instrument was found [23]. A study looking to evaluate the frequency of musculoskeletal pain in professional orchestral musicians with regard to their instrument affiliation found female gender and performance anxiety to be predictors of PRMD [24]. Paarup et al. performed a cross-sectional questionnaire study of 441 symphony orchestra musicians investigating the prevalence, duration, and consequences of musculoskeletal symptoms [5]. On an annual basis, 14% more women than men experienced musculoskeletal symptoms in the following anatomical regions: neck, upper and lower back, shoulders, elbows, hands, and wrists. These investigators found that 19% more women than men reported more than 7 days of daily musculoskeletal pain [5]. The presence of regional pain among British symphony musicians and its relationship to environment and mental health suggested a higher risk of reported PRMDs among women than men. Another cross-sectional study assessing 59 classical orchestra musicians reviewed potential correlations between biomechanical, environmental, psychosocial, and personal risk factors and PRMDs. No significant gender difference in PRMD incidence was found in regard to age and gender [24].

Dystonia, a potentially career-ending condition, affects men more frequently than women [25]. The Sound Practice project found that female musicians reported more anxiety and depression than male musicians [26]. Similar to recorded substance use in the United States, male musicians have a higher tendency to use substances than female musicians [27]. Nodal osteoarthritis (OA) of the intraphalangeal finger joints and the base of thumbs is more common in females [28]. OA of the second and third metacarpophalangeal (MCP) joints more commonly affect older men than women [29]. It should be mentioned, however, that comprehensive analysis of these studies indicates that the greatest risk of developing PRMDs is multifactorial [30]. The type of instrument chosen by female musicians may be a better predictor of injury risk. This is best exemplified in a study showing that string instruments are more often chosen by female musicians; therefore the choice of instrument rather than gender may be the most important factor in determining the risk of PRMD [31].

Overall Fitness

Based on current literature, there is a lack of education regarding overall health and fitness as musicians enter their practice. The limited formal education regarding rest after injury, lifestyle modifications, and early identification of injury puts musicians at unnecessary risk for PRMDs [9, 32]. Although poor health has been associated with more musculoskeletal pain/symptoms in musicians, most data derive from cross-sectional studies with limited consistency [16, 33, 34].

Lack of general physical conditioning, joint hypomobility or laxity, and previous injuries are risk factors for PRMDs. Each musician has independent limiting variables making these risk factors modifiable or non-modifiable. An example is joint laxity due to a previous injury or underlying condition such as Ehlers–Danlos syndrome. Individuals affected by this syndrome may not improve regardless of treatment. A 2011 study by Wilke et al. has demonstrated a lower rate of perceived exertion during rehearsal in musicians who regularly engaged in physical activity compared to those who were sedentary [35]. A vigorous and lasting career in performing arts has been linked to having good overall fitness by taking part in regular cardiovascular and resistance training [36]. Other studies have shown conflicting evidence with insufficient prevention of PRMDs in musicians who participate in generic aerobics and strengthening programs [37]. The American College of Sports Medicine recommends that, in order to improve cardiovascular fitness, the healthy adult should partake in five sessions of moderate-intensity exercise per week for at least 30 minutes or three sessions of high-intensity exercise per week for 20 minutes per session [38]. Examples of moderate-intensity exercise include brisk walking, low resistance cycling, swimming, and jogging. Based on the same guidelines, muscular conditioning could be improved with two sessions a week of resistive exercise. Ideally one should perform 2–3 sets of 10–20 repetitions with 90 seconds of rest between each set, with a goal of targeting 8–10 muscle groups weekly. Unlike competitive athletes, no purpose-designed exercise plan for the prevention of PRMDs for musicians exists. Given the similarities between sports athletes and musicians, designing and implementing goal-directed programs may be cost-effective and beneficial at improving functional outcomes [39].

Exercise regimens aimed to target specific body regions and to increase the endurance of distinct musculature do exist and should be utilized for improving motor function and movement patterns [40]. An example in the athletic population includes the use of exercise-based knee injury prevention programs for the prevention of anterior cruciate ligament (ACL) injuries in appropriate individuals. A reduction in the frequency and severity of PRMDs in musicians could be achieved with the use of 12-week targeted exercise regimens to strengthen and support commonly injured musculature [41]. The benefits of these regimens on reported pain declined after 6 months. As in any population, consistency and compliance are limiting factors in the health-promoting benefits of an exercise program. Musical play is time-consuming, and many variables are present which may represent a significant challenge to successful implementation of regular exercise programs. If individual exercise is not possible, considering group exercise prior to or following rehearsals should be entertained.

Nutrition/Hydration

Similar to athletes, proper hydration and nutrition above that required by the general population are essential for the prevention of PRMDs and successful recovery [42]. Since no formal nutrition and hydration advice exists for musicians, following the advice to sports athletes may provide injury prevention and recovery improvement in the music-making population. Instrument play is an intense endurance activity that requires strategic timing of daily meals and snacks composed of the appropriate amounts of carbohydrate, fats, proteins, vitamins, and minerals to sustain optimal performance [42]. Proper hydration prior to, during, and following rehearsals and performances is essential. Recommendations should be individualized depending on body habitus, comorbid conditions (e.g., diabetes), medication use (e.g., diuretics), and environment (e.g., temperature). Musicians should be educated with regard to the prevention and signs of dehydration in addition to the adverse effects of cognitive and physical function in the presence of impaired hydration status. Although outside the scope of this chapter, eating disorders and disordered eating patterns should be suspected in at-risk musicians. Severe nutritional depletion is a hazard to musculoskeletal health. Similar to sports athletes who have a high degree of personal and external stressors and perfectionism, eating disorders are common and should be treated appropriately.

Psychological and Psychosocial Risk Factors

Psychological risk factors that may predispose musicians to injury consist of a wide array of psychiatric symptoms and conditions including performance anxiety, depression, mood disorders, social phobias, and extreme personality traits or personality disorders such as somatization and hypochondriasis. Psychosocial factors that should be considered include financial status and potential burden, external perfectionism, and other sources of external pressure including institutional, employment, educational, and peers. Traits of extreme perfectionism can also be a contributing force in poor injury reporting and management [43].

Prior to the Sound Practice project, which assessed eight professional Australian orchestras over a 5-year period [26], there has been limited research over the past 2 decades evaluating the mental health of professional musicians. The Sound Practice project demonstrated an inverse affiliation between psychological factors and PRMDs [26]. Among the participants, 33% of musicians met the criteria for social phobia, and 22% screened positive for post-traumatic stress disorder (PTSD) and 32% for depression. Clearly, there was an association with psychological issues and reported PRMD discomfort levels [26].

Reported hearing deficits of musicians have been associated with psychological symptoms, impaired psychosocial environment, and perceived stress [43]. The Sound Practice Project found that among 63% of survey participants, 43% believed they had hearing loss, and 64% used earplugs at least intermittently. With the high risk of noise-induced hearing loss in orchestra musicians, physical and psychological assessment should be considered as impairments may affect PRMDs [26]. Performance anxiety and work-related stress seemed to be positively related with musculoskeletal disorders in musicians although current evidence is limited and sometimes incongruent. The relationship between psychological and physical prosperity is complex, and more research and recommendations for screening, prevention, and treatment in the musician population are warranted.

Substance Misuse

Lifestyle choices such as substance use and misuse of prescription drugs can affect general health and ultimately increase the risk and impair recovery from PRMDs. Use of marijuana and illicit drugs once or more on an annual basis was reported by musicians, which is higher than the reported use of the general population (28%) [27]. A study investigating the consumption of caffeinated energy drinks in 226 New York musicians aged 18–45 found that frequency of energy drink use was positively associated with heavy use of alcohol and misuse of prescription drugs; however, the role of caffeine as a univariate factor was not investigated [44]. In a study assessing strategies to cope with musical performance anxiety (MPA), more than 30% of those surveyed reported using a substance in order to cope with MPA [45]. Although substance use is not directly linked to musculoskeletal disorders, it is known to impair an individual's general health [45]. Future research is needed to better define the prevalence and predictive risk of substance use in musicians in order to educate, prevent, and effectively treat affected musicians.

Posture and Biomechanics

Poor posture and biomechanics in addition to incorrect instrument technique are potentially modifiable risk factors that should not be overlooked in musicians. Appropriate posture is a body position that allows for controlled, harmless loading of the body, while maintaining the ability for flexible movement in an efficient energy system [46]. Maintaining correct posture while playing an instrument can be challenging as many instruments require distinct alterations in anatomical position during use [47]. Required alterations in posture for extended periods of time while activating muscles and repetitively loading the musculoskeletal system places musicians at increased risk for PRMDs [48].

Biomechanical analysis provides an interactive assessment of an individual during dynamic activities. Literature on music performance biomechanics is limited, but, given the success of this science in sports medicine, evidence-based studies on the mechanisms and prevention of injury should be summoned for the welfare of musicians [49]. Although the literature is inconsistent regarding the exact risk associated with poor posture and biomechanics as well as anthropometric factors, health-care providers caring for musicians should perform an in-depth physical exam and use its findings to guide further management. Both musculoskeletal and nerve function should be examined in addition to other body systems as indicated (e.g., pulmonary function studies in wind players). An individual's degree of mobility should be evaluated, and tools, such as the Beighton Score for the assessment of hyperlaxity, should be utilized if needed (see section Hypermobility Syndrome). Musicians should be encouraged to bring their instrument to clinical visits to allow direct observation of posture, fit, and technique. Due to lack of adequate research, our current understanding of risk factors for PRMD in musicians is limited which only gives us an indication of hypothetical relationships.

Pathology of Injuries

In general, there are two types of injuries chronic and acute. Acute injuries that occur in an instant are possible in musicians; chronic injuries are due to repetitive traumas to soft tissues and develop slowly. Overuse is the most common cause of injury in musicians [50]. Overuse injuries can affect the following soft tissue structures: tendons, muscle-tendon structures, bursa, nerve tissue, bone, periosteum cartilage, and soft tissue compartments. Musicians are at risk of such injuries when tissues become damaged due to repetitive stress beyond its normal function.

When musicians are not appropriately trained for repetitive motions required to play their instruments, the involved soft tissues become damaged and require time to undergo repair.

Excessive stress on the musculoskeletal system eventually leads to pain. If a musician does not acknowledge this pain, a cycle of compensation, muscle tension, contracture formation, and inflammation may ensue. Aside from pain/discomfort, signs of overuse injuries include erythema, impaired function, warmth of the affected area, and potential swelling. The progression of overuse injury is commonly elucidated into four stages. Pain in the affected area following physical activity defines stage one. Stage two is characterized by pain that occurs during physical activity but does not impair performance, whereas the pain associated with stage three does impede performance. When pain is an unremitting event at rest, overuse injuries are considered to be in stage four.

Repetitive strain on body tissue resulting in overuse injuries is most commonly caused by errors in instrumental play, similar to errors in training causing injury in athletes [51]. Engaging in instrumental play without the appropriate muscle strength and endurance, imbalances in muscles, biomechanical limitations, inflexibility, faulty playing technique, ill-suited instruments or other equipment, and insufficient recovery in addition to practicing errors can all predispose a musician to develop overuse injuries [51].

Tendinopathy

A tendon is a stable, although flexible, tissue that attaches muscle to bone [52]. When a tendon is being overused, pain and swelling occur. Damaged and/or diseased tendons are unable to withstand loads similar to those of healthy tendons leading to decreased biomechanical functioning of the body. Overuse tendinopathy in musicians can diminish or tarnish music playing and sometimes even end a career if symptoms are ignored [53].

Healthy tendons are composed of collagen fibers and extracellular matrix with nerves and vessels networked in between. Under healthy physiological conditions of nutrition and blood flow, exercise strengthens a tendon's ability to withstand weight loads up to a given threshold. When this is exceeded, tendinopathy ensues. The pathophysiology of tendinopathy has been mostly investigated in animal models as human tendons are surgically explored only when patients are symptomatic and not in the early stages of tendinopathy. In such models, a constellation of complex changes, ultimately leading to degeneration of the tendon, occurs [54]. Overused tendons undergo a microdisruption of fibers, an injury that triggers release of growth factors and activation of collagen-producing cells or fibroblasts aimed at repairing the injured tissue [54]. However, mediators of inflammation and microvascularization are also generated and stimulate the synthesis of enzymes, the so-called matrix metalloproteinases, that degrade the extracellular matrix of the injured tendon resulting in degeneration and weakening of this structure. Other tissue fac-

Table 13.1 Extrinsic and intrinsic risk factors of tendinopathy

Extrinsic risk factors	Intrinsic risk factors
Loading: Excessive volume, speed, magnitude Training: Abrupt changes in load amount or type, faulty equipment	Age Body structure Gender Genetics

Table 13.2 Medical conditions and medications associated with tendinopathy

Medical condition	Rheumatoid disease Psoriasis, gout, pseudogout Inflammatory bowel disease (Crohn's disease, ulcerative colitis) Infections Malignancy Thyroid disease Diabetes Cushing's syndrome Dyslipidemias Tobacco abuse Obesity Poor nutrition
Medications	Cholesterol-lowering medications (statins) Antimicrobials (fluoroquinolones) Corticosteroids

tors are also generated and produce a concomitant growth of nerve fibers whose irritation of is responsible for the generation of pain and further sustained inflammation [54].

Risk factors for developing tendinopathy can be intrinsic and/or extrinsic. Intrinsic factors include gender, age, genetics, and biomechanics, whereas extrinsic factors are associated with body demands or movement errors. Table 13.1 provides examples of intrinsic and extrinsic risk factors of tendinopathy. Various medical conditions and medications are thought to be associated with the development of tendinopathy (Table 13.2). Musicians diagnosed with a tendinopathy-related medical condition or associated medication should be educated and managed appropriately [55–60].

Tendinopathy is separated into tendinitis and tendinosis [61]. This distinction, albeit not universally accepted, is necessary when considering potential treatment options. Tendinitis is described as an acute overload from a sudden or massive load to the tendon causing micro-injury to the tissue matrix. Tendinosis is a degenerative process where the collagen makeup of tendon tissue is subjected to a faulty healing response and continuous overuse [62]. The continual biomechanical demands faced by musicians place them at higher risk for tendinosis rather than tendinitis [62].

Given the inflammatory changes that occur during tendinitis, treatment should be directed to reducing inflammation. Treatment options used to decrease inflammation include corticosteroids and nonsteroidal anti-inflammatories, both of which are avoided in tendinopathy due to potential negative effects on collagen repair.

Tendinitis generally resolves within 6 weeks, whereas tendinosis may heal after a longer time, sometimes up to 9 months, commensurate to collagen production by fibroblasts [61]. Tendinosis treatment should begin with rest, necessary biomechanical and ergonomic adjustments, stretching, cryotherapy, eccentric strengthening, optimizing nutrition, and manual therapy [63].

Although tendinopathy can affect various anatomical regions, musicians are most often affected in their upper extremities. Determining which movements are used most frequently and/or inappropriately during instrument playing will help to define anatomical locations most at risk for the development of tendinopathy. As an example, there is great potential for the development of tendinopathy of the left or right wrist and thumb, right elbow, and left shoulder in fiddle players due to the body positioning during play.

Specific Tendinopathy Affecting Musicians

Epicondylitis of the Elbow

The elbow is constructed of a lateral and medical epicondyle. The wrist extensors attach to the lateral epicondyle, whereas the flexors of the wrist insert on the medial epicondyle. Injury to the wrist extensors, most commonly the extensor carpi radialis brevis muscle (ECRB), occurs in lateral epicondylitis. Injury to the pronator teres and flexor carpi radialis muscles constitutes medial epicondylitis. In spite of its name, epicondylitis represents the chronic process of tendinosis and not acute inflammation. Repetitive motions requiring the wrist to move outside of its normal position, while the muscle–tendon junction is contracting, may increase the risk for epicondylitis. Various studies have established a relationship between occupational injuries and epicondylitis, but none have focused specifically on instrumental musicians.

Information obtained from biomechanical studies addressing faulty techniques performed by tennis players [64] can apply to musicians. Continuous contraction or excessive extension of the wrist extensors, excessive forearm pronation, and extreme supination with ulnar deviation of the wrist are biomechanical faults that may place musicians at risk for the development of lateral epicondylitis. Outside of the general treatment recommendations for tendinopathy, a counter force brace placed approximately 6–10 cm above the elbow joint may decrease strain at the musculotendon junction, therapeutically decreasing pain and improving function. Guidance from a trained physical or occupational therapist to facilitate a progressive eccentric strengthening program may be advantageous.

De Quervain's Tenosynovitis

At the location of the first dorsal compartment, the abductor pollicis longus (APL) and extensor pollicis brevis (EPB) tendons glide through a tunnel constructed of fibrous tissue and osseous structures. Thickening of these tendons due to overuse makes them difficult to pass through this anatomical tunnel. Musicians who require prolonged extension and abduction of the thumb are at higher risk of developing de Quervain's tendinopathy. Symptoms are often localized to the radial aspect of the wrist and are exacerbated by instrument play in addition to other activities requiring thumb and wrist movement. Musicians seeking conservative treatment can use a forearm-based thumb spica splint, while allowing the intraphalangeal joints to remain moveable, although musical performance may be restricted or impossible with its use [65].

Intersection Syndrome

A condition called Drummer's wrist or more formally known as intersection syndrome commonly affects the wrists of instrumentalists. Intersection syndrome occurs when extensor tendons in the forearm experience friction due to repetitive movements with simultaneous tension. Repetitive resisted wrist extension can affect the point at which the abductor pollicis longus and extensor pollicis brevis muscles cross over the extensor carpi radialis brevis and extensor carpi radialis longus tendons. This condition is often misdiagnosed as de Quervain's syndrome but can be distinguished by its more dorsal location of pain [65].

Upper Extremity Peripheral Nerve Compression and Entrapment Syndromes

Upper extremity peripheral nerve damage can lead to multiple disorders and should be considered in instrumental musicians presenting with sensory loss, weakness, and/or pain involving the hand, arm, or shoulder. Even though multiple disorders and mechanisms can affect nerve function, compression or nerve entrapment syndromes are the most common cause of nerve pathology in the upper extremity. The suspected incidence of nerve entrapment disorder appears to range from 4% to 48% [66]. It is reasonable to assume that the demand of placing the body in persistent abnormal anatomical positions during instrument play is a substantial risk factor for the development of PRMDs. If musicians are misdiagnosed or ignore symptoms of mild neuropathy, progression to more severe symptoms may end a career.

To date, there is no consensus on the most common neuropathies affecting instrumental musicians. Carpal tunnel syndrome, a mononeuropathy affecting the median nerve in the wrist, has been a frequently reported upper extremity peripheral nerve syndrome in instrumental musicians [67]. Ulnar neuropathy at the elbow and cervical radiculopathy, due to compression of the spinal nerves at the cervical spine, are also common. A study by Lederman in 2006 found that the thoracic outlet is more common in musicians than carpal tunnel syndrome, cervical radiculopathy, and ulnar neuropathy [68].

Clinical Signs and Symptoms

In the beginning stages, intermittent nerve compression, which is often due to positioning in instrumental musicians, compromises blood flow to the nerve. Continued restriction of blood flow to the nerve eventually leads to demyelination and symptoms of pain and weakness that eventually become unremitting. With prolonged and untreated compression, the distal nerve segment may degenerate further and possibly undergo a process called transection. Transection, also known as neurotmesis, is a complete severing of the nerve. Transection may also follow acute traumatic injury to the nerve (e.g., laceration from a knife). Other causes of nerve damage include vascular inflammation (e.g., vasculitis), atherosclerosis, infections (e.g., herpes simplex), radiation exposure, and metabolic disorders (e.g., diabetes).

The presentation of peripheral nerve pathology depends on which nerve is being compromised. In general, nerve damage leads to numbness, burning, tingling, weakness, and paresthesia of the affected anatomic region. Nerves function as either motor, sensory, or both. When motor nerves are affected, muscle weakness (e.g., decreased grip strength) and sometimes atrophy can result. In cases of sensory nerve damage, symptoms include less weakness and more discomfort, pain, and loss of sensation (e.g., inability to distinguish temperature changes). When an instrumental musician presents with upper extremity numbing and pain, a nerve compression syndrome should be suspected.

The career of instrumental musicians can be temporarily or permanently halted by the functional impairment and disability of upper limb nerve entrapment disorders. A change in playing duration, frequency, instructor, or instrument type and technique can lead to nerve ailments. The development of a nerve compression disorder could also be related to the type of instrument being played. Musicians who play the violin are required to place their left forearm into supination, while having their wrist and elbow in flexion. This position may compress nerves of the upper extremity, particularly those in the elbow [69]. Violinists and harpists may be subjected to the development of cervical radiculopathy attributable to their neck positioning during play [70, 71].

Diagnosis

Inspection, palpation, assessment of range of motion, and provocative testing should be performed by clinicians who are assessing musicians for potential nerve entrapment disorders. Even though the physical exam can provide valuable diagnostic information, some of these tests have low sensitivity and specificity which minimize their diagnostic value [72]. Observing musicians while playing their instrument offers a dynamic element to the assessment and may be helpful to modify their technique.

Cervical neck instability, loss of disc space, osseous abnormalities, and alterations of the normal cervical lordosis of the spine may be visualized with plain radiographs of the cervical spine. Plain radiographs are however often not beneficial in diagnosing peripheral nerve disorders.

Electrodiagnostic studies (EDS), including electromyography (EMG) and nerve conduction studies (NCS), are the most commonly used and effective diagnostic tools to distinguish upper extremity peripheral nerve disorders. EMG/NCS can be helpful in confirming nerve demyelination. Nerve demyelination is distinguished on EMG/NCS as conduction velocity with conduction blocks across affected nerve segments. EMG/NCS are also useful for the detection of focal nerve entrapments (e.g., median nerve in carpal tunnel) rather than plexopathies affecting multiple nerves stemming from a specific region such as the brachial plexus [71]. EDS is less suitable for diagnosing mild or acute nerve entrapments, and clinicians should be aware that a normal EDS does not exclude an asymptomatic nerve compression.

When a musician presents with signs and symptoms of cervical spine disease, an MRI may be warranted as it provides specific etiology information such as disc degeneration, herniation, and compression of nerve roots. MRI is particularly useful in acute cases of peripheral nerve pathology as an obstructing lesion may be the culprit. Imaging by computerized axial tomography (CT) holds value in the assessment of osseous structures and in the presence of implantable devices (e.g., pacemaker) that preclude the use of MRI. More recently the use of high-resolution ultrasonography has shown promising advantages in the diagnosis of peripheral neuropathies of the upper extremity. This imaging technique is a noninvasive, cost-effective tool that can visualize areas of nerve enlargement suggestive of nerve compression and may also be useful in the detection of traumatic nerve pathology and inflammatory nerve changes. It should be mentioned that most of the above diagnostic modalities may not be needed in obvious focal neuropathies caused by habitual nerve compression (e.g., instrument play).

In rare situations, a musician's medical history or exam may prompt serological testing. Some peripheral nerve syndromes are more common in individuals who have thyroid abnormalities (e.g., altered levels of thyroid stimulating hormone), diabetes (e.g., abnormal fasting blood glucose and hemoglobin A1C), infectious diseases (e.g., positive Lyme disease titers), or genetic conditions (e.g., hereditary neuropathy). Timely and accurate diagnosis is necessary in the musician population in order to clarify injury severity, determine prognosis, prevent surgical intervention, and institute a treatment plan.

General Management

Both conservative and nonconservative modalities for the management of upper extremity peripheral nerve entrapment syndromes exist. Heat treatment approach depends on the needs and goals of the musician, syndrome severity, financial/insurance situations, as well as on individual barriers and demands. Modifying instrument technique, improving posture, lifestyle alterations, managing medical conditions, and changing playing schedules should be initial approaches. When playing performance is markedly impaired, a musician may seek a more permanent treatment. Splinting, physical therapy, drug therapy with dietary supplements, anti-inflammatory therapy, and oral glucocorticoids are sometimes used in the initial stages of treatment. Local glucocorticoid injections as well as orthobiologic modalities are also options. The decision to pursue surgical intervention should be made on an individual basis. Various surgical techniques exist, but musicians should be aware that technique and outcomes vary depending on which nerve is affected.

Specific Peripheral Nerve Syndromes Affecting Musicians

Carpal Tunnel Syndrome (Median Neuropathy)

Pathogenesis Carpal tunnel syndrome (CTS) develops when the median nerve in the wrist is compressed by surrounding anatomical structures [72]. Within the wrist, the median nerve travels along with several tendons through a tunnel made up of eight carpal bones. If tendons traveling within the tunnel enlarge (e.g., thickening due to tendinopathy) or in cases where the tunnel narrows (e.g., arthritis), the median nerve can become compressed. Compression of the median nerve can also occur due to injury or fracture of the wrist, underlying medical conditions (e.g., systemic lupus erythematosus, rheumatoid arthritis), pregnancy, endocrine disorders (diabetes, hypothyroidism, acromegaly), and osteoarthritis as well as frequent use of vibrating devices [73]. Repetitive, prolonged, forceful motion while the wrist is flexed is the most frequent cause of median nerve entrapment in instrumental musicians.

Instrumental musicians should be aware of risk factors associated with the development of CTS. Among the general population, women are three times more likely to develop CTS than men. This gender trend may be related to the fact that females have smaller carpal tunnels than men as well as certain conditions being more prevalent in the female population (e.g., pregnancy, rheumatoid arthritis). However, no data exist demonstrating that female musicians are at higher risk of developing CTS when compared to male instrumental musicians. Other risk factors include being middle-aged, obese, genetics, and tobacco use.

Symptoms CTS symptoms usually develop gradually in instrumental musicians; as the condition worsens, these symptoms may progress to affect not only sensation but also strength and dexterity. The hallmark symptom of CTS is paresthesia (numbness and tingling) or pain along the anatomical distribution of the median nerve. The median nerve is both a motor and sensory nerve that regulates sensation in the thumb, index finger, and radial (thumb) side of the ring finger in addition to muscle control stemming from the base of the thumb [73]. Although symptoms most commonly localize to the wrist, extension to the shoulder is possible. Instrumental musicians are affected by their symptoms during play, but typically symptoms are worse at night [73]. CTS can occur bilaterally, but this may be less likely in the music-making population as only one wrist is generally affected as opposed to a typist who subjects both wrists to compression.

In cases of mild symptoms or lack of electrodiagnostic evidence, it is reasonable for musicians to begin with conservative treatment modalities. Depending on the musician's goals, initial treatment can begin with splinting, splinting with a glucocorticoid injection, or glucocorticoid injection alone [74, 75]. Combination therapy may be more effective than either modality alone. Splinting the affected wrist in a neutral position, to inhibit prolonged flexion or extension, is thought to minimize compression of the median nerve within the carpal tunnel. Splints are available over the counter or can be custom made by an occupational therapist or other qualified specialists. Full-time splinting is nearly impossible for most instrumental musicians; night-only splinting may be a better option as this provides similar benefit in symptom relief [75]. Oral or locally injected glucocorticoids may offer short-term improvement of CTS symptoms, but no trial has been conducted directly comparing these two treatment modalities. Similar symptomatic relief at 6 months has been found for splinting and injection, but an injection offers better acute relief [76]. Additional nonsurgical options for the treatment of CTS include carpal bone mobilization, yoga, ultrasound therapy, nerve gliding, laser/magnetic/electrical, anti-inflammatories, and other oral medications, but the evidence is limited and of low quality to recommend with assurance. Surgical intervention has shown to be more effective than splinting and/or glucocorticoid injections for long-term relief [77, 78]. Musicians who are symptomatic, failed conservative treatment, and have evidence of serious nerve damage based on electrodiagnostic studies (EMG/NCS) should strongly consider surgical interventions including surgical decompression. In severe cases of CTS, a musician may decide to forgo conservative treatment attempts and proceed directly to surgery to expediate return to instrument play. Up to approximately 90% of individuals with carpal tunnel syndrome fail conservative treatment and require surgical intervention [79]. Algorithms based on various clinical and diagnostic grading scales exist to help determine the appropriate treatment. Between 70% and 90% of individuals with CTS who undergo splinting or surgical decompression show improvement of symptoms after 12 months. There are no data assessing the prognosis of instrumental musicians diagnosed with CTS.

Thoracic Outlet Syndrome (TOS)

Pathogenesis Thoracic outlet syndrome is an umbrella term for three different pathological entities: neurogenic (nTOS), venous (vTOS), and arterial (aTOS). In general TOS is a constellation of symptoms caused by abnormal compression of the neurovascular bundle [80]. The neurovascular bundle is a network of nerve and vascular structures that are located in an area termed the thoracic outlet. The thoracic outlet is bordered by the first rib and situated behind the clavicle. In addition to the cervical 8 and thoracic 1 nerve roots, within the neurovascular bundle exists the brachial plexus, a network of sensory and motor nerves that innervate the shoulder and arms. The vascular structures that exist within the thoracic outlet include the subclavian artery and vein [81, 82].

This chapter focuses on neurogenic TOS as the musician population is at great risk for developing this type of TOS. Neurogenic TOS results from alterations of the thoracic outlet due to trauma, muscular impairments (e.g., postural weakness or changes), and congenital abnormalities (rib abnormalities) [83]. Musicians are required to endure strenuous and abnormal postural positions for extended periods of time, placing constant tension on the shoulder. These static postures and repetitive arm movements can contribute influence to nTOS. To date, no data exist on a relationship between the risk of developing nTOS and instrument type, gender, or other characteristics of musicians.

Clinical signs and symptoms Symptoms of neurogenic TOS are similar to nerve entrapment syndromes. Musicians may experience upper extremity paresthesia, pain, and weakness in the shoulder, arm, or hand. Potential development of difficulty performing fine motor tasks, cramping, and atrophy can be detrimental to a musician's career. Interrelated terms, signs, and symptoms make the diagnosis of nTOS challenging [83]. Diagnosis can usually be made by a seasoned clinician through history and physical exam, but electrodiagnostic testing is beneficial to rule out other etiologies.

General management Musicians diagnosed with nTOS should initially be treated with physical therapy to include mobilization or manipulation with intention to decrease thoracic outlet compression by strengthening, retraining, and moving hypomobile involved structures. In musicians who do not respond to conservative treatment, surgical intervention including thoracic outlet decompression may be necessary. Although initial success rates following surgery is around 90%, benefit declines over time [84, 85].

Cubital Tunnel Syndrome (Ulnar Nerve Entrapment Syndrome)

Pathogenesis The ulnar nerve is commonly known as "musicians' nerve" as it serves to control fine finger movements. Normally, it originates from the C8-T1 nerve roots of the brachial plexus and travels posteromedially to the humerus before it passes behind the medial epicondyle of the elbow in the cubital tunnel. Moving distally, the ulnar nerve passes superficial to the flexor retinaculum of the hand as it enters into the wrist via an area termed Guyon's canal. The ulnar nerve and its branches provide sensory innervation of the fifth digit, medial half of the fourth digit, anterior skin, and nails of the palm. Additionally, the ulnar nerve and its branches provide innervation to the flexor muscles of the forearm and hand as well as smaller lumbrical muscles used for fine finger movements.

The ulnar nerve is not only susceptible to entrapment syndromes via compression at the elbow and wrist, but, as it courses distally in the upper extremity, it is unprotected by muscles and bones making it vulnerable to superficial injury. Followed by median nerve entrapment in CTS, the ulnar nerve is the next most commonly diagnosed mononeuropathy [86, 87]. While the incidence and prevalence of ulnar entrapment are unknown, compression most commonly occurs at the elbow followed by the wrist [88, 89]. Other etiologies of ulnar nerve entrapment can occur at the axilla (e.g., crutches), abnormal anatomical structures (e.g., tumors, fractures, vascular anomalies) in addition to genetic and infectious syndromes.

Musicians are at risk of ulnar entrapment from aberrations at the elbow and wrist. There is limited knowledge regarding risk factors for the development of ulnar neuropathy in musicians as well as the general population. Two large studies have suggested a positive association of ulnar neuropathy at the elbow with smoking [90, 91]. Body weight, gender, alcohol use, trauma, and comorbid conditions such as hypertension and diabetes do not seem to be risk factors. Exclusive studies with musicians have not been conducted, but musicians who smoke and play an instrument requiring continual elbow flexion may be at greater risk of developing ulnar neuropathy [92].

Clinical signs and symptoms Entrapment of the ulnar nerve initiated from the elbow ordinarily presents with pain at the elbow, paresthesia affecting the fourth and fifth digits, and worsening of symptoms at night. When the ulnar nerve impairment initiates from the wrist, weakness and atrophy of the hand, decreased dexterity, and sensory changes transpire. Playing a musical instrument requires the use of intrinsic hand muscles (i.e., the lumbricals and interossei) for precise finger control as well as larger muscles of the forearm and hand which control functional movements necessary for grip and carrying objects. Regardless of whether the entrapment occurs at the elbow or at the wrist, loss of these functions is detrimental to musicians. Similar to other focal nerve entrapment syndromes, electrodiagnostic testing (NCS and EMG) is an accepted tool used for the diagnosis of ulnar neuropathies. Ultrasonography and magnetic resonance imaging (MRI) may be useful to rule out other causes (e.g., ganglion cysts) [93].

General management Treatment of ulnar neuropathy depends on symptom severity as well as on the goals of the affected musician. Intermittent and persistent symptoms reported as mild to moderate should be initially managed conservatively. Musicians with mild impairment may find spontaneous resolution of symptoms with appropriate rest, adjustment of playing technique, and avoidance of proactive actions such as leaning on the elbow/wrist (e.g., while driving, typing, cycling) and perpetual elbow/wrist flexion (e.g., talking on the phone). Splinting the elbow in limited flexion, continuously or only at night, may result in improvement of mild cases. The success of conservative treatment modalities for ulnar neuropathy occurring at the wrist is less promising [94, 95]. Surgical intervention may be unavoidable in instrumental musicians who fail 6 months of conservative treatment, in those who initially present with well-defined clinical and electrodiagnostic evidence of moderate to severe neuropathy, and in those who have progressive symptoms. Musicians ought to be aware that general poor health and symptoms of more than 2 years may not benefit from surgical treatment [96]. Seeking immediate medical care for symptoms of ulnar nerve neuropathy may avoid career-altering or career-ending injury.

Cervical Radiculopathy

Pathogenesis Cervical radiculopathy is defined as a pathological process affecting one or more cervical nerve roots [97]. The cervical spine is formed by seven cervical vertebrae (C1–C7) and eight cervical nerve roots. Each vertebra has four nerve roots, two on each side that branch off from the spinal cord. Two types of nerve roots exist: the ventral root carries motor signals to a specific group of muscles, and the dorsal root provides sensory information to designated skin regions. Cervical spinal nerves provide sensory and functional control to various parts of the body depending on the spinal level to which they correspond. Rotational movements of the head are controlled by the upper cervical spine, whereas head flexion and extension are regulated by lower cervical segments [98].

The etiology of cervical radiculopathy can be degenerative or nondegenerative. Degenerative causes of cervical radiculopathy are compressive in nature and often due to cervical disc herniation or cervical spondylosis. Situated between two cervical vertebrae lies an intervertebral disc composed of an inner surface called the nucleus pulposus, an outer ligamentous structure termed the annulus. Damage to the intervertebral disc can lead to tearing of the annulus resulting in prolapse of the nucleus pulposus which can consequentially compress the corresponding nerve root. A more common cause of compressive cervical radiculopathy is cervical spondylosis, a general term for degenerative changes of the spine that seem to worsen with age. The etiology of cervical spondylosis is not fully understood, but degenerative changes of the vertebrae, osteophyte formation, and desiccation of the vertebral disc play a role. Cervical spondylosis can lead to narrowing of the cervical spine, and this is defined as cervical stenosis. Although less common, nondegenerative causes of cervical radiculopathy should be considered and include vascular, malignant, and infectious causes. Axial neck pain (pain originating from neck muscles/ligaments/joints) may mimic or coexist with cervical radiculopathy especially among instrumental musicians [99]. During play, musicians often have increased antero-positioning of the head resulting in spine and neck pathology. Violinist and violists are accustomed to maintaining a position of elbow flexion, prolonged wrist and forearm supination in addition to holding the instrument between their chin and shoulder all while using their right arm for bowing. These complex movements, overtime or when altered due to fatigue following a demanding repertoire, can place violinists and violists at risk of neck, shoulder, and upper extremity injury. Inappropriate posture, poor training, and muscle misuse/overuse can lead to poor scapula stabilization. This myriad of situations can lead to multiple conditions including cervicalgia, costoclavicular compression syndrome, and myalgia of the trapezius. Correction of anatomical deformity and retraining are favorable to the prevention and treatment of spine/neck pathology seen in instrumentalists.

Epidemiological studies assessing cervical radiculopathy in the general population are dated, and no studies have been conducted evaluating risk factors for this condition in instrumental musicians. Advancing age, Caucasian race, tobacco use, and previous lumbar radiculopathy have been mentioned as plausible risk factors among current literature. Heavy lifting, various sports (golf, platform and springboard diving), and consistent use of vibrating tools are also suggested risk factors [97].

Clinical signs and symptoms The presentation of cervical radiculopathy varies depending on cervical nerve root involvement. Instrumental musicians with cervical radiculopathy may report neck pain, with ipsilateral radiation of arm pain, sensory deficits, paresthesia, and possibly weakness. Danger signs for more serious pathology include fever, chills, unexplained weight loss, upper motor neuron signs (gait disturbance, hyperreflexia, difficult with fine motor tasks), muscle atrophy, and Lhermitte's phenomenon (a shock-like paresthesia that occurs with neck flexion). Radiculopathy can be differentiated from axial neck pain by the presence of unilateral arm symptoms as described above [99].

General management As with all PRMDs occurring in musicians, treatment of cervical radiculopathy should be a collaborative decision that considers multiple variables. Optimal management for compressive cervical radiculopathy has yet to be established, and there are no studies assessing the outcomes of treatment in instrumental musicians with cervical radiculopathy. Conservative treatment should be attempted initially in musicians with a clear diagnosis of cervical radiculopathy in the absence of more serious pathology. Oral analgesics, prednisone and nonsteroidal anti-inflammatory drugs, immobilization, physical therapy, manipulation, exercise, and avoiding activities that exacerbate symptoms should be considered. Instrumental musicians should revise their playing technique and schedule and consider using instrument-specific adaptive devices (e.g., chin rest in a violinist). In cases of severe or disabling symptoms or when conservative treatment fails, cervical epidural steroid injections have shown to be helpful in some cases [100].

Currently, there are limited high-quality data examining the long-term outcomes of cervical radiculopathy. A systematic literature review has shown significant spontaneous improvement of symptoms after 4–6 months [100]. After initial symptom resolution, one-third of patients may experience recurrence. If symptoms remain similar to those at initial presentation, conservative treatment can be reinstated. There is no clearly established length of time for nonoperative treatment before considering surgery [100]. Musicians with refractory signs and symptoms of cervical radiculopathy, evidence of nerve root compression consistent with clinical presentation, and progressive motor deficits should discuss surgical interventions with a medical provider.

Bursitis

A bursa is a saclike structure filled with fluid that serves to protect and improve function of various musculoskeletal structures. Bursae are present throughout the body, both in deep and superficial anatomical locations. Deep bursae allow muscles to glide over bone, whereas superficial bursae have a cushion-like function separating bone and skin. In its pathological context, an injured bursa is termed bursitis. Although this term infers that the pathology is inflammatory in nature, no true inflammatory process exists [101]. For the purpose of this text, focus will be placed only on bursitis locations prevalent in the musician population.

Forms of bursitis are classified as chronic aseptic, septic, or acute traumatic; they may result from prolonged pressure, direct injury or trauma, overuse activities, as well as medical conditions including inflammatory disease (e.g., rheumatoid arthritis), crystal-induced arthropathy (e.g., gout), and infectious causes (e.g., septic arthritis). Prolonged direct pressure of specific superficial bursae (e.g., leaning on elbow) and overuse activities affecting structures in close proximity (e.g., instrument play) to bursae are common among instrumental musicians. Medical conditions that have shown an association with bursitis include gout, diabetes, rheumatological disease (e.g., rheumatoid arthritis), HIV, and alcoholism. This chapter focuses on the following upper extremity bursitis: subacromial bursitis, olecranon bursitis, and scapulothoracic bursitis.

Subacromial bursitis The subacromial bursa functions to separate the supraspinatus muscle and tendon from the bony acromion process of the scapula. Subacromial bursitis is included under the spectrum of shoulder pathology termed subacromial impingement syndrome (SAIS) which is discussed in more depth elsewhere in this chapter (see section "Subacromial Impingement Syndrome (SAIS)").

Olecranon bursitis Similar to the general population, the most frequently reported superficial bursitis in instrumentalists is that affecting the elbow. Olecranon bursitis occurs when the bursa positioned posteriorly over the olecranon process of the ulna in the elbow has an abnormal increase in the fluid volume within its sac. The superficial location of this bursa allows it to freely glide under the skin during elbow extension and flexion but also makes it more susceptible to injury. The bursa is also poorly vascularized making it vulnerable to both infection and inflammation. Numerous etiologies for olecranon bursitis have been reported, but the most common culprit is minor, repetitive trauma [102].

Scapulothoracic bursitis This bursitis results from mechanical friction between the ribs and superior-medial angle of the scapula. Instrumental musicians are susceptible to scapulothoracic bursitis due to repetitive movements requiring repeated elevation of the upper extremity. Scapula rotation during upper extremity elevation is directed upward and externally as it tilts posteriorly. Abnormal scapula movement patterns due to weak or dysfunctional scapular musculature, impaired posture, and relating muscles/tendon fatigue increase the risk for scapulothoracic bursitis. Pianists who use improper biomechanics for instrument play or are at risk of overuse injuries may be subjected to scapular abnormalities. Changes in scapular kinematics can develop from overuse as well as improper instrument technique. Clinical symptoms of scapulothoracic bursitis include pain located in the posterior shoulder, as well as crepitus and local tenderness at its anatomical location [103].

Treatment Noninfectious causes of bursitis are usually self-limiting. In most instances, treatment is based on symptom relief which include protection of the joint, analgesics, and intrabursal injections of glucocorticoids. Instrument technique must be adjusted if the musician is placing direct pressure over the effected bursa [104, 105].

The management of subacromial bursitis is discussed later in this chapter (see section "Subacromial Impingement Syndrome (SAIS)"). Olecranon bursitis is managed by avoiding pressure on the area or using specific devices as a barrier. Elbow orthosis should be made by an occupational therapist; this device should not restrict the range of motion and fit comfortably by having the inner surface constructed with soft padding. Fluid aspiration is needed to test for infection or crystal arthropathy in appropriate cases and to sometimes decompress the bursal sac to allow for better fitting protective equipment. As in all types of bursitis, the use of anti-inflammatory medication, if not contraindicated, may offer benefit. Surgical treatment of chronic olecranon bursitis, in etiologies other than rheumatoid arthritis, has been shown to provide benefit [104, 105].

Scapulothoracic bursitis usually spontaneously resolves in the general population, but this may not be the case in musicians who continue to pursue movements that may exacerbate this condition. Conservative treatment utilizing physical therapists to guide scapular strengthening exercises, in addition to anti-inflammatory drugs, may be beneficial. In cases of failed physical therapy, a glucocorticoid injection may be beneficial, but this injection requires a trained sports medicine physician or equivalent skilled in imaging techniques such as ultrasonography. Image assistance during the injection will promote proper needle placement and avoid upper chest wall structures that could become injured and cause complications (e.g., pneumothorax, nerve injury).

Shoulder Conditions Affecting Musicians

Subacromial Impingement Syndrome (SAIS)

Subacromial impingement syndrome (SAIS) is a spectrum of shoulder pathologies varying from tears to tendinopathy of the rotator cuff. Repetitive shoulder abduction between 60 and 120 degrees is a common requirement of instrumental musicians. Constant movement of the shoulder within this range can however lead to SAIS. SAIS is the most commonly reported disorder of the shoulder [106, 107].

The cause of subacromial impingement is a multifactorial clinical picture affected by the kinematics of the glenohumeral joint and scapulothoracic articulation in addition to abnormal anatomical variants. Normal abduction of the shoulder compresses structures around the glenohumeral joint. Structures include the four rotator cuff muscles (supraspinatus, infraspinatus, teres minor, and subscapularis), labrum, subacromial bursa, and the long head of the biceps' tendon. When this motion occurs repetitively, the glenohumeral joint becomes unstable. When pathology or anatomical variants are present (e.g., osteoarthritis, acromion morphology, decreased distance between the humeral head and undersurface of the acromion), there is a risk for shoulder impingement of the rotator cuff muscles and tendons as these pass though the subacromial space [106, 107]. Instruments that involve increased shoulder abduction (e.g., flute, violinists, violists) make surrounding structures vulnerable to impingement. Musicians with weakness or dysfunction of the shoulder stabilizing muscles (shoulder joint capsule, tendons, muscular structures, and ligaments) are at increased risk for SAIS.

SAIS can lead to subacromial bursitis, rotator cuff tendinopathy, and rotator cuff tears. Similar to SAIS, no definite pathophysiology for rotator cuff tendinopathy has been universally accepted. Insult to the rotator cuff tendon(s) through overuse, degeneration, or acute injury may compromise the normal vascular system of rotator cuff. Overloading the tendon with excessive overhead activity, in addition to older age and other comorbidities (e.g., traumatic fall, rheumatoid disease, arthritis, Ehlers-Danlos syndromes, and diabetes), are factors contributing to injury [106, 107].

The signs and symptoms of shoulder impingement are similar to those of rotator cuff tendinopathy, thus making diagnosis challenging. Overhead activities often cause pain around the lateral arm and deltoid region. Symptoms seem to be nocturnal and worse while lying on the affected shoulder. Similar pain patterns to SAIS and rotator cuff tendinopathy are reported in those with rotator cuff tearing. The degree of weakness is dependent on the extent of tearing. Of note, shoulder pain may also originate from other neck conditions (e.g., cervical radiculopathy) [106, 107].

Musculoskeletal ultrasound is becoming the gold standard for initial imaging of rotator cuff pathology. Although this tool is operator-dependent, it is more cost-effective than MRI and also serves as a therapeutic option.

There is limited evidence supporting treatments for SAIS. Symptomatic partial and chronic rotator cuff tears should be initially treated conservatively with physical therapy. The goal of this therapy is to modify the musicians' biomechanics by enhancing flexibility through shoulder capsular stretching and strengthening of shoulder muscles including deltoid, periscapular, and rotator cuff. Detailed assessment of a musician's playing technique will offer insight into the causative source of the impairment and also help to direct a personalized management approach toward recovery. In addition to cryotherapy, glucocorticoid injections may over short term offer relief of pain. Repetitive glucocorticoid injections can be detrimental to the integrity of the tendon in the long term. At least 6 weeks of physical therapy, with or without one or two glucocorticoid injections, are recommended before surgical intervention is considered.

Surgical intervention, with arthroscopic decompression, when compared to conservative treatment with primarily physical therapy for SAIS showed no significant benefit in a 2019 meta-analysis of 13 randomized control trials [108]. When compared to conservative treatment, patients who underwent surgery for isolated shoulder impingement (without rotator cuff tear) had no significant reduction in pain or function at 1-year follow-up. Three months of physical therapy should be the initial treatment for musicians with isolated shoulder impingement [108]. Surgical intervention may be needed in musicians who fail conservative treatment for partial or chronic rotator cuff tears. The current literature recommends immediate surgical repair for acute, full-thickness rotator cuff tears in healthy patrons. Elderly individuals and those who are not good surgical candidates (e.g., serious comorbidities) should pursue nonoperative treatment for acute rotator cuff tears.

Adhesive Capsulitis

Adhesive capsulitis, also known as frozen shoulder, is a condition characterized by limited passive and active range of motion. The etiology of adhesive capsulitis is often idiopathic. Although the pathophysiology is not fully understood, the condition is associated with thyroid disease, autoimmune disease, diabetes, Parkinson's disease, and surgery [109]. The pathology of adhesive capsulitis is characterized by initial inflammation around the shoulder joint capsule and surrounding structures followed by fibrotic, adhesive changes of the synovial fluid as well as subsequent thickening and contraction of the shoulder joint's capsule. This process leads to substantial loss of shoulder motion, the hallmark of adhesive capsulitis [109]. The nondominant shoulder is more likely to be affected. Even slight limitations of external rotation seen in adhesive capsulitis can make instrument playing impossible. Shoulder-related injuries can be debilitating to musicians both in daily activities of life and while making music [110]. Symptoms generally progress through three phases. The first phase is the most painful and is described similarly to the pain associated with SAIS. At the end of the first phase and the initial part of the second phase, the shoulder joint becomes notably stiffer. As the syndrome progresses through the second phase, motion restriction worsens, while pain decreases. The third and final phase is depicted by a gradual return in shoulder range of motion. Adhesive capsulitis is a self-limiting condition, but its lengthy duration can be damaging to an instrumental musician's career, sometimes restricting play completely. Although ultrasonography and MRI imaging may demonstrate characteristic changes associated with adhesive capsulitis, diagnostic imaging is generally not needed [111].

To date, no unanimous approach to treatment has been reached. A rapid return to musical play is an understandable desire, but forceful physical therapy during the initial phases may prolong recovery; therefore gentle shoulder exercises emphasizing mobility are recommended. More aggressive exercises can be introduced as shoulder range of motion improves. When symptoms are moderate or severe, an intra-articular glucocorticoid injection may be beneficial. The data are limited, but a combination of a progressive physical therapy program and glucocorticoid injection may provide the most benefit [112]. Another semi-conservative treatment approach is an intra-articular dilation injection [113]. A large volume of nonsteroidal fluid (e.g., saline) is injected intra-articularly with the purpose of shoulder joint capsular distention. Currently, no randomized control trials comparing conservative treatment and surgical intervention exist. Surgical options include shoulder manipulation under general anesthesia to stretch the capsule and arthroscopic surgical release of the capsule [113, 114]. Observational data suggests that surgery may not offer a significant benefit [115].

Miscellaneous Conditions

Osteoarthritis

Osteoarthritis (OA) is also called degenerative joint disease. The variability in OA is noteworthy as the age of onset, specific location, progression, and reported severity of pain as well as loss of function make this condition highly individualized and difficult to treat. The cushion-like tissue surrounding bones, termed cartilage, is broken down in OA inhibiting normal joint movement and causing pain or discomfort. As cartilage breakdown progresses, the entire joint becomes affected including the subchondral bone, synovial tissue, and structures such as the meniscus (a fibrocartilaginous tissue that separates some joint spaces) [116]. The pathogenesis and etiology of OA includes a complex and multifactorial constellation of anatomic, genetic, molecular, and lifestyle variables [117].

Although no studies have been conducted on musicians, joint dislocation, ligament strains/tears, and cartilage injury predispose individuals to OA. Trauma-related sports injuries can negatively affect joints, but the role of overuse injury (e.g., instrument play by musicians) in OA is poorly understood. Age is one of the most common risk factors of OA with most affected individuals being over the age of 65 [117]. As obesity continues to become a worldwide problem, the relationship between OA and obesity has become more understood [118, 119]. There appears to be a correlation of persistent body inflammation, possibly due to aging and comorbid conditions such as diabetes, with the development of OA [120]. Although further data is needed, a genetic predisposition for the development of OA is accepted [120].

Symptoms associated with OA are related to the particular joint involved. OA of the cervical and thoracic spine, first carpometacarpal (CMC) joint and interphalangeal joints of the fingers/wrist, shoulder joint, and less commonly the elbow joint is of concern to musicians. Oboists and clarinetists use their right thumb, specifically the metacarpophalangeal joint, to play their instruments and therefore are at higher risk of OA symptom exacerbation [121]. Generally symptoms of OA include pain, tenderness, bony swelling, joint deformity, and instability of the joint. OA can affect a single joint or multiple joints. Conditions such as rheumatoid arthritis, fibromyalgia, hemochromatosis, psoriatic arthritis, and crystalline arthritis can be overlooked as these entities share similarities. Imaging studies are usually not required for the diagnosis of OA. Peripheral OA can be diagnosed if the following three parameters are met: (1) age over 45, (2) morning stiffness more than or equal to 30 minutes, and (3) persistent joint pain in one or few joints [122].

Hand Osteoarthritis

When OA affects the hand joint, symptoms are usually symmetrical and bilateral with the distal interphalangeal (DIP) joints and thumb bases being most commonly affected [123]. Even in the absence of pain, joint stiffness may limit the musicians' ability to perform. Nodal osteoarthritis is characterized by Heberden's and/or Bouchard's nodes along the intraphalangeal joints of the fingers. This subset of OA is more common in females and has a strong genetic predisposition. Progression of nodules can cause lateral deviation of the joints and impair normal finger dexterity. OA affecting the base of thumbs is more common in the older female population and can result in limited pinching and gripping motions. OA of the thumb's base can lead to significant functional impairment and may require surgery in musicians who fail conservative treatment but desire to continue musical play [28]. OA of the second and third metacarpophalangeal (MCP) joints is less common, but a condition called Missouri metacarpal syndrome, affecting older men with occupations requiring demanding use of their hands, has been described [29].

The goals of OA treatment in the musician population are to control pain, improve function, and prevent further joint damage. If risk factors such as obesity or diabetes are coexistent, these should be addressed and managed appropriately. Physical therapy, weight management, adaptive devices (e.g., specialized brace for CMC OA that minimizes thumb abduction), and changes in playing technique should be considered by the musician. Although multiple studies exist on dietary supplements for the purpose of OA, these studies are low yield and inconsistent; however, such supplements can be considered also due to a low risk for adverse effects. Topical nonsteroidal anti-inflammatory medications and capsaicin can be administered locally to the site of pain. Multiple algorithms exist for a stepwise approach to pharmacological treatment options for OA. NSAIDs, acetaminophen, and duloxetine are recommended, but opiate medications are usually avoided due to their addictive nature and high side effect profiles. Intra-articular glucocorticoids are also largely avoided, due to short-term benefits and possible worsening of joint integrity if used to frequently. Orthobiologics accelerate tissue healing (see section Hypermobility Syndrome) and may be of benefit to OA, but the majority of related studies have been conducted on knee OA rather than the anatomical locations of concern to musicians. Surgical treatment with joint replacement and/or fusion essentially depends on symptoms, failed treatment response, individual's goal, and particular joint affected. Restricted range of motion following surgical intervention is of greatest concern in musicians as this limitation is permanent.

Trigger Finger (Stenosing Flexor Tenosynovitis)

Trigger finger is the most common cause of hand pain in adults, and its prevalence in musicians may be at least similar or even higher [123]. Flexor tendons of the finger allow for efficient and forceful production of movement. This motion is maximized by a retinacular sheath that normally functions as a pulley system. The flexor tendon runs through a fibrous tunnel of multiple pulleys. The most common location of pathology is at the A1 pulley where the highest dynamism and tension occur. Repetitive, prolonged finger flexion and extension are essential parts of the biokinetics needed for instrument play but make instrumental musicians vulnerable to flexor tendon swelling. Hypertrophy and inflammation of the flexor tendon cause a disproportion in the surrounding pulley scaffold and tendon size [124]. As the flexor tendon catches, smooth finger movements are challenged and can lead to critical restrictions in musical performance.

With trigger finger, musicians will often experience a loss of smooth motion and deficits in dexterity, while playing their instrument and sometimes at rest. Initially, the condition is painless but often progress both in pain and loss of motion. The pain is most commonly located over the metacarpophalangeal (MCP) joint, which is on the volar side of the hand and specific for the A-1 pulley. Clinical history and exam are efficient to diagnosis trigger finger. Various conditions other than trigger finger can cause pain, motion loss, swelling, locking, and discomfort; these include Dupuytren's contracture, tenosynovitis, tendon sheath infection, and calcification around the joints and/or tendons. Although conservative treatment is suggested for the initial management of trigger finger, symptoms may completely restrict instrument performance. Waiting for symptoms to resolve with activity modification, splinting, and anti-inflammatory medications for 4–6 weeks may not be practical during a musician's career. Even though a local glucocorticoid injection should not be the first option, this approach may be necessary in cases of persistent pain and finger locking. If symptoms do not resolve or decrease by at least 50% after a first injection, a repeat injection in 6 weeks may be warranted. If conservative and semi-conservative treatments fail, musicians should seek surgical interventions as these are effective [125–128]. Although complications from surgery are rare, musicians should consider that infection, nerve/tendon injury, and tendon scarring are possibilities and could potentially restrict their music playing capabilities. When surgical outcomes are good, musicians can expect to return to daily activities of life (e.g., dressing, eating) within days and to more strenuous activities (e.g., instrument play) within 1–2 weeks [129].

Dupuytren's Contracture

Dupuytren's contracture is a condition that begins with a progressive thickening of the palmar fascia, causing contracture and eventually loss of finger extension. The impact of this condition on musicians is unknown, but limitations of motion can be assumed to affect musical performance. As the condition evolves, nodules begin to form on the fascia resulting in finger contracture in a fixed flexed position. The exact cause of Dupuytren's contracture is unknown, but excessive fibroblast growth and abnormal deposition of collagen are thought to bring about fascial thickening. Repetitive movements or previous injury does not appear to play a role in the development of this condition. There have been reports of increased risk in individuals required to use vibratory hand tools for occupational purposes, but this connection is tenuous. Specific genes have been associated with the development of Dupuytren's contracture, and there is a higher incidence in those of northern European descent. Musicians should be aware that diabetes, in addition to tobacco and alcohol use, may increase the risk for Dupuytren's contracture and therefore may want to modify their lifestyle.

The goal of treatment for instrumental musicians is to optimize finger flexibility. Without treatment about half of cases will progress, but sadly no treatment has been shown to stop disease progression [130]. The benefit of splinting, occupational hand exercises, and massage is limited [131]. Nonoperative treatments exist for flexion contraction of proximal interphalangeal joint, although the benefit of these options including splinting, occupational hand exercises, and massage is limited. Injecting glucocorticoids into the fibrotic lesion may resolve local pain or slow growth of the nodule. One study found clostridial collagenase injections to have similar symptom improvement as surgical interventions at 5 years [132]. More data is needed but this less invasive option should be considered. No controlled trials have been conducted on prophylactic external beam radiation, but future research might lead toward recommending this as a feasible treatment option for this condition [133]. Unfortunately for those with severe and limiting symptoms, surgery may be the necessary treatment. The choice of surgical technique is dependent on surgeon preference in addition to individual disease features. Since this condition may not impact hand/finger movements for many years and a small chance does exist for spontaneous regression, musicians should consider surgery only when symptoms are intolerable.

Ganglion Cysts

Tendon sheaths, joint capsules, bursae, and ligaments are made of connective tissue. Herniation from this tissue forms a ganglion cyst characterized as a fluid-filled sac containing a gelatinous, mucinous substance [134]. Ganglion cysts are the most common soft tissue, tumorlike, lesions of the hand. The pathogenesis of ganglion cysts remains poorly unknown as is the causative role of overuse or repetitive movement. It is not yet clear whether ganglion cysts of the wrist and/or hand correlate with pain or restriction of movements during musical performance. Similar to the general population, female musicians especially those in the second to forth decades of life may be at higher risk of cyst development. Ganglion cysts are not limited in their location, but most commonly occur on the dorsal side of the wrist. Clinically, ganglion cysts are palpable, firm, rubbery, sometimes tender masses that may be associated with pain [135]. Large or strategically placed cysts can interfere with musical play if the wrist range of motion is altered. Seldom, cysts can compress a nerve and may cause motor and/or sensory loss hindering music production.

In questionable cases, ultrasonography or MRI and fine needle aspiration biopsy can discern these benign cysts from other masses of the wrist and hand (e.g., epidermoid cysts, lipomas, infectious tenosynovitis, tenosynovitis giant cell tumors, rheumatoid nodules, and sarcomas) [136]. Given their benign nature, observation and reassurance of ganglion cysts are appropriate as these cysts will resolve spontaneously in over half of cases [137]. If the cysts are symptomatic, musicians may consider using a brace but only temporarily as prolonged immobilization can lead to muscle atrophy and playing limitations [138]. Large or obstructing cysts can limit a musician's wrist flexion which is problematic particularly in string instrumentalists. Aspiration of ganglion cysts may be necessary in such cases to allow for unrestricted range of motion. Aspiration of cysts on the dorsal aspect is less precarious than those located on the volar wrist. Neurovascular structures such as branches of the median nerve and radial artery must be avoided during aspiration of volar cysts. This can be successfully performed by a musculoskeletal specialist familiar with ultrasonography. Aspiration may offer immediate relief of symptoms but recurrence is common. Small trials have been conducted evaluating the recurrence of ganglion cysts; some of these trials have demonstrated no recurrence within 1 year, while others have found that over 50% of cysts return within the same timeframe [139]. No added benefit has been found with the injection of glucocorticoids into ganglion cysts, and there is a risk of skin discoloration secondary to atrophy of the subcutaneous fat [129]. Surgical intervention is recommended in musicians with recurrent symptoms following aspiration and in those with continued symptoms. Overall, surgery with removal of all cystic components has a rate of recurrence at approximately 10% [140].

Hypermobility Syndrome

Joint hypermobility syndrome (JHM) is one of the most common hereditary connective tissue disorders affecting approximately 10–20% of the general population. Females, Asians, West Africans, children, and adolescents tend to be more affected by JHM [141]. The presence of JHM is usually scored by the Beighton score [141]. Limited studies exist gauging the association of hypermobility syndromes and PRMDs in musicians, but preliminary evidence suggests that these performing artists, particularly females, have a higher incidence of JHM [142]. Chronic wrist pain experienced by musicians may increase the risk for JHM. Musicians with untreated JHM are at risk for recurrent and/or persistent diffuse musculoskeletal pain, fatigue, soft tissue injuries, and impaired overall physical condition. The vague nature of this condition paired with limited diagnostic testing capabilities often leads to misdiagnosis. JHM syndrome remains a conundrum to clinicians as it is indistinguishable from other connective tissue disorders specifically the hypermobility variant of Ehlers-Danlos syndrome [143]. Early diagnosis in young musicians may prevent future PRMDs and allow career progression. Education is the cornerstone for effective management. Physical therapy with a therapist experienced in JHM is also essential in acute cases as well as to long-term management. In addition to suitable exercises, therapists can direct musicians to appropriate adaptive devices and splints.

Dystonia

While various neuromuscular disorders can affect a musician's practice, performance, and career, this chapter focuses on dystonias. Dystonias are a class of movement disorders characterized by intermittent or sustained contractions of muscles causing abnormal, often repetitive, movements or postures or both [144]. With approximately 16 per 100,000 individuals in the general population being affected by primary dystonia, this condition is one of the most common movement disorders [145]. A more recent literature search comparing the prevalence of focal dystonia in the general population with dystonia in musicians found respective differences of 1:6600 to 1:100; task-specific movement disorders exhibited differences of 1:80000 to 1:100 in this study [146]. Dystonias have been described by their clinical features or proposed etiology. Dystonias affecting the musician population are generally referred to as focal task-specific movement dystonia (FTSPD). FTSDs generally result from a specific action and are isolated to a specific anatomical region. FTSDs affect also other occupations including typists, hairdressers, painters, tailors, and shoemakers that require similar sustained repetitive use of isolated body structures. Sports-related FTSDs are also reported by athletes such as pistol shooters and golfers as these individuals similarly utilize small repetitive movements [147].

Diagnosing dystonia disorders in musicians can be challenging due to the lack of validated assessment tools. Despite the multiple tools that exist for assessing primary dystonia, scales for task-specific dystonia evaluation are limited. The Arm Dystonia Disability Scale (ADDS) is known as a useful means to assist in the diagnosis of FTSD [148].

For the purpose of this chapter, musicians' dystonia will be subdivided into hand dystonia and *embouchure* dystonia. Hand dystonia affects those musicians who perform demanding repetitive movements involving the use of their hand(s). Hand dystonia has been noted to occur in musicians playing a variety of instrument types. Movements depend on the specific muscle activation required by an instrument. For instance, required hand movements in pianists, such as abnormal flexion, are more frequently disturbed. Due to the use of lumbrical activation in brass and woodwind players, abnormal finger extension is common [14]. Brass and woodwind players are also affected by *embouchure* dystonia, which is defined as abnormal involuntary lip and face movements such as tremors and jaw clenching [149].

The etiology of FTSD remains to be determined but a multifactorial origin has been accepted. Multiple studies have shown a genetic predisposition ranging from 20% to 25% of individuals with FTSD having an affected family member. Although no specific mutation within the genome has been established, there is an association of FTSD with the arylsulfatase G (ARSG) gene [150, 151]. Abnormal motor networks, inhibitory circuits, and impaired neural plasticity are pathophysiological factors associated with the development of FTSD. Table 13.3 provides more details regarding the pathophysiology of FTSDs. Musician's environment, personality traits, and anthropometric factors are also thought to play a role in the development of FTSDs. The development of FTSD shows a gender association with

Table 13.3 Proposed pathophysiology of FTSDs [14, 154–161]

Inhibition	Plasticity	Motor networks
Decreased short intracortical inhibition (SICI) Impaired surrounded inhibition Reduced excitability of cortical inhibitory circuits	Maladaptive neural plasticity Plasticity is thought to be necessary for learning, but certain musicians may not have appropriate inhibition of new neural networks Decreased short latency afferent inhibition	Impaired sensorimotor integration Hyperactivation of basal ganglia (identified on fMRI studies) Abnormal cortical representations of digits in the homunculus (identified on fMRI and PET studies) Cerebellar dysfunction Impaired connections between the basal ganglia and cerebellum Mechanism is less understood

men being four times more affected than females. Perfectionism, specific anxiety, and personality traits in addition to over-practicing more difficult repertoires and techniques may also be potential triggers [152, 153].

Existing treatments for dystonia consist of conservative and invasive options including the use of oral medication, physical therapy, chemodenervation, and surgical intervention. Oral medications such as baclofen, phenytoin, primidone, and trihexyphenidyl (an anticholinergic agent) have inconsistent results regarding efficacy, and their use is less desirable because of significant side effects.

Chemodenervation with botulinum neurotoxin (BoNT) is the first choice in dystonia therapy [160]. Botulinum acts by reducing specific muscle contractures by inhibiting acetylcholine at neuromuscular junctions. Types A–G BoNT degrade peripheral cholinergic neurons by acting on the specific SNARE protein. These target-specific actions prevent the release of acetylcholine at the neuromuscular junction, thus resulting in muscle paralysis lasting for several months [161]. BoNT may also reduce afferent sensory input from muscles to the central nervous system, in addition to its involvement in cell life cycles, gene expression, and neuritogenesis (formation of neuronal axons and dendrites) [162]. Although multiple types of BoNT exist, only serotypes A and B are approved for clinical use. BoNT type A is permitted for the treatment of all FTSD, while BoNT type B is approved only for cervical dystonia [162]. BoNT has shown successful reduction in dystonic symptoms, but the risk of motor function loss and interference with musical play is possible. The risk and benefits of BoNT as a treatment option must be discussed in depth with musicians.

Neuromuscular retraining is a therapeutic option thought to reduce dystonic movements and improve playing ability in musicians. Current literature gauging the benefit of retraining programs varies in evidence levels. Sensorimotor retraining that selectively immobilizes the affected body part, while providing transcranial direct current stimulation to the motor cortex, is a hopeful treatment option but requires further investigation [163]. Motor control retraining when combined with constraint-induced therapy (CIMT), a specialized task-oriented approach to improve control of affected extremity, has shown positive outcomes not only in individuals affected by brain injuries (e.g., traumatic brain injuries or cerebrovascular injuries) but also in musicians struggling with FTSDs [164]. This type of combination therapy is facilitated through the use of splint immobilization of the non-pathological limb in order to promote the use of the impaired limb [164]. Sensorimotor retraining (SMR) is a technique that immobilizes one or more digits, other than the dystonic finger, using splints, while having the impaired finger perform specific sequential finger exercises. SMR has proven beneficial in pianists and guitarists [164]. Learning-based sensorimotor retraining is another treatment modality to consider for the treatment of FTSD in musicians. This treatment involves imagining normal movements to promote somatosensory retraining with and without the use of an instrument. Practing in a "slow-downed" manner with gradual increases in speed of play may also serve as a remedy for musician FTSD. Although current literature demonstrates moderate evidence to suggest positive effectiveness of neuromuscular education programs for the treatment of FTSD in musicians, studies with validated outcome measures are needed.

Gamma knife thalamotomy and deep brain stimulation have shown promising results, but due to the potential critical adverse effects of these treatments, they are considered on an individual basis only in refractory cases. Although, substantial gains have been made in recent years regarding the pathophysiology, risk factors, and therapeutic options for FTSD, more advanced research is needed toward a better management of affected musicians.

Injuries Related to Type of Instrument

All musicians, regardless of instrument, are susceptible to the development of PRMDs. Required bodily movements share similarities between musculoskeletal problems associated with those of other occupations. In theory, musculoskeletal injuries experienced by musicians should be based on the anatomical location and on the particular types of instrument being played. Current literature shows minimal variations in symptoms and clinical consequences among mostly orchestra musicians playing different instruments. This section will acknowledge several relationships that instrumental musicians and clinicians should be familiar with.

As previously mentioned, on average 80% of instrumental musicians suffer a PRMD during their career [1, 5, 15]. Multiple studies have revealed higher reporting of musculoskeletal complaints among musicians than nonmusicians [21]. Acute PRMD (within the past year) was reported more often in musical students compared to medical students; reported chronic pain was also higher in musician students (36%) compared to medical students (10.3%) [21]. Another study addressing chronic PRMD found that over 50% of surveyed Australian orchestra musicians reported musculoskeletal pain lasting for more than 12 weeks [26]. Among the various studies, risk factors for the development of PRMD were related to biomechanical factors, perceived physical environment, playing duration and loads, instrument weight, previous musculoskeletal injuries, performance anxiety, high stress levels, and insufficient recovery [15, 24, 26].

When considering PRMD based on anatomical location, the literature displays inconsistent results. A study addressing PRMD in Israeli orchestra musicians found the shoulder (60%), lower back (50%), upper back (40%), and neck (35%) to be the most concerning sites of pain [24], whereas pain was reported in the neck (14%), left upper limb (15%), right upper limb (22%), and back (25%) among surveyed Australian orchestra musicians [26]. Frequent or permanent neck pain and lower back and shoulder pain are commonly reported, but inconsistency between studies makes defining specific anatomical locations challenging [5, 23].

Uncovering associations between instrument type and location of PRMD has also proven too be difficult. Upper string musicians are more likely to be affected by PRMDs in comparison to other instrumentalists with violinists being more likely to report pain than other instruments in this category [23]. The majority of PRMDs reported by upper and lower string instrumentalists was related to the left upper extremity [26]. Lower string instrumentalists had more face/lip injuries compared to those playing upper string instruments [26]. When compared to string instrumentalists, woodwind instrumentalists noted more neck, wrist, and hand musculoskeletal pain [5]. Brass players reported less elbow, wrist/hand, and lower back pain compared to other string instrumentalists [5], while percussionists reported back followed by upper extremity injuries more frequently.

Despite numerous epidemiological assessments, a confident association between used instrument type and risk for PRMDs remains elusive. To assist instrumental musicians and those clinicians caring for their musculoskeletal needs, known relationships between instrument type, biomechanics, and musculoskeletal injury have been outlined in Table 13.4.

Table 13.4 Injuries by instrument groups

Instrument type	General biomechanics required to play instrument	Most common injuries
Woodwind Piccolo Recorder Bassoon	Lumbrical activation, abnormal finger extension is common Repetitive mouth movements	Hand dystonia Embouchure dystonia
Flute	Require a non-ergonomic playing shoulder abduction position	Left-sided neck pain Subacromial impingement syndrome (SAIS) Wrist pain
Clarinet Oboe	Hold their instruments mostly with their right thumbs	Right thumb especially at the metacarpophalangeal joint CMC joint osteoarthritis
Stringed Bass Harp Dulcimer	Majority of orchestra players play in the sitting position Similarly string instruments require that the right hand be used to hold and move a bow to make a sound The left fingertips are placed on the fingerboard to determine the pitch	Tendinopathy – wrist, hand, elbow Tenosynovitis (trigger finger)

Table 13.4 (continued)

Instrument type	General biomechanics required to play instrument	Most common injuries
Violin Viola	Can be sitting or standing The instrument is placed between chin and shoulder. Requires prolonged, extreme supination of the forearm and wrist, elbow flexion, and repetitive bowing with the right arm The left hand holds the instrument, as left fingers needs to move freely The bow is gripped by the right thumb, middle, and ring finger, while the index and little finger are placed gently on the bow Appropriate technique requires the extension of the right thumb	Subacromial impingement syndrome (SAIS); left shoulder Nerve entrapment syndromes Hand dystonia If extended, injury to right thumb is possible
Cello	Always sitting The body of the cello is placed between the musician's knees The endpin (spike) is located at the bottom of the cello and makes contact with the floor. This serves to support the instrument Finger biomechanisms are similar to violin/viola. The fingerboard is located left to the head	Similar to conditions seen in violinists/violas
Contrabass	Sometimes considered string or wind instrument Larger instrument requiring the musician to stand or sit on a high stool Requires prolonged flexion of the cervical, thoracic, and lumbar spine String grip is different from other string instruments. The forearm is supine when gripping the bow	Cervical, thoracic, and lumbar back pain
Brass Trumpet Trombone Tuba French horn Cornet Saxophone Bugle	Lumbrical activation, abnormal finger extension is common Repetitive mouth movements Prolonged stabilization of spine while leaning forward	Hand dystonia Embouchure dystonia Cervical neck and back pain
Electronic Keyboard Guitar		Hand dystonia
Percussion Drums Cymbals Triangle Chimes Tam-tam Glockenspiel Timpani Bells Xylophone	Repeated snapping of the wrists and fingers	Intersection syndrome Epicondylitis
Piano	Abnormal flexion in the right hand Overuse of wrist Posture affected scapula biomechanics	Hand dystonia De Quervain's tenosynovitis; CMC joint arthritis Scapulothoracic bursitis

Orthobiologics

The use of orthobiologics for the management of musculoskeletal injuries is a relatively recent practice. Orthobiologics are biological substances that promote ligament repair, tendon healing, regeneration of cartilage, and bone formation. Biological substances that are commonly used in modern orthopedic practices include platelet-rich plasma (PRP), stem cells, bone grafts, hyaluronic acid, and autologous blood products [165–169].

General consensus on the benefit of orthobiologics is still lacking, but their minimally invasive nature (e.g., injection) suggests an appealing therapeutic role [166]. Insurance may however not cover or supplement the cost of orthobiologics for the treatment of musculoskeletal conditions.

PRMDs affecting instrumental musicians are mostly influenced by hyaluronic acid and platelet-rich plasma orthobiologics. Hyaluronic acid (HA) is a substance that is normally present in the extracellular matrix of tissues. Its molecular structure is characterized by a network of non-sulfated glycosaminoglycan with viscoelastic properties [166]. HA is most widely studied in the treatment of joint disorders and osteoarthritis but is also used in tendon pathologies (e.g., trigger finger) and other soft tissue conditions (e.g., ganglion cysts) [167, 168]. The proposed beneficial mechanism of HA includes analgesic effect, anti-inflammatory effect, and protection of chondrocytes (cartilage-producing cells) and subchondral bone. Its use for tendon injury is not well established, but increased collagen production has been suggested in rotator cuff disease, a reasonable consideration for musicians wanting to pursue conservative treatment options. HA has shown to be useful in other treatments of the shoulder including adhesive capsulitis and glenohumeral joint osteoarthritis. HA has been less successful in osteoarthritis of the elbow; however, based on one randomized control trial, it may have a role in the treatment of elbow epicondylitis [167]. HA has yet to show superior benefit to placebo or corticosteroid injections in the treatment of injured small joints (e.g., hand joints). Newer techniques for the prevention of ganglion cyst recurrence following aspiration include injected hyaluronidase into the cyst [167]. Studies are however not promising as they show a 77% recurrence in the hyaluronidase group compared to 24% in the surgery group [167]. HA injections are well-tolerated, and adverse effects are infrequent, and previously reported serious adverse events were not related to this agent [168].

Platelet-rich plasma (PRP) is a high-platelet volume substance fractioned by different methodologies from autologous blood and with reasonable safety profile [169]. PRP is used in a variety of musculoskeletal pathologies, but for the intent of this chapter, focus is placed on PRP prolotherapy of musculoskeletal conditions affecting the upper extremities in instrumental musicians. Prolotherapy is a regenerative type of injection therapy aimed at ameliorating pain and function in tendinopathies. Recovery from damaged tendons can be a slow and tedious process, frustrating and detrimental to a musician's performance. PRP may stimulate a healing response by enhancing the secretion of growth factors, by increasing synthesis of collagen and glycosaminoglycan, and by activating specific genes that may accelerate tendon repair [170]. Epicondylitis and rotator cuff injuries are common among instrumental musicians. Clinical trials and meta-analyses studies have however shown results inconsistent with those derived from experimental models. To date, three clinical trials have not provided a strong evidence for PRP as an effective option for epicondylitis, while a systemic review and meta-analysis study of randomized clinical trials found improvement in pain, when comparing PRP with autologous blood and glucocorticoid injection [171]. PRP may be considered in refractory cases of lateral epicondylitis in musicians desiring conservative treatment options [172].

Conclusions

Musicians are at high risk for developing playing-related musculoskeletal disorders including overuse injuries, neuropathies, and motor control disorders. Discomfort and dysfunction can seriously affect and even end the career of instrumental musicians.

Longitudinal studies assessing both incidence and prevalence are needed to better identify risk factors for PRMDs in musicians. Much of the literature assessing PRMD in these performing artists is centered around retrospective questionnaires where accuracy of information may be affected by errors of recall. A variety of better testing methods are needed to obtain more definitive data. Further studies to assess differences in PRMDs among musicians based on gender, age, and other nonmusician populations are also needed. Understanding the role that genetics plays in PRMDs may offer further insight into better prevention and treatment of PRMDs. Expanding investigations on preventative strategies through educational programs for instrumental musicians is essential. Adapting educational, prevention, and *nutrition* programs as well as therapy regimens directed to sports athletes may provide an additional tool to the current care of instrumentalists with PRMDs. More information on orthobiologics and their use in the treatment of PRMD would be also highly beneficial to musician desiring to avoid nonconservative treatment options that may be associated with loss of motion.

It is imperative that professionals caring for instrumentalists appreciate that music making may not only be a beloved hobby but a committed profession that is also a financial source of income. Recognition of musculoskeletal conditions and early intervention are essential to care for the musician population effectively. Instrumental musicians deserve customized research studies directed to determining how they are affected by PRMDs in addition to tailored education programs, therapy regimens, and treatment approaches.

References

1. Lederman RJ. Neuromuscular and musculoskeletal problems in instrumental musicians. Muscle Nerve. 2003;27(5):549–61. https://doi.org/10.1002/mus.10380.
2. Hoppmann R. Musculoskeletal problems of instrumental musicians. In: Sataloff RT, Brandfonbrener AG, Lederman RJ, editors. Performing arts medicine. 3rd ed. Narberth, PA: Science and Medicine Inc; 2010.
3. Holder N, Clark H, DiBlasio J, Hughes C, Scherpf J, Harding L, Shepard K. Cause, prevalence, and response to occupational musculoskeletal injuries reported by physical therapists and physical therapist assistants. Phys Ther. 1999;79(7):642–52.
4. Steinmetz A, Scheffer I, Esmer E, Delank K, Peroz I. Frequency, severity and predictors of playing-related musculoskeletal pain in professional orchestral musicians in Germany. Clin Rheumatol. 2014;34(5):965–73.
5. Paarup H, Baelum J, Holm J, Manniche C, Wedderkopp N. Prevalence and consequences of musculoskeletal symptoms in symphony orchestra musicians vary by gender: a cross-sectional study. BMC Musculosket Disord. 2011;12(1):223–36.
6. Leaver R, Harris E, Palmer K. Musculoskeletal pain in elite professional musicians from British symphony orchestras. Occup Med. 2011;61(8):549–55.
7. Kenny D, Ackermann B. Performance-related musculoskeletal pain, depression and music performance anxiety in professional orchestral musicians: a population study. Psychol Music. 2013;43(1):43–60.
8. Myer GD, Jayanthi N, Difiori JP, Faigenbaum AD, Kiefer AW, Logerstedt D, Micheli LJ. Sports specialization, part II: alternative solutions to early sport specialization in youth athletes. Sports Health. 2016;8(1):65–73.
9. Zaza C, Farewell V. Musicians' playing-related musculoskeletal disorders: an examination of risk factors. Am J Ind Med. 1997;32(3):292–300.
10. Guptill C. The lived experience of working as a musician with an injury. Work. 2011;40(3):269–80.
11. Guptill C. Injured professional musicians and the complex relationship between occupation and health. J Occup Sci. 2012;19(3):258–70.
12. Raymond D, Romeo J, Kumke K. A pilot study of occupational injury and illness experienced by classical musicians. Workplace Health Saf. 2012;60(1):19–24.
13. Jiandani M, Mhatre B. Physical therapy diagnosis: how is it different? J Postgrad Med. 2018;64(2):67–92.
14. Altenmüller E, Jabusch H. Focal dystonia in musicians: phenomenology, pathophysiology and triggering factors. Eur J Neurol. 2010;17:31–6.
15. Baadjou VAE, Roussel NA, Verbunt JAMCF, Smeets RJEM, Bie RAD. Systematic review: risk factors for musculoskeletal disorders in musicians. Occup Med. 2016;66(8):614–22.
16. Watson A. What can studying musicians tell us about motor control of the hand? J Anat. 2006;208(4):527–42.
17. Hoenig K, Müller C, Herrnberger B, Sim E, Spitzer M, Ehret G, et al. Neuroplasticity of semantic representations for musical instruments in professional musicians. Neuroimage. 2011;56(3):1714–25.
18. Chan C, Ackermann B. Evidence-informed physical therapy management of performance-related musculoskeletal disorders in musicians. Front Psychol. 2014;5:706–19.
19. Kannus P, Parkkari J, Järvinen T, Järvinen T, Järvinen M. Basic science and clinical studies coincide: active treatment is needed after a sports injury. Scand J Med Sci Sports. 2003;13:150–4.
20. Lee SH. Performing arts medicine collaborative: prevention and rehabilitation. Invited panel symposium: DIVA: Drum Corp, Disney, and Dystonia: Exploring Performing Arts Medicine. American College of Sports Medicine 66th annual meeting. Orlando, Florida, May 29–June 1, 2019.

21. Järvinen T, Järvinen T, Kääriäinen M, Äärimaa V, Vaittinen S, Kalimo H, et al. Muscle injuries: optimizing recovery. Best Pract Res Clin Rheumatol. 2007;21(2):317–31.
22. Kok L, Vlieland T, Fiocco M, Nelissen R. A comparative study on the prevalence of musculoskeletal complaints among musicians and non-musicians. BMC Musculoskelet Disord. 2013;14(1):9–15.
23. Kok L. The high prevalence of playing-related musculoskeletal disorders (PRMDs) and its associated factors in amateur musicians playing in student orchestras: a cross-sectional study. PLoS One. 2018;13(2):e0191772.
24. Kaufman-Cohen Y, Ratzon N. Correlation between risk factors and musculoskeletal disorders among classical musicians. Occup Med. 2011;61(2):90–5.
25. Stahl C, Frucht S. Focal task specific dystonia: a review and update. J Neurol. 2016;264(7):1536–41.
26. Ackermann B, Kenny D, O'Brien I, Driscoll T. Sound practice improving occupational health and safety for professional orchestral musicians in Australia. Front Psychol. 2014;5:973–83.
27. Miller K, Quigley B. Sensation-seeking, performance genres and substance use among musicians. Psychol Music. 2011;40(4):389–410.
28. Bijsterbosch J, Watt I, Meulenbelt I, Rosendaal FR, Huizinga TWJ, Kloppenburg M. Clinical and radiographic disease course of hand osteoarthritis and determinants of outcome after 6 years. Ann Rheum Dis. 2010;70:68–73.
29. Williams WV, Cope R, Gaunt WD, Adelstein EH, Hoyt TS, Singh A, Pressly TA, English BR, Ralph HS, Walker SE. Metacarpophalangeal arthropathy associated with manual labor (Missouri metacarpal syndrome). Clinical, radiographic, and pathologic characteristics of an unusual degenerative process. Arthritis Rheum. 1987;30:1362–71.
30. Christensen J, Johansen S, Knardahl S. Psychological predictors of change in the number of musculoskeletal pain sites among Norwegian employees: a prospective study. BMC Musculoskelet Disord. 2017;18:140–52.
31. Dommerholt J. Performing arts medicine – instrumentalist musicians part I – general considerations. J Bodyw Mov Ther. 2009;13(4):311–9.
32. Berque P, Gray H, McFadyen A. Playing-related musculoskeletal disorders among professional orchestra musicians in Scotland – a prevalence study using a validated instrument: the musculoskeletal pain intensity and interference questionnaire for musicians (MPIIQM). Med Probl Perform Art. 2016;31(2):78–86.
33. Bekerom MPVD, Struijs PA, Blankevoort L, Welling L, Dijk CNV, Kerkhoffs GM. What is the evidence for rest, ice, compression, and elevation therapy in the treatment of ankle sprains in adults? J Athl Train. 2012;47:435–43.
34. Shafer-Crane G. Repetitive stress and strain injuries: preventive exercises for the musician. Phys Med Rehabil Clin N Am. 2006;17:827–42.
35. Wilke C, Priebus J, Biallas B, Froböse I. Motor activity as a way of preventing musculoskeletal problems in string musicians. Med Probl Perform Art. 2011;26(1):24–9.
36. Foxman I, Burgel BJ. Musician health and safety. AAOHN J. 2006;54:309–16.
37. Smidt N, de Vet H, Bouter L, Dekker J. Effectiveness of exercise therapy: a best-evidence summary of systematic reviews. Aust J Physiother. 2005;51(2):71–85.
38. Thomas DT, Erdman KA, Burke LM. American College of Sports Medicine Joint position statement: nutrition and athletic performance. Med Sci Sports Exerc. 2016;48:543–68.
39. Ko K-J, Ha G-C, Kim D-W, Kang S-J. Effects of lower extremity injuries on aerobic exercise capacity, anaerobic power, and knee isokinetic muscular function in high school soccer players. J Phys Ther Sci. 2017;29:1715–9.
40. Chan C, Driscoll T, Ackermann B. Development of a specific exercise programme for professional orchestral musicians. Inj Prev. 2012;19:257–63.
41. Chan C, Driscoll T, Ackermann B. Exercise DVD effect on musculoskeletal disorders in professional orchestral musicians. Occup Med. 2012;64:23–30.
42. Popkin BM, Danci KE, Rosenberg IH. Water, hydration, and health. Nutr Rev. 2010;68(8):439–58.

43. Hasson D, Theorell T, Liljeholm-Johansson Y, Canlon B. Psychosocial and physiological correlates of self-reported hearing problems in male and female musicians in symphony orchestras. Int J Psychophysiol. 2009;74:93–100.
44. Miller KE, Quigley BM. Energy drink use and substance use among musicians. J Caffeine Res. 2011;1:67–73.
45. Hernández SO, Zarza-Alzugaray FJ, Casanova O. Music performance anxiety. Substance use and career abandonment in Spanish music students. Int J Music Educ. 2018;36:460–72.
46. Hansson KG, Kendall HO, Kendall FP, Boynton DA. Posture and pain. JBJS. 1956;38(2):474–3.
47. O'Sullivan K, O'Sullivan P, O'Sullivan L, Dankaerts W. What do physiotherapists consider to be the best sitting spinal posture? Man Ther. 2102;7:432–7.
48. Price K, Watson A. Effect of using Ergobrass ergonomic supports on postural muscles in trumpet, trombone, and French horn players. Med Probl Perform Art. 2018;33(3):183–90.
49. Lundborg B, Grooten W. Resistance training for professional string musicians: a prospective intervention study. Med Probl Perform Art. 2018;33(2):102–10.
50. Windt J, Gabbett TJ. How do training and competition workloads relate to injury? The workload—injury aetiology model. Br J Sports Med. 2016;51:428–35.
51. Chéron C, Le Scanff C, Leboeuf-Yde C. Association between sports type and overuse injuries of extremities in adults: a systematic review. Chiropr Man Therap. 2017;25:4. https://doi.org/10.1186/s12998-017-0135-1.
52. Scott A, Backman LJ, Seed C. Tendinopathy: update on pathophysiology. J Orthop Sports Phys Ther. 2015;45:833–41.
53. Cook JL, Rio E, Purdam CR, Docking SI. Revisiting the continuum model of tendon pathology: what is its merit in clinical practice and research? Br J Sports Med. 2016;50:1187–91.
54. Abate M, Gravare-Silbernage K, Siljeholm C, Di Iorio A, De Amicis D, Salini V, Werner S, Paganelli R. Pathogenesis of tendinopathies: inflammation or degeneration? Arthritis Res Ther. 2009;11:235–51.
55. Dean BJF, Lostis E, Oakley T, Rombach I, Morrey ME, Carr AJ. The risks and benefits of glucocorticoid treatment for tendinopathy: a systematic review of the effects of local glucocorticoid on tendon. Semin Arthritis Rheum. 2014;43:570–6.
56. Khaliq Y, Zhanel GG. Fluoroquinolone-associated tendinopathy: a critical review of the literature. Clin Infect Dis. 2003;36:1404–10.
57. Kirchgesner T, Larbi A, Omoumi P, Malghem J, Zamali N, Manelfe J, Lecouvet F, Berg BV, Djebbar S, Dallaudière B. Drug-induced tendinopathy: from physiology to clinical applications. Joint Bone Spine. 2014;81:485–92.
58. Marie I, Delafenêtre H, Massy N, Thuillez C, Noblet C. Tendinous disorders attributed to statins: a study on ninety-six spontaneous reports in the period 1990–2005 and review of the literature. Arthritis Rheum. 2008;59:367–72.
59. Lundgreen K, Lian ØB, Scott A, Nassab P, Fearon A, Engebretsen L. Rotator cuff tear degeneration and cell apoptosis in smokers versus nonsmokers. Arthroscopy. 2014;30:936–41.
60. Khan K. Management of tendinopathy. Yearbook Sports Med. 2010;2010:55.
61. Evelyn Bass LMT. Tendinopathy: why the difference between tendinitis and tendinosis matters. Int J Ther Massage Bodywork. 2012;5(1):14–7.
62. Khan KM, Cook JL, Taunton JE, Bonar F. Overuse tendinosis, not tendinitis. Phys Sportsmed. 2000;28:38–48.
63. Chaitow L. Massage therapy: a profession in search of future directions? J Bodyw Mov Ther. 2013;17(3):269–70.
64. Chatterjee R, Vyas J. Diagnosis and management of intersection syndrome as a cause of overuse wrist pain. BMJ Case Rep. 2016;2016. https://doi.org/10.1136/bcr-2016-216988.
65. Wilson RJ, Watson JT, Lee DH. Nerve entrapment syndromes in musicians. Clin Anat. 2014;27:861–5.
66. Dawson DM. Entrapment neuropathies: clinical overview. Hosp Pract. 1995;30:37–44.

67. Radhakrishnan K, Litchy WJ, Ofallon WM, Kurland LT. Epidemiology of cervical radiculopathy. Brain. 1994;117:325–35.
68. Lederman RJ. Focal peripheral neuropathies in instrumental musicians. Phys Med Rehabil Clin N Am. 2006;17(4):761–79.
69. Jho H. Microsurgical anterior cervical foraminotomy for radiculopathy: a new approach to cervical disc herniation. J Neurosurg. 1996;4(2):155–60.
70. Dahlin LB, Wiberg M. Nerve injuries of the upper extremity and hand. EFORT Open Rev. 2017;2(5):158–70.
71. Nardin RA, Patel MR, Gudas TF, Rutkove SB, Raynor EM. Electromyography and magnetic resonance imaging in the evaluation of radiculopathy. Muscle Nerve. 1999;22:151–5.
72. Bland J. Carpal tunnel syndrome. Curr Opin Int Med. 2005;4(6):578–82.
73. Bickel KD. Carpal tunnel syndrome. J Hand Surg. 2010;35:147–52.
74. Muller M, Tsui D, Schnurr R, Biddulph-Deisroth L, Hard J, Macdermid JC. Effectiveness of hand therapy interventions in primary management of carpal tunnel syndrome: a systematic review. J Hand Ther. 2004;17:210–28.
75. Walker WC, Metzler M, Cifu DX, Swartz Z. Neutral wrist splinting in carpal tunnel syndrome: a comparison of night-only versus full-time wear instructions. Arch Phys Med Rehabil. 2000;81:424–9.
76. Gooch CL, Mitten DJ. Treatment of carpal tunnel syndrome: is there a role for local corticosteroid injection? Neurology. 2005;64:2006–7.
77. Ly-Pen D, Andréu J-L, Blas GD, Sánchez-Olaso A, Millán I. Surgical decompression versus local steroid injection in carpal tunnel syndrome: a one-year, prospective, randomized, open, controlled clinical trial. Arthritis Rheum. 2005;52:612–9.
78. O'Connor D, Marshall S, Massy-Westropp N. Non-surgical treatment (other than steroid injection) for carpal tunnel syndrome. Cochrane Database Syst Rev. 2003;2003(1):CD003219.
79. Verdugo R, Salinas R, Castillo J, Cea G. Surgical versus non-surgical treatment for carpal tunnel syndrome. Cochrane Database Syst Rev. 2008;8(4):CD001552.
80. Waldman SD. Thoracic outlet syndrome. In: Atlas of common pain syndromes. St. Louis: Elsevier/Saunders; 2012. p. 77–9.
81. Wojcik G, Sokolowska B, Piskorz J. Epidemiology and pathogenesis of thoracic outlet syndrome. Curr Issues Pharm Med Sci. 2015;28:24–6.
82. Klaassen Z, Sorenson E, Tubbs R, Arya R, Meloy P, Shah R, et al. Thoracic outlet syndrome: a neurological and vascular disorder. Clin Anat. 2013;27(5):724–32.
83. Kuhn JE, Lebus GF, Bible JE. Thoracic outlet syndrome. J Am Acad Orthop Surg. 2015;23:222–32.
84. Axelrod DA, Proctor MC, Geisser ME, Roth RS, Greenfield LJ. Outcomes after surgery for thoracic outlet syndrome. J Vasc Surg. 2001;33:1220–5.
85. Franklin GM, Fulton-Kehoe D, Bradley C, Smith-Weller T. Outcome of surgery for thoracic outlet syndrome in Washington state workers compensation. Neurology. 2000;54:1252–8.
86. Newington L, Harris EC, Walker-Bone K, et al. Carpal tunnel syndrome and work. Best Pract Res Clin Rheumathol. 2015;29:440–53.
87. Bachoura A, Jacoby SM. Ulnar tunnel syndrome. Orthop Clin North Am. 2012;43:467–74.
88. An TW, Evanoff BA, Boyer MI, Osei DA. The prevalence of cubital tunnel syndrome. J Bone Joint Surg. 2017;99:408–16.
89. Chen S-H, Tsai T-M. Ulnar tunnel syndrome. J Hand Surg. 2014;39:571–9.
90. Latinovic R. Incidence of common compressive neuropathies in primary care. J Neurol Neurosurg Psychiatry. 2006;77:263–5.
91. Frost P, Johnsen B, Fuglsang-Frederiksen A, Svendsen SW. Lifestyle risk factors for ulnar neuropathy and ulnar neuropathy-like symptoms. Muscle Nerve. 2013;48(4):507–15.
92. Campbell W. Ulnar neuropathy at the elbow. Muscle Nerve. 2000;23(4):450–2.
93. Svernlöv B, Larsson M, Rehn K, Adolfsson L. Conservative treatment of the cubital tunnel syndrome. J Hand Surg. 2009;34:201–7.

94. Shah C, Calfee R, Gelberman R, Goldfarb C. Outcomes of rigid night splinting and activity modification in the treatment of cubital tunnel syndrome. J Hand Surg. 2013;38(6):1125–30.
95. Szabo R, Kwak C. Natural history and conservative management of cubital tunnel syndrome. Hand Clin. 2007;23(3):311–8.
96. Padua L, Aprile I, Caliandro P, Foschini M, Mazza S, Tonali P. Natural history of ulnar entrapment at elbow. Clin Neurophysiol. 2002;113(12):1980–4.
97. Iyer S, Kim HJ. Cervical radiculopathy. Curr Rev Musculoskelet Med. 2016;9:272–80.
98. Lee H-S, Park HY, Yoon JO, Kim JS, Chun JM, Aminata IW, Cho W-J, Jeon I-H. Musicians medicine: musculoskeletal problems in string players. Clin Orthop Surg. 2013;5:155–60.
99. Wong JJ, Côté P, Quesnele JJ, Stern PJ, Mior SA. The course and prognostic factors of symptomatic cervical disc herniation with radiculopathy: a systematic review of the literature. Spine J. 2014;14(8):1781–9.
100. Fouyas I, Sandercock P, Statham P, Nikolaidis I. How beneficial is surgery for cervical radiculopathy and myelopathy? BMJ. 2010;341(jul13 2):c3108.
101. Aaron DL, Patel A, Kayiaros S, Calfee R. Four common types of bursitis: diagnosis and management. J Am Acad Orthop Surg. 2011;19:359–67.
102. Blackwell JR, Hay BA, Bolt AM, Hay SM. Olecranon bursitis: a systematic overview. Shoulder Elbow. 2014;6:182–90.
103. Cools AM. Evaluation of isokinetic force production and associated muscle activity in the scapular rotators during a protraction-retraction movement in overhead athletes with impingement symptoms. Br J Sports Med. 2004;38:64–8.
104. Kerr DR, Carpenter CW. Arthroscopic resection of olecranon and prepatellar bursae. Arthroscopy. 1990;6:86–8.
105. Stewart NJ, Manzanares JB, Morrey BF. Surgical treatment of aseptic olecranon bursitis. J Shoulder Elbow Surg. 1997;6:49–54.
106. Koester MC, George MS, Kuhn JE. Shoulder impingement syndrome. Am J Med. 2005;118:452–5.
107. Watts AR, Williams B, Kim SW, Bramwell DC, Krishnan J. Shoulder impingement syndrome: a systematic review of clinical trial participant selection criteria. Shoulder Elbow. 2016;9:31–41.
108. Khan M, Alolabi B, Horner N, Bedi A, Ayeni O, Bhandari M. Surgery for shoulder impingement: a systematic review and meta-analysis of controlled clinical trials. CMAJ Open. 2019;7(1):E149–58.
109. Hani Zreik N, Malik R, Charalambous C. Adhesive capsulitis of the shoulder and diabetes: a meta-analysis of prevalence. Muscles Ligaments Tendons J. 2019;6(01):26–34.
110. Wong C, Levine W, Deo K, Kesting R, Mercer E, Schram G, Strang B. Natural history of frozen shoulder: fact or fiction? A systematic review. Physiotherapy. 2017;103:40–7.
111. Hand C, Clipsham K, Rees JL, Carr AJ. Long-term outcome of frozen shoulder. J Shoulder Elbow Surg. 2008;17:231–6.
112. Carette S, Moffet H, Tardif J, et al. Intraarticular corticosteroids, supervised physiotherapy, or a combination of the two in the treatment of adhesive capsulitis of the shoulder: a placebo-controlled trial. Arthritis Rheum. 2003;48:829–38.
113. Buchbinder R, Green S, Youd J, Johnston R, Cumpston M. Arthrographic distension for adhesive capsulitis (frozen shoulder). Cochrane Database Syst Rev. 2008;23(1):CD07005.
114. Mun SW, Baek CH. Clinical efficacy of hydrodistention with joint manipulation under interscalene block compared with intra-articular corticosteroid injection for frozen shoulder: a prospective randomized controlled study. J Shoulder Elbow Surg. 2016;25:1937–43.
115. Rill BK, Fleckenstein CM, Levy MS, Nagesh V, Hasan SS. Predictors of outcome after non-operative and operative treatment of adhesive capsulitis. Am J Sports Med. 2010;39:567–74.
116. Chen D, Shen J, Zhao W, Wang T, Han L, Hamilton J, et al. Osteoarthritis: toward a comprehensive understanding of pathological mechanism. Bone Res. 2017;5(1):16044.

117. Loeser RF, Goldring SR, Scanzello CR, Goldring MB. Osteoarthritis: a disease of the joint as an organ. Arthritis Rheum. 2012;64:1697–07.
118. Anandacoomarasamy A, Caterson I, Sambrook P, Fransen M, March L. The impact of obesity on the musculoskeletal system. Int J Obes (Lond). 2007;32:211–22.
119. Appleton T. Year in review – osteoarthritis biology. Osteoarthr Cartil. 2017;25:S7.
120. Identification of new susceptibility loci for osteoarthritis (arcOGEN): a genome-wide association study. Lancet. 2012;380:815–23.
121. Bedson J, Croft P. The discordance between clinical and radiographic knee osteoarthritis: a systematic search and summary of the literature. BMC Musculoskelct Disord. 2008;9(1):116–26.
122. Gillis J, Calder K, Williams J. Review of thumb carpometacarpal arthritis classification, treatment and outcomes. Can J Plast Surg. 2011;19(4):134–8.
123. Moore JS. Flexor tendon entrapment of the digits (trigger finger and trigger thumb). J Occup Environ Med. 2000;42:526–45.
124. Sbernardori M, Bandiera P. Histopathology of the A1 pulley in adult trigger fingers. J Hand Surg. 2007;32(5):556–9.
125. Saldana MJ. Trigger digits: diagnosis and treatment. J Am Acad Orthop Surg. 2001;9:246–52.
126. Makkouk AH, Oetgen ME, Swigart CR, Dodds SD. Trigger finger: etiology, evaluation, and treatment. Curr Rev Musculoskelet Med. 2007;1:92–6.
127. Rozental T, Zurakowski D, Blazar P. Trigger finger: prognostic indicators of recurrence following corticosteroid injection. J Bone Joint Surg. 2008;90(8):1665–72.
128. Wojahn R, Foeger N, Gelberman R, Calfee R. Long-term outcomes following a single corticosteroid injection for trigger finger. J Bone Joint Surg. 2014;96(22):1849–54.
129. Ryzewicz M, Wolf JM. Trigger digits: principles, management, and complications. J Hand Surg. 2006;31:135–46.
130. Arn KGGR. Eighteen years follow-up study of the clinical manifestations and progression of Dupuytren's disease. Scand J Rheumatol. 2001;30:31–4.
131. Larocerie-Salgado J, Davidson J. Nonoperative treatment of PIPJ flexion contractures associated with Dupuytren's disease. J Hand Surg. 2011;37:722–7.
132. Peimer CA, Blazar P, Coleman S, Kaplan FTD, Smith T, Lindau T. Dupuytren contracture recurrence following treatment with collagenase clostridium histolyticum (CORDLESS [collagenase option for reduction of Dupuytren long-term evaluation of safety study]): 5-year data. J Hand Surg. 2015;40:1597–605.
133. Ball C, Izadi D, Verjee L, Chan J, Nanchahal J. Systematic review of non-surgical treatments for early Dupuytren's disease. BMC Musculoskelet Disord. 2016;17(1):345–61.
134. Giard M-C, Pineda C. Ganglion cyst versus synovial cyst? Ultrasound characteristics through a review of the literature. Rheumatol Int. 2014;35:597–605.
135. Salerni G, González R, Alonso C. Dermatoscopic pattern of digital mucous cyst: report of three cases. Dermatol Pract Concept. 2014;4(5):65–7.
136. Beaino ME, Araujo DM, Lazar AJ, Lin PP. Synovial sarcoma: advances in diagnosis and treatment identification of new biologic targets to improve multimodal therapy. Ann Surg Oncol. 2017;24:2145–54.
137. Suen M, Fung B, Lung C. Treatment of ganglion cysts. ISRN Orthop. 2013;2013:1–7.
138. Varley GW, Needoff M, Davis TRC, Clay NR. Conservative management of wrist ganglia. J Hand Surg. 1997;22:636–7.
139. Kang L, Akelman E, A-PC W. Arthroscopic versus open dorsal ganglion excision: a prospective, randomized comparison of rates of recurrence and of residual pain. J Hand Surg. 2008;33:471–5.
140. Bontempo NA, A-PC W. Arthroscopic excision of ganglion cysts. Hand Clin. 2014; 30:71–5.
141. Grahame R. Hypermobility: an important but often neglected area within rheumatology. Nat Clin Pract Rheumatol. 2008;4:522–4.

142. Lederman R. Alice G. Brandfonbrener, MD—a personal remembrance. Med Probl Perform Art. 2014;29(3):123–4.
143. Castori M, Dordoni C, Valiante M, et al. Nosology and inheritance pattern(s) of joint hypermobility syndrome and Ehlers-Danlos syndrome, hypermobility type: a study of intrafamilial and interfamilial variability in 23 Italian pedigrees. Am J Med Genet. 2014;164:3010–20.
144. Albanese A, Bhatia K, Bressman SB, et al. Phenomenology and classification of dystonia: a consensus update. Mov Disord. 2013;28:863–73.
145. Steeves TD, Day L, Dykeman J, Jette N, Pringsheim T. The prevalence of primary dystonia: a systematic review and meta-analysis. Mov Disord. 2012;27:1789–96.
146. Rozanski VE, Rehfuess E, Bötzel K, Nowak D. Task-specific dystonia in professional musicians. A systematic review of the importance of intensive playing as a risk factor. Dtsch Arztebl Int. 2015;112:871–7.
147. Adler CH, Crews D, Hentz JG, Smith AM, Caviness JN. Abnormal co-contraction in yips-affected but not unaffected golfers: evidence for focal dystonia. Neurology. 2005;64:1813–4.
148. Albanese A, Sorbo FD, Comella C, et al. Dystonia rating scales: critique and recommendations. Mov Disord. 2013;28:874–83.
149. Frucht SJ, Fahn S, Greene PE, Obrien C, Gelb M, Truong DD, Welsh J, Factor S, Ford B. The natural history of embouchure dystonia. Mov Disord. 2001;16:899–906.
150. Stojanović M, Cvetković D, Kostic VS. A genetic study of idiopathic focal dystonias. J Neurol. 1995;242:508–11.
151. Bäumer T, Schmidt A, Heldmann M, et al. Abnormal interhemispheric inhibition in musicians dystonia – trait or state? Parkinsonism Relat Disord. 2016;25:33–8.
152. Leijnse JNAL, Hallett M, Sonneveld GJ. A multifactorial conceptual model of peripheral neuromusculoskeletal predisposing factors in task-specific focal hand dystonia in musicians: etiologic and therapeutic implications. Biol Cybern. 2014;109:109–23.
153. Ioannou CI, Altenmüller E. Psychological characteristics in musician's dystonia: a new diagnostic classification. Neuropsychologia. 2014;61:80–8.
154. Beck S, Richardson SP, Shamim EA, Dang N, Schubert M, Hallett M. Short intracortical and surround inhibition are selectively reduced during movement initiation in focal hand dystonia. J Neurosci. 2008;28(41):10363–9.
155. Hallett M. Neurophysiology of dystonia: the role of inhibition. Neurobiol Dis. 2011;42:177–84.
156. Sohn YH, Hallett M. Disturbed surround inhibition in focal hand dystonia. Ann Neurol. 2004;56:595–9.
157. Bäumer T, Demiralay C, Hidding U, Bikmullina R, Helmich RC, Wunderlich S, Rothwell J, Liepert J, Siebner HR, Münchau A. Abnormal plasticity of the sensorimotor cortex to slow repetitive transcranial magnetic stimulation in patients with writer's cramp. Mov Disord. 2007;22:81–90.
158. Meunier S, Garnero L, Ducorps A, Mazières L, Lehéricy S, Montcel STD, Renault B, Vidailhet M. Human brain mapping in dystonia reveals both endophenotypic traits and adaptive reorganization. Ann Neurol. 2001;50(4):521–7.
159. Candia V, Schäfer T, Taub E, Rau H, Altenmüller E, Rockstroh B, Elbert T. Sensory motor retuning: a behavioral treatment for focal hand dystonia of pianists and guitarists. Arch Phys Med Rehabil. 2002;83:1342–8.
160. Ashkenazi A, Silberstein SD. Botulinum toxin and other new approaches to migraine therapy. Annu Rev Med. 2004;55:505–18.
161. Matak I, Lacković Z. Botulinum neurotoxin type A: actions beyond SNAP-25? Toxicology. 2015;335:79–84.
162. Bentivoglio AR, Del Grande A, Petracca M, Ialongo T, Ricciardi L. Clinical differences between botulinum neurotoxin type A and B toxins. Toxicon. 2015;93:S8–9.
163. Furuya S, Nitsche MA, Paulus W, Altenmüller E. Surmounting retraining limits in musicians dystonia by transcranial stimulation. Ann Neurol. 2014;75:700–7.
164. Enke A, Poskey G. Neuromuscular re-education programs for musicians with focal hand dystonia: a systematic review. Med Probl Perform Art. 2018;33:137–45.

165. Dhillon M, Patel S, Shetty V, Behera P. Orthobiologics and platelet rich plasma. Indian J Orthop. 2014;48(1):1–9.
166. Frizziero A. Six-months pain relief and functional recovery after intra-articular injections with hyaluronic acid (mw 500-730 kda) in trapeziometacarpal osteoarthritis. Muscles Ligaments Tendons J. 2014;4:256–61.
167. Jagers OP, Akkeruis M, Van Der Heuden M, Brink P. Hyaluronidase versus surgical excision of ganglia: a prospective, randomized clinical trial. J Hand Surg. 2002;27(3):256–8.
168. Oliveras-Moreno J-M, Hernandez-Pacheco E, Oliveras-Quintana T, Infante-Cossio P, Gutierrez-Perez J-L. Efficacy and safety of sodium hyaluronate in the treatment of Wilkes stage II disease. J Oral Maxillofac Surg. 2008;66:2243–6.
169. McCarrel T, Minas T, Fortier L. Optimization of leukocyte concentration in platelet-rich plasma for the treatment of tendinopathy. J Bone Joint Surg. 2012;94(19):e143(1–8).
170. Jo CH, Kim JE, Yoon KS, Shin S. Platelet-rich plasma stimulates cell proliferation and enhances matrix gene expression and synthesis in tenocytes from human rotator cuff tendons with degenerative tears. Am J Sports Med. 2012;40:1035–45.
171. Arirachakaran A, Sukthuayat A, Sisayanarane T, Laoratanavoraphong S, Kanchanatawan W, Kongtharvonskul J. Platelet-rich plasma versus autologous blood versus steroid injection in lateral epicondylitis: systematic review and network meta-analysis. J Orthop Traumatol. 2015;17:101–12.
172. Saltzman BM, Jain A, Campbell KA, Mascarenhas R, Romeo AA, Verma NN, Cole BJ. Does the use of platelet-rich plasma at the time of surgery improve clinical outcomes in arthroscopic rotator cuff repair when compared with control cohorts? A systematic review of meta-analyses. Arthroscopy. 2016;32:906–18.

Chapter 14
Experiences in Music Performance Anxiety: Exploration of Pedagogical Instruction Among Professional Musicians

Julia A. Clearman

Introduction

Since its identification during 1970–1985, music performance anxiety (MPA) has stayed a fairly misunderstood topic in the performance careers of professional musicians [1]. Exploration and research of MPA have been pursued mainly within the academic realm. Consequently, there is a void between what is known in academic research and the practical application of that research knowledge among musicians. MPA has remained widespread among performing musicians with as many as 50–70% of musicians admitting to experiencing MPA at some point in their careers [2–5].

Music performance anxiety, often known as "stage fright," is most commonly understood as a fear of live musical performance [2]. When the musician thinks about, or engages in, a live performance that is perceived as threatening or feared, the natural physiological "fight–flight–freeze" response is triggered [3]. Due to the work of Charles Darwin in the mid-nineteenth century, it is commonly understood that a fearful or threatening situation engages the autonomic nervous system preparing the victim to respond quickly with a "fight," "flight," or "freeze" response [6, 7]. This immediate response triggers the sympathetic nervous system signaling a release of additional adrenaline to the body to increase the chance of survival [7]. At this point, the victim chooses to fight the feared situation ("fight"), flee ("flight"), or stay still and hope for camouflage protection ("freeze"). When a performance initiates a feeling of fear within the brain of a musician, the automatic physiological reaction is to engage the "fight," "flight," or "freeze" response which often results in a debilitating impairment during musical performance [2]. This negative performing experience then strengthens the musician's fear of performing instigating a

J. A. Clearman (✉)
Wheaton College Graduate School, Wheaton, IL, USA

S.-H. Lee et al. (eds.), *Perspectives in Performing Arts Medicine Practice*,
https://doi.org/10.1007/978-3-030-37480-8_14

seemingly unbreakable cycle of MPA. The devastating consequence of a natural protective agency not only is troublesome for performing musicians but can also lead to a decision to end their careers in music far too early [2, 7, 8].

There are many possible reasons why live music performances could be perceived as threatening to the musician. The exact triggers for this fear vary widely between musicians and musical genres indicating that there is no single root cause for MPA. One study done by Perdomo-Guevara examined MPA in different genres and found that those who perform in nonclassical musical traditions, such as jazz, pop, folk, or rock, experience less performance anxiety than those performing in the classical musical tradition [9]. Nagel suggested that for some the experiences of MPA could stem from a fear of either success or failure [10]. Nagel further elucidated that parental expectations of success and failure could be a root cause for fearing performance. The performing musician might be more successful than the parents, inadvertently shaming the parents for their lack of success. The fear of failure might stem from the inability to meet parental expectations in performance causing a loss of love or affection from one or both parents. Additional studies suggest that triggers for MPA mainly emanate from both external and internal triggers with an internal "pressure from self" being the most prevalent [6]. Even these few studies illustrate the wide variation in academic research between explanations of what triggers MPA.

In their book *Psychology for Musicians*, Lehmann, Sloboda, and Woody expanded on what triggers MPA [11]. They grouped possible triggers into three distinct categories: "the person" (i.e., internal triggers), "the situation" (i.e., external triggers from either relaxed or pressurized performances), and "the musical task" (i.e., external triggers from either the difficulty of the music or the level of preparedness) [11]. The first category ("the person") is deeply rooted in what the individual musician brings to the performing situation. Items in this category often show similarity to trait anxiety (anxiety that comes from within a person) [12, 13], perfectionism [11], social anxiety (it is important to note here that MPA and social anxiety disorder differ distinctly in the duration of anxiety with social phobia being more continuous and MPA being more episodic) [14], and parental interaction affecting a musician's performance [5]. The second category ("the situation") emphasizes the impact of the actual performance with pressurized situations, such as juries, competitions, and auditions typically being agreed upon as being the most stressful types of performance situations [7, 15]. These types of performances are typically more stressful for young developing musicians who may lack experience and who have their new career dependent on being successful in these performances [16–18]. The third category ("the musical task") encompasses the actual technical skill of the musician performing. Factors in this type of category would be the musical preparedness of the musician, the difficulty of music being played, memory, and the developed experience of the musician to handle collaborative performances. This category parallels the idea of test anxiety which is a task- oriented anxiety. Measurable outcomes, pressure to perform well, and the possibility of negative results often reinforce a fear response within the individual during the test-taking experience. Consequently, this increases the level of anxiety attributed to thinking about and actually completing future tests [19, 20].

A succinct way of understanding the most common manifestations of MPA is to further elaborate the three categories identified by Lehmann, Sloboda, and Woody [20]. Internal characteristics, such as trait anxiety, perfectionism, emotional dysregulation, and parental interactions, may coincide with physiological challenges (nervousness, shaking, shortness of breath, nausea, rapid heart rate, sweating, hot flashes, and an inability to breathe). Situational or external factors may lead to negative thoughts, cognitive fog, fear of failure or success, dread of the public, and panic over a highly pressurized performance situation. Factors regarding musical ability and the musical task can produce memory loss, performance stress, an inability to articulate well-practiced music, worry over unchangeable performance factors, and the lack of opportunity to rehearse on the instrument or warm up before the performance. Within these different categories, the experiences of MPA often result in a chaotic mess of physiological, psychological, and emotional distress and can cause the musician to perform well below his or her ability [3].

Historical treatment of MPA can be classified in four different areas: drug or medical treatment, psychotherapy, body awareness (such as Alexander Technique or biofeedback), and skill acquisition training. The first treatment, and probably the most widely accepted treatment therapy for MPA, is the administration of a beta-blocker by a licensed physician [21, 22]. Beta-blockers are used predominantly because they block the uptake of epinephrine (adrenaline) subsequently maintaining a consistent heart rate and calming physiological sensations [23]. For many years, *propranolol* has been the preferred beta-blocker for treating MPA because of its rapid reduction of physical symptoms [23–26]. The second treatment is psychotherapy and more specifically cognitive-behavioral therapy (CBT). CBT has been successful in reducing some anxiety, particularly anxiety that originates from a more cognitive foundation [26–28]. Additionally, psychoanalytic therapy has been found to be helpful in some cases where the trigger for MPA is deeply interpersonal [29, 30]. The third treatment is body awareness through Alexander Technique and biofeedback. This treatment encourages musicians to become familiar with and engage relaxation during the stress, ultimately leading to higher proficiency in performance [31–33]. The fourth and final area for MPA treatment is skill acquisition training. The aim of skill acquisition training is to empower musicians to modify their own MPA through learning mental skills, memory techniques, and anxiety management. This has been found to successfully reduce experiences of MPA and increase performance proficiency [34–36].

With MPA being so intertwined with live performance, one wonders what is being done pedagogically to help reduce the experiences of MPA in the lives of musicians. The relationship between student and teacher is innately personal [37, 38]. Many music students look up to their teachers as role models in the music profession to provide support and guidance in the issues that will be faced in a music career [37]. In this unique role, the music teacher has the opportunity to deeply influence how developing musicians perceive music performance. However, only a few studies have examined how pedagogy could be used as an intervention for MPA [39, 40]. Picard concluded that certain aspects of cognitive processes could be isolated during the experiences of MPA and that teachers could influence these cognitive processes by helping the students come face to face with their MPA, ultimately "reframing" the negative cognitive patterns of MPA in students [39]. Robertson and Eisensmith suggested that teachers use their inimitable influence by using a "scratch pad pop-up model" to teach attention control techniques and thus eliminate distracted cognitions which could factor into MPA [40].

While these intervention ideas are helpful, there is a gap between the academic literature and established evidence-based pedagogy to address MPA. Teachers have an influential role in their student's performance development, and therefore it is important to develop informed pedagogical interventions for MPA. Interdisciplinary studies between psychologists and music teachers can bridge the gap toward reducing experiences of MPA, as well as prevent further enervating experiences of MPA. The purpose of the current study was to examine whether or not professional musicians had experienced a pedagogical intervention for MPA in their training and to what extent the intervention had influenced their MPA experience. The results of this study may help formulate a foundation to guide future pedagogical intervention strategies.

Method

Site of Study

This research study was conducted in a major city in the USA. Professional musicians from a large community music school and a private college were contacted via a mass faculty email. All musicians had completed higher education in music and had spent at least 5 years in a career of music performance and teaching. Those who self-identified as having experiences with music performance anxiety (MPA) were invited to volunteer for the study. Over 200 faculty were contacted and 20 responded by volunteering to participate. Six musicians were selected based on availability during end-of-semester concerts and recitals. Each participant was given a pseudonym for identification.

Participants

Evan With a family background in music, Evan played a brass instrument all throughout his childhood. He chose to pursue an undergraduate degree in music performance and went on to earn a graduate degree as well. Now, Evan is an accomplished brass player and performs frequently as a professional musician with orchestras and ensemble groups in the local community. A musician with natural charisma, Evan described music as "part of my identity" during his interview.

Ithaca Also growing up in a family that supported musical achievement heavily, Ithaca began her music lessons at a young age and spoke of her deep love of the violin as something that made her "feel good" about herself. She discovered a passion for teaching as a high school student, went on to get an undergraduate degree in music, and is now a professional music teacher at a local community arts school where she frequently performs in ensemble concerts.

Matt Growing up, Matt was placed in piano lessons by his parents but did not really dive into his musical learning until a bit later in life. He originally began his undergraduate degree under a different instrument, but ultimately switched to piano by the time he started graduate studies. Now as a professional pianist, Matt prefers accompanying over solo performance.

Jasmine Juggling clarinet and piano lessons all throughout high school, Jasmine is now an active performer in ensembles. She changed teachers frequently during those formative years and had intended to pursue something besides piano in college. Eventually, studies in music education and piano playing won out over her other interests. Jasmine maintains her professional performing career, while also teaching a substantial studio of young pianists.

Analise Her parents were aspiring musicians, and Analise's childhood memories are filled with music continuously flooding her home. She pursued music education in college and then went on to earn dual master's degrees. She now spends her time teaching a full-time studio of piano students and playing organ for her church.

Yanna For Yanna, piano lessons began with the "lady down the street" at a young age, and she grew up performing for recitals and festivals. She pursued both piano and music education during her undergraduate studies and then focused on performance studies during her master's degree. A dedicated musician, Yanna has more recently split her professional career between directing band classes for a local school, teaching piano lessons to her home studio, and being an adjunct professor at a college nearby.

Data Collection and Interview Questions

Participants were asked to take part in a 30-minute in-depth interview in person with the researcher. The interviews were audio recorded and then subsequently transcribed for analysis. At the beginning of the interview, the participants were told that the research was twofold: (1) exploring how individual musicians experience MPA and (2) inquiring into the presence of pedagogical assistance for MPA during pre-professional music education. Following an interview prompt script, the exploration into individual MPA experiences sample questions were as follows:

1. Can you tell me a little about your experience with MPA?
2. How have you seen MPA affect your performances (perhaps via emotional, physical, cognitive disruptions)?
3. Were there any specific triggers that seemed to increase or decrease your experiences with MPA?

After individual experiences of MPA were examined, the focus of the interview switched to inquiring about pedagogical interventions with questions like the following:

1. Can you think of a time when your teacher introduced ideas or discussed MPA with you during your lessons?
2. If yes, could you tell me more about what he or she said? If no, do you have any ideas on why that topic was avoided during lessons?
3. If you were given instruction on how to cope with MPA, what were some of those ideas, thoughts, or instructions and did you find these ideas helpful?

At the end of each interview, the participants were allowed to openly discuss other areas in which MPA had impacted their personal life and musical career.

Data Analysis

Interpretative phenomenological analysis (IPA) seeks to analyze qualitative data in a way that highlights personal experience and can be used in a single case study or in a multi-perspective research design that connects multiple relationships through a shared phenomenon [41]. IPA also allows participants the freedom to explore deeper understanding of their own experiences as they express to the researcher their personal views, experiences, and understood life stories [42–44]. The process of IPA begins by grounding the analysis in the narrative nature of the data. It then moves beyond the data into different levels of interpretive and psychological conceptualization often by discovering interconnected emergent themes [45]. IPA has been used widely across disciplines, from understanding the personal stories behind addiction treatment to illustrating the sufferings of Parkinson's disease, with each use of IPA organizing findings into explanatory themes [46, 47]. Integrating IPA into understanding individual musical experiences has previously been used in studies covering topics of music therapy, amateur keyboard players, and experiences of MPA in undergraduate music students [48–50]. For this study, IPA was applied directly to experiences of MPA in post-education, professional musicians and to experiences of pedagogical interventions utilized to ameliorate performance success.

IPA was done in six steps. Step one included an initial auditory review of the interview recordings during which four emergent themes were observed. Step two was the transcription of the audio files during which personal statements and direct references to the four emergent themes were highlighted for future review. Step three gathered all data related to the emergent themes and reviewed each statement carefully to ensure compatibility with the specific theme. In step four, emergent theme data were coded separately, and connections to specific themes across all data were observed. In step five, each interview transcript was reviewed case by case to ensure that individual differences were not overlooked. The final step six organized the categorical data into a new conceptualized model of IPA for understanding individual experiences of MPA. This new conceptualization model was titled *Four Systems Model of Interpretative Phenomenological Analysis for Music Performance Anxiety* (4SM of IPA for MPA).

Results

Four Systems Model of Interpretative Phenomenological Analysis for Music Performance Anxiety

The development of 4SM of IPA for MPA identified four themes that were present in all participants' recollection of MPA experiences (Fig. 14.1). The four themes were (1) *initial onset*; (2) *rehearsed anxiety*; (3) *physical, psychological, and emotional manifestations of MPA*; and (4) *a lack of helpful pedagogical assistance*. During the first theme, *initial onset*, the musician could usually point back to a specific time or memory where MPA was felt for the first time. After the initial onset, the same initial anxiety would resurface and sometimes intensify in subsequent performances leading to the second theme of *rehearsed anxiety*. Each time MPA would appear in a performance, the anxiety response would be rehearsed in the mind of the musician solidifying and conditioning this anxiety response into music performance. Additionally, the third theme, *physical, psychological, and emotional manifestations of MPA*, produced a myriad of different symptoms that would attach to the rehearsed anxiety response

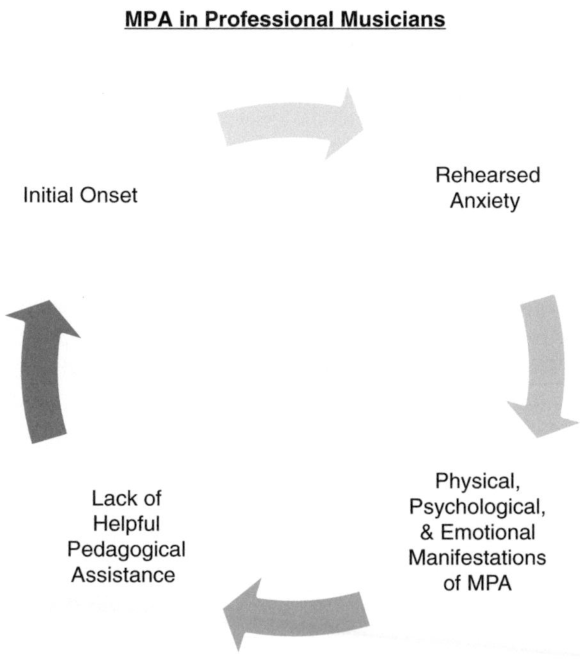

Fig. 14.1 Four systems model of interpretative phenomenological analysis for music performance anxiety (4SM of IPA for MPA)

initiating a visceral response. Taken together, the rehearsed anxiety and the physical, psychological, and emotional manifestations of MPA could consequently produce an additional anxiety response to the uncomfortable symptomatic manifestations of MPA causing the musician to both fear the performance and the symptoms of MPA that were initiated by the performance. Wrapped in a cycle of MPA, the first line of defense would be to turn to the musician's teacher to find guidance or advice to seek professional psychological and medical help for MPA suffering. However, turning to the music teacher to seek help for MPA most frequently did not provide an adequate source of assistance even if the music teacher tried to intervene. This phenomenon suggested that music educators may not be fully equipped to support students who experience MPA either in private lessons or by directing students to professional psychological and/or medical intervention. This concept developed the fourth and final theme of a *lack of helpful pedagogical assistance.*

Theme One: Initial Onset

The initial onset of MPA took several different forms in the participant musicians but was most typically one of the following: a shameful or humiliating event in high school or college, a new high-pressured performance, or comparative anxiety (anxiety that arises due to comparing oneself with an idealized standard or person). For both Matt and Jasmine, the onset of MPA happened at a specific traumatic event. In the following, Matt's memory vividly illustrates what a humiliating performance experience leading to an initial onset of MPA can look like:

> **Matt**: I remember one masterclass that I was accompanying [*in college*]. I really didn't know what I was doing. It was some Brahms song. This was before YouTube, and you had to go to the library and get the album. I don't know if I even ever listened to it, and we played it, and this was probably the most humiliating thing that ever happened to me in my life. The presenter of the masterclass just tapped me on the shoulder and said, "Do you mind?" He moved me off the bench and then he accompanied her [*the singer*] and it was a completely different song [*at*] a completely different tempo. I didn't even recognize what he was playing! I was mortified. I held it together, but on the way back to my apartment, I just lost it. And that was [*when*] the "you can't play, you weren't prepared" [*thoughts started*] and then the self-doubt would come [*with a*] "you aren't very good" [*recurring thought*].

Matt's memory of humiliation during performance began a pattern of negative thoughts laced with anxiety that eventually became entrenched in the idea of performance. This experience for Matt is what triggered the initial onset of MPA.

The initial onset of MPA for Yanna, Ithaca, and Analise came through the experiences of pressurized performances during which some type of consequential outcome is connected with how successful the performance is completed. Examples of pressurized performances are peer performances, juries, auditions, and professional performances. When one does not perform as well as expected, pressurized performances can trigger the onset of performance anxiety. In the words of Yanna:

> **Yanna**: I started feeling [*MPA*] most once I got to college and was tackling harder pieces; the stakes seemed to be higher with juries, and more frequent performances. We [*are*] talking about Friday music hours where you were playing in front of your peers, and then I did

a couple of competitions. At that point, and I blew it, like I played just poorly. It was one of those "I can't believe I played like this" moments. I was prepared, I had worked hard, this had never happened before. What happened? It was like I was in there and then I would blank. I would forget, panic, all those terrible feelings, and then the problem with that was that I carried all that baggage to each performance with this fear of like, "I could completely lose it" and then I would, basically.

Evan's initial onset of MPA was different than the other participants and came through comparative anxiety. In his memory, he felt MPA for the first time while in high school because he compared himself to a peer player and did not measure up to the perceived high standard of this peer's playing. In all six of the participants' stories, the initial onset of MPA happened in a unique way often after many years of music performances where no MPA had previously been experienced.

Theme Two: Rehearsed Anxiety

Rehearsed anxiety is a concept that was developed during the data analysis of this study. The conceptualization of rehearsed anxiety follows a similar process of music performance from the selection of a specific song to the full realization of that selection during live performance. The musician identifies a selection, becomes familiar with it, and then rehearses it until it is able to be executed with full mastery during performance. Rehearsed anxiety operates the same way. MPA surfaces through an initial onset (selection), is identified in the central nervous system as being a valid anxiety response to performance (familiarization), and then is rehearsed (rehearsal) with each subsequent performance culminating in perpetual experiences of MPA. Each continued anxiety-ridden performance makes the response of rehearsed anxiety stronger even if the initial factors which caused the onset of that anxiety are no longer present. The rehearsed anxiety then solidifies the physiological, psychological, and emotional symptoms which often alter the musician's perception of performance into a new pattern of expected MPA at each performance. All participants indicated that this conceptualization of rehearsed anxiety described some part of their experiences of MPA. Evan's story is particularly salient as he explains his interactions with rehearsed anxiety in the following:

Evan: [*During my undergraduate degree*], I remember starting to get really bad dry-mouth. I couldn't breathe. I would like shake when I play[*ed*]. I would get this sort of fake vibrato with my [*instrument's*] sound. And that was a little detrimental to some of my auditions. I remember walking away from it being like, "I didn't play like me. This is not how I sound!" [*As I went on*] it would sort of ebb and flow. Some performances were exceptional, and I would be happy. And some performances, mostly auditions or studio class performances where I was in front of my peers, I would get that shake and it would always manifest itself in sort of constant, sort of a tremor, and my air just couldn't… I couldn't hold my [*instrument*] steady and my air wouldn't be steady, and that all came to a head, I think, at my senior recital, when I remember, I worked so hard and I was ready. I remember getting out there and my mouth just went dry, and my first piece was a complete disaster, like, I remember it was one of the most traumatic things that has ever happened. I went back out for the second one, and I was like, "okay, that happened and I've got an hour left of music let's just go," and the rest of it went okay, but everything sort of went back to that after that [*moment*].

Theme Three: Physical, Psychological, and Emotional Symptoms of MPA

Symptomatic MPA manifests in physical, psychological, and emotional symptoms that often negatively disrupt music performance. Physical symptoms include inability to focus, shaking, dry mouth, increased heart rate, constricted breathing, loss of hearing awareness, feeling hot or cold, or being nauseated. Psychological symptoms can be disillusionment with perceived musical ability, attention and memory loss, cognitive fog, being unable to control cognitions, and distracting thoughts during performance. Emotional symptoms of MPA can be fear, worry, distress over anticipated mistakes, self-questioning, or self-doubt. These emotional symptoms can have far-reaching effects as musicians may blame themselves for a failed performance and carry that shame with them long after the performance has ended. These lingering feelings of blame and shame can further interfere with the self-identity and feelings of self-worth that the musician accepts individually [51, 52].

It should be noted that the symptomatic expression of MPA is very rarely experienced in distinct physical, psychological, and emotional categories, but rather the experience of symptomatic MPA is usually a chaotic conglomeration of physical, psychological, and emotional symptoms. Whatever the original symptom is, it can trigger a chain of other symptoms activating all three categories resulting in a complete catastrophe. Each participant acknowledged experiencing some form of symptomatic MPA. A few of the participants were able to work with the symptoms in a way that did not completely hinder the performance. Other participants were not able to bring their symptoms under control. Jasmine and Yanna personally shared their experiences with symptomatic MPA with pristine clarity in the following:

> **Jasmine**: I remember accompanying and my foot being just like totally out of control, like shaking, and trying to pedal. I am sure my hands were hot and cold all that kind of stuff. I don't remember feeling so paralyzed when I was younger as I do now, because, like, now that is one of the common things. I feel like I am losing control. I feel like concrete.

> **Yanna**: I think the cognitive fog is a big one because it feels like I am a different person when I am trying to get myself ready. Then I get hyper aware of everything that is going on around me, but then, I get very tense, my muscles get very tense. The anxiety does happen there, but yeah, I do get the increased heart rate definitely and the perspiration happens. I don't necessarily shake, that's great, but it's just the other stuff when I am panicking. It feels like your mind is working so fast, but everything is in slow motion as it is going by.

Theme Four: Lack of Helpful Pedagogical Assistance for MPA

The second initiative of the current study was to inquire into whether or not pedagogical intervention for MPA had been employed in the lives of the participants. The relationship between a music student and music teacher is complex, and yet students often look to the music teacher for guidance in how to perform well [37, 38]. This relationship allows for the music teacher to intervene at crucial times when MPA is wreaking havoc in the performances of students. Music teachers can use their influence to increase awareness for available resources of professional psychological and medical assistance for MPA along with encouraging skill acquisition during lessons for performance. Unfortunately, pedagogical instruction often remains solely in the realm of musical and artistic development. This leaves the emotional and psychological skills necessary for performance as untouched tools for the unsuspecting and unguided student to discover when MPA is already entrenched inside the experience of performance.

Three expressions of pedagogical assistance emerged from the data: (1) meaningful pedagogical assistance, (2) weak pedagogical assistance, and (3) no pedagogical assistance for MPA. Some of the advice received by participants were not always directed specifically toward addressing MPA but rather sought to correct technical or focus-based issues. In some cases, this instruction was helpful for the participants and in other cases it was not. Three out of the six participants reported having received some kind of pedagogical assistance for addressing MPA in performance, but only one reported that the assistance addressed MPA in an effective way.

Ithaca: In college my teacher addressed [*MPA*]. I remember her giving me concrete suggestions on what to try and I had so many opportunities to try it because I was performing every week. I think that was helpful. I liked the fact that she was being so concrete about what to try and then analyzing, "Did it work?" [*She*] not only [*gave*] me one concrete suggestion, but then waited weeks to see if [*it*] worked, not just try it once, "oh, that didn't work let's try something else."

The remaining three participants did not receive pedagogical assistance in handling MPA. Their stories were full of distress and frustration over past performances gone wrong without personally knowing how to end the cycle of MPA. Jasmine and Analise expressed their frustration in the following:

Jasmine: Just a lot of making yourself go through the agony and then living through it. Through that constant exposure starting to feel like you could [*perform, it brought*] confidence. But, even with doing all that, it got pretty severe. I couldn't eat; I lost so much weight. I don't remember ever discussing it [*performance anxiety*] other than having my teacher suggest, "playing for your friends that are kind and aren't getting critical."

Analise: A bunch of us friends read the book, something about tennis playing. We all read that, and that was supposed to apply to music. Well, I didn't think it applied at all. That was like the only time [*where MPA came up*].

Discussion

The six participants included in this research study showed similar themes in their stories when the *Four Systems Model of Interpretative Phenomenological Analysis for Music Performance Anxiety* was applied to the data explaining an understanding of individual experiences with MPA. In each story, the four notable themes were (1) *initial onset*; (2) *rehearsed anxiety*; (3) *physical, psychological, and emotional symptoms of MPA*; and (4) *a lack of helpful pedagogical assistance*. As an exploratory study, there were several ideas highlighted by the results that should be given more consideration. For musicians, more awareness of MPA and its potential effects on their lives is needed. For music educators, awareness and understanding of MPA and the possible negative effects on students are essential [13]. For medical and health professionals, using a multidimensional approach to incorporate all symptomatic effects of MPA in addition to collaborating with the musician's teacher may increase the effectiveness of the selected treatment.

Musicians seeking higher education in music will likely spend some, if not a majority, of their time after graduation performing for an audience. As such, it is suggested that more attention during collegiate education be given to teaching students how to handle this aspect of their performing careers. This need for more performance training during education is affirmed in a study done by Clark and Lisboa [36]. They suggested that, like any other performance-based careers (i.e., sports), the cognitive and emotional skills for handling a career in music performance should be fundamental in the instruction of a pre-professional musician along with the muscle and musical skills being taught. This increased education could be done through workshops, lectures, or continuing education; however, it would be most effective if awareness of MPA and management skills were integrated into early musical development.

As the first line of defense for students, music educators can create an environment where open communication about MPA can be explored. Secondarily, music educators should make an effort to develop a network of medical and health professionals who can act as resources for students who could be of assistance for students experiencing MPA. This acceptance of and collaboration between teachers and medical or health professionals could increase student commitment to treatment plans and enhance performance skills training.

Ideas for medical and health professionals come through a thorough understanding of the complexities of MPA in the lives of musicians and the necessity to instigate interdisciplinary collaboration with music educators to include health awareness in music education. Knowing that the physiological symptoms are often only a side effect of a much deeper psychological or emotional issue, medical and health professionals should look beyond symptomatic MPA to determine a treatment plan that adequately addresses the varied aspects of MPA.

While it is important to avoid over-generalizing findings, the results of this study suggest that a deeper understanding of individual MPA can be gathered through the *Four Systems Model of Interpretative Phenomenological Analysis for Music Performance Anxiety.* Ideas suggested here should be taken mainly as suggestions for additional research into the subjective experiences of MPA in the lives of professional musicians. The intent of this article is to raise a deeper awareness for how continued research of MPA can promote performance quality in the musical industry by increasing mental health awareness in the experiences of MPA.

Notes There is no conflict of interest.

This paper is based on a presentation at the *Third USF-PAMA Southeast Regional Conference: Lifecycle of the Performing Artist*, June 1–3, 2018, Tampa, Florida, and *36th Annual Performing Arts Medicine Association International Symposium: Glamour and Grit: Building an Entourage for Health*, June 30–July 3, 2018, Orange, California.

References

1. Fogle D. Toward effective treatment for music performance anxiety. Psychotherapy (Chic). 1982;19:368–75.
2. Wesner R, Noyes R, Davis T. The occurrence of performance anxiety among musicians. J Affect Disord. 1990;18:177–85.
3. Kirchner J. A qualitative inquiry into musical performance anxiety. Med Probl Perform Art. 2003;18:78–82.
4. James I. Western orchestral musicians are highly stressed. Resonance Inter Music Counc. 1998;26:19–20.
5. Marchant-Haycox S, Wilson G. Personality and stress in performing artists. Personal Individ Differ. 1992;13(10):1061–8.
6. Kenny D. The psychology of music performance anxiety. New York: Oxford University Press, Inc; 2011. p. 92–3, 264.
7. Wilson G, Roland D. Performance anxiety. In: Parncutt R, McPherson G, editors. The science and psychology of music performance. New York: Oxford University Press, Inc; 2002. p. 47–62.
8. Nideffer R, Hessler N. Controlling performance anxiety. Coll Music Symp (Coll Mus Symp). 1978;18:146–53.
9. Perdomo-Guevara E. Is music performance anxiety just an. Individual problem? Exploring the impact of musical environments on performers' approaches to performance and emotions. Psychomusicology. 2014;24:66–74.
10. Nagel J. Performance anxiety and the performing musician: a fear of failure or a fear of success? Med Probl Perform Art. 1990;5:37–40.
11. Lehmann A, Sloboda J, Woody R. Psychology for musicians. New York: Oxford University Press, Inc; 2007. p. 146.
12. Kenny D, Davis P, Oates J. Music performance anxiety and occupational stress amongst opera chorus artists and their relationship with state and trait anxiety and perfectionism. J Anxiety Disord. 2004;18:757–77.
13. Papageorgi I, Hallam S, Welch G. A conceptual framework for understanding musical performance anxiety. Res Stud Music Educ (RSME). 2007;28:83–107.
14. Osborne M, Franklin J. Cognitive processes in music performance anxiety. Aust J Psychol. 2002;54:86–93.
15. Cox W, Kenardy J. Performance anxiety, social phobia, and setting effects in instrumental music students. J Anxiety Disord. 1993;7:49–60.
16. Boucher H, Ryan C. Performance stress and the very young musician. J Res Music Educ (JRME). 2011;58:329–45.
17. Nusseck M, Zander M, Spahn C. Music performance anxiety in young musicians: comparison of playing classical or popular music. Med Probl Perform Art. 2015;30:30–7.
18. Ryan C. Exploring musical performance anxiety in children. Med Probl Perform Art. 1998;13:83–8.
19. Kirkland K, Hollandsworth J. Effective test taking: skills-acquisition versus anxiety-reduction techniques. J Consult Clin Psychol. 1980;48:431–9.
20. Segool N, Carlson J, Goforth A, Embse N, Bartherian J. Heightened test anxiety among young children: elementary school students' anxious responses to high-stakes testing. Psychol Sch. 2013;50:489–99.
21. Brandfonbrener A. Beta blockers in the treatment of performance anxiety. Med Probl Perform Art. 1990;5:23–6.
22. Lehrer P. A review of the approaches to the management of tension and stage fright in music performances. J Res Music Educ (JRME). 1987;35:143–53.
23. Patston T, Loughlan T. Playing with performance: the use and abuse of beta-blockers in the performing arts. Vic J Music Educ. 2014;1:3–10.

24. Kenny D, Driscoll T, Ackermann B. Psychological well-being in professional orchestral musicians in Australia: a descriptive population study. Psychol Music. 2014;42(2):210–32.
25. Branfonbrener A. Beta blockers in the treatment of performance anxiety. Med Probl Perform Art. 1997;5(1):23–6.
26. Kenny D. A systematic review of treatments for music performance anxiety. Anxiety Stress Coping. 2005;18(3):183–208.
27. Kendrick M, Craig K, Lawson D, Davidson P. Cognitive and behavioral therapy for musical-performance anxiety. J Consult Clin Psychol. 1982;50:353–62.
28. Nagel J, Himle D, Papsdorf J. Cognitive-behavioral treatment of musical performance anxiety. Psychol Music. 1989;17:12–21.
29. Kenny D, Arthey S, Abbass A. Intensive short-term dynamic psychotherapy for severe music performance anxiety: assessment, process, and outcome of psychotherapy with a professional orchestral musician. Med Probl Perform Art. 2014;18:78–82.
30. Plaut E. Psychotherapy of performance anxiety. Med Probl Perform Art. 1990;5:58–63.
31. Thurber M. Effects of heart-rate variability biofeedback training and emotional regulation on music performance anxiety in university students. 2007. https://digital.library.unt.edu/ark:/67531/metadc5428/m2/1/high_res_d/dissertation.pdf. Assessed 12 Nov 2018.
32. Valentine E, Fritzgerald D, Gorton T, Hudson J, Symonds E. The effect of lessons in the Alexander technique on music performance in high and low stress situations. Psychol Music. 1995;23:129–41.
33. Wells R, Outhred T, Heathers J, Quintana D, Kemp A. Matter over mind: a randomized-controlled trial of single-session biofeedback training on performance anxiety and heart rate variability in musicians. PLoS One. 2012;7(10):e46597.
34. Hoffman S, Hanrahan S. Mental skills for musicians: managing music performance anxiety and enhancing performances. Sport Exerc Perform Psychol. 2012;1(1):17–28.
35. Clark T, Williamon A. Evaluation of a mental skills training program for musicians. J Appl Sport Psychol. 2011;23(2):342–59.
36. Clark T, Lisboa T. Training for sustained performance: moving toward long-term musician development. Med Probl Perform Art. 2013;28:159–68.
37. Presland C. Conservatoire student and instrumental professor: the student perspective on a complex relationship. Br J Music Educ. 2005;22:237–48.
38. Davidson J, Moore D, Sloboda J, Howe M. Characteristics of music teachers and the progress of young instrumentalists. J Res Music Educ (JRME). 1998;46:141–60.
39. Picard A. Qualitative pedagogical inquiry into cognitive modulation of music performance anxiety. Bull Counc Res Music Educ. 1999;140:62–76.
40. Robertson D, Eisensmith K. Teaching students about performance anxiety: the scratch pad pop-up model. Music Educ J. 2010;97:31–5.
41. Larkin M, Shaw R, Flowers P. Multiperspectival designs and processes in interpretative phenomenological analysis research. Qual Res Psychol. 2019;16(2):182–98.
42. Smith J, Flowers P, Larkin M. Interpretative phenomenological analysis: theory, method, and research. London: SAGE Publications, Ltd; 2012.
43. Larkin M, Thompson A. Interpretative phenomenological analysis in mental health and psychotherapy research. In: Harper D, Thompson AR, editors. Qualitative research methods in mental health and psychotherapy: a guide for students and practitioners. Malden: WileyBlackwell; 2012. p. 101–16.
44. McCoy LK. Longitudinal qualitative research and interpretative phenomenological analysis: philosophical connections and practical considerations. Qual Res Psychol. 2017;14(4):442–58.
45. Smith J. Reflecting on the development of interpretative phenomenological analysis and its contribution to qualitative research in psychology. Qual Res Psychol. 2004;1(1):39–54.
46. Rácz J, Kassai S, Pintér J, Benedeczki P, Dobó-Nagy Z, Horváth Z, et al. The therapeutic journeys of recovering helpers – an interpretative phenomenological analysis. Int J Ment Heal Addict. 2015;13:751–7.

47. Bramley N, Eatough V. The experience of living with Parkinson's disease: and interpretative phenomenological analysis case study. J Psychol Health. 2005;20(2):223–34.
48. Lee J, McFerran KS. Applying interpretative phenomenological analysis to video data in music therapy. Qual Res Psychol. 2015;12(4):367–81.
49. Taylor A. Using interpretative phenomenological analysis in a mixed methods research design to explore music in the lives of mature age amateur keyboard players. Music Educ Res. 2015;17(4):437–52.
50. Robinson G, Nigbur D. Experiences of musical performance anxiety in final-year undergraduate music students: an interpretative phenomenological analysis. Soc Psychol Rev. 2018;20(1):18–32.
51. Chesky K, Hipple J. Performance anxiety, alcohol-related problems, and social/emotional difficulties of college students: a comparative study between lower-division music and non-music majors. Med Probl Perform Art. 1997;12:126–32.
52. Kemp A. The musical temperament: psychology and personality of musicians. Oxford: Oxford University Press; 1996.

Chapter 15
Distilling Dart: Minding Bodily Approaches to Performance Through a Framework for Integration and the Alexander Technique

Elizabeth Johnson

Introduction

The Dart Procedures are a developmental movement sequence born from scientific, somatic, therapeutic, and dance histories advanced by anatomist and anthropologist Raymond Dart and Alexander Technique teachers Joan and Alex Murray [1]. Located primarily in Alexander Technique and dance practices, the Dart Procedures "devolve" the mover in a reverse evolutionary sequence from standing, to anthropoidal postures such as creeping and crouching, eventually returning to standing [1–3] (Fig. 15.1). Applied concepts from this sequence deepen bodily awareness and call attention to habits and interferences in coordination across all manner of performance disciplines. It is crucial for performing artists to understand the physical and mental habits that interfere with their technical and artistic achievement.

Since as a physical practice, the Dart Procedures have remained mainly in the context of the Alexander Technique, the benefits of that century-old educational method permeate and are perhaps even amplified in their doing. This is relevant for performing artists in particular as F.M. Alexander's eponymous technique was born from his struggles with vocal failure in theater performance [4]. Many prominent arts training institutions and practices are aware of the benefits of the Alexander Technique and look to it as a method for addressing physical and mental stress habits that impede technical and aesthetic freedom [5]. The Juilliard School offers a range of courses in the Alexander Technique in dance, music, and theater; first-year dance students are required to take the introductory course [6–8]. Multiple studies suggest that, practiced regularly or even in a limited series of lessons, the Alexander Technique significantly reduces neck and lower back pain, may improve respiratory function and body use, and gives performers psychophysical skills to cope better

E. Johnson (✉)
School of Theatre and Dance, Nadine McGuire Theatre and Dance Pavilion, University of Florida, Gainesville, FL, USA
e-mail: ejohnson@arts.ufl.edu

S.-H. Lee et al. (eds.), *Perspectives in Performing Arts Medicine Practice*,
https://doi.org/10.1007/978-3-030-37480-8_15

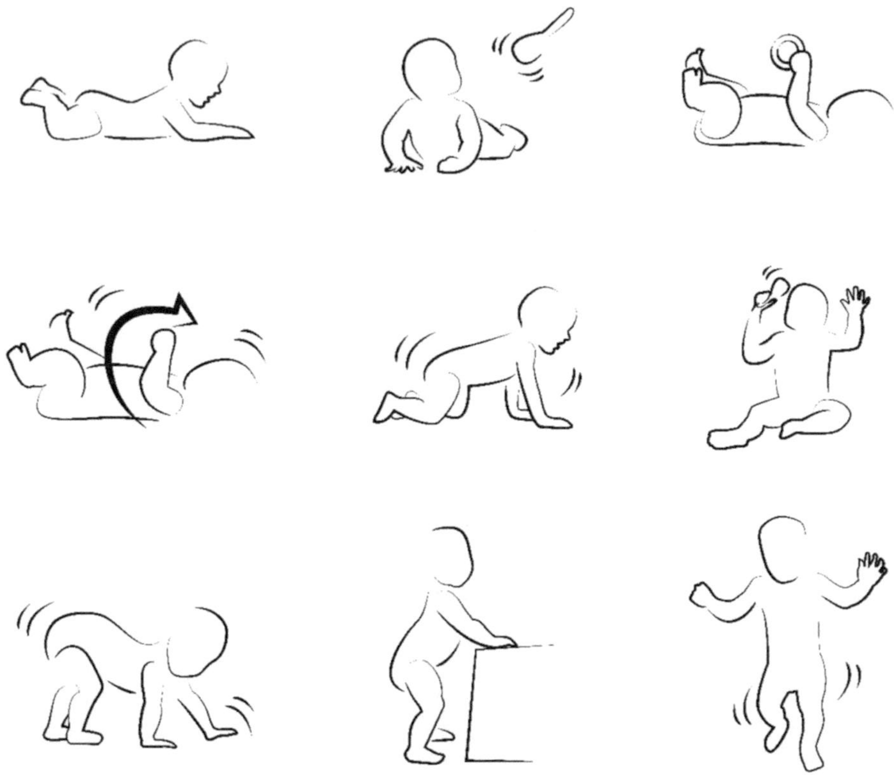

Fig. 15.1 Ontogenetic: Toddler milestones and motor development during the first year. (Source: Jennylipet/Shutterstock.com)

with performance anxiety [4, 5, 9]. As an outgrowth of those underlying benefits, exploring the Dart Procedures and the subsequently distilled Framework for Integration concepts can help performers of all backgrounds to become more aware and coordinated and to adopt new practices that facilitate ease in performance.

Raymond Dart

In order to understand the story of the Dart Procedures and their importance in the canon of developmental movement, it is important to know a little more about Raymond Dart. Australian born in 1893 and educated in London, Dart was a paleoanthropologist, neuroanatomist, doctor, and educator [1]. By 1922, at the young age of 29, he was already Chair of the Anatomy Department at the University of Witwatersrand in Johannesburg, South Africa [10]. He stayed at the University of South Africa and eventually served as Dean until 1958. As quoted by Nettl-Fiol and Vanier, his paleontological claim to fame was the 1924 discovery of *Australopithecus*

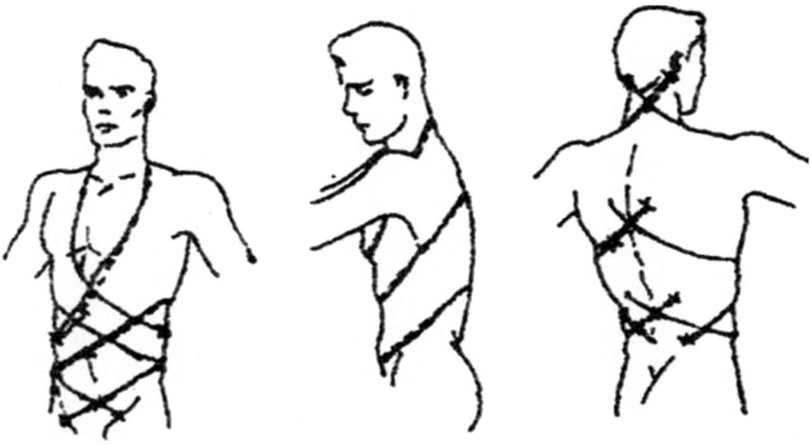

Fig. 15.2 Dart's spiral musculature as featured in 1968 Institutes for the Achievement of Human Potential (IAHP). (Photo permission: Alex Murray)

africanus, the "missing link" or Taung Child [1]. In his book, *Adventures with the Missing Link*, Dart said the Taung Child was a new species marking the evolution between our primate ancestors and modern humans evidenced in postural and other physical attributes [1, 10]. Also germane to the development of the Dart Procedures was his identification of the double spiral arrangement of the human musculature [2] (Fig. 15.2).

The procedures' story entered into personal and therapeutic territory when Dart sought out Alexander Technique lessons from Irene Tasker, a well-known teacher who worked in South Africa from 1935 to 1944 [11]. For 2 years, Dart employed Tasker (who had studied extensively with both F.M. Alexander and Maria Montessori) to work with his son Galen, born prematurely and suffering cyanotic episodes that left him brain injured/spastic [1, 11]. Dart later moved to Philadelphia to serve as a professor at the Institutes for the Achievement of Human Potential (IAHP), dedicated to the rehabilitation and treatment of brain-injured children [1, 10]. The IAHP was originally established by physical therapist Glenn Doman and educational psychologist Carl Delacato and drew on the ideas of Temple Fay, neurosurgeon and head of neurosurgery at Temple University [1, 10].

Still resonant in the movements in the Dart Procedures is Fay's idea that the infant brain develops—as does the evolution of the human species—through stages that mirror those of fish, reptiles, and mammals, until finally recognizably human [1]. These ideas originate with German bio-geneticist Ernst Haeckel's 1866 biogenetic law: "the stages an animal embryo undergoes during development are a chronological replay of that species' past evolutionary forms" or "ontogeny recapitulates phylogeny" [12]. The idea that human development directly echoes the phylogenetic past has been debunked by modern science, but the pioneers of developmental movement (Dart, Irmgard Bartenieff, Bonnie Bainbridge Cohen, etc.) explored deeply how strongly human ontogeny still bears resemblance to so much of that evolutionary and phylogenetic history (e.g., moving through development from crawling to walking, babies embody similar crawling patterns to reptiles) [13].

Dart's Collaboration with Alex and Joan Murray

Raymond Dart experienced an in-person lesson with the founder of the Alexander Technique (AT), F.M. Alexander [11]. From that experience forward, he remained a lifelong enthusiast of the technique and over years, worked in continued collaboration with other teachers. First-generation British Alexander Technique teacher, Walter Carrington, trained AT teachers Alex and Joan Murray [1, 2]. Upon his suggestion, Alex read Dart's article *The Postural Aspect of Malocclusion* and discovered that Dart delineated postures very similar to those in the Alexander Technique [1, 2]. Murray began a process of embodying them as exactly as possible, with wife and fellow teacher Joan organizing the in-between transitions and movement sequencing [1]. In 1967, Dart and the Murrays established contact and began a dynamic partnership that would bear significant fruit over the next 6 years. Integrated into this continuing work was Joan's embodied knowledge as a professional dancer, her experience of her infant daughter's developmental stages, and her cumulative observations of all the babies brought to the Alexander Technique teacher-training course in which she and Alex taught for five decades [1, 2]. The formal outcome of Dart and the Murray's rich association has become known as a developmental movement sequence called the Dart Procedures.

The Dart Procedures

In *Dance and the Alexander Technique: Exploring the Missing Link,* the authors emphasize that the Murrays believed, "The 'procedures' themselves are merely a starting point for investigation, rather than being a fixed idea or sequence" and "… in hindsight, the Murrays would have preferred the term 'process'" … "because evolution and child development are processes, and so is the Alexander Technique" [1, p.31]. To encapsulate, "The Dart Procedures contain a series of positions that, when linked, become a movement sequence that retraces the path of developmental and evolutionary patterns" [1, p.32]. It is important to emphasize that because the Murrays were working from the perspective of applying Alexander Technique principles, learning or performing the sequence is only a first step in recognizing movement patterns; the ultimate importance would be attending to what Alexander called psychophysical use [1, 2]. As with many developmental and repatterning sequences, the Dart Procedures reveal to the mover habits, movement preferences (especially in spinal patterning), interferences in simple coordination, challenges to range of motion, etc.

Dart Procedures Sequence

The Dart Procedures sequence that emerged from the Dart–Murray collaboration featured in their book [1, 2] as well as online [3] is generally performed in the order shown here, but it can be started, finished, or explored more fully at any point.

1. *Standing on toes*: Mover rises to toes facing the back of a chair—from here will descend all the way to the floor in a devolution from mammalian, to reptilian, to fishlike movements [1, 2, 3].
2. *Shallow monkey position*: Facing back of a chair and sometimes assisted, the mover bends hips and knees toward a very shallow squat and slightly inclined over the chair. The Alexander Technique uses this posture quite a lot; it is often called a position of "mechanical advantage" [2, p.163].
3. *Hands on the back of the chair*: In the shallow squat, the mover grasps the back of the chair with the long fingers and thumbs.
4. *Anthropoidal*: The mover places knuckles on the back of the chair while maintaining the inclined squat position.
5. *Deeper anthropoidal*: The chair is turned around to face the mover who then descends into a deeper squat with knuckles on chair seat.
6. *Tarsoid*: The mover descends into an even deeper squat until back of the hands to wrists rest on the chair seat.
7. *Anthropoidal*: The chair is moved away, and mover bends into deepest squat resting knuckles on floor with hips up—this is a very gorilla/primate-like posture.
8. *Creeping-quadrupedal*: The mover descends to all fours in a table top on hands and knees.
9. *Kowtow*: The mover sits back onto heels, bending into deep flexion of the torso, hips, and knees with a rounded back as in the yoga "Child's Pose."
10. *Pentapodal*: Here there are five points of support touching the floor as the mover rolls to top of the head with the cranial globe, elbows, and knees all touching floor.
11. *Pre-fetal*: In pentapodal, the mover crosses ankles and arms with forearms across upper chest and hands wrapped around the neck.
12. *Fetal crouch*: With assistance, the mover retreats to a full fetal position back toward heels in deepest hip, knee, and spinal flexion.
13. *Rolling to semi-supine*: This step includes spirals in the fetal crouch which entail turning the head to look left and right, while ankles and arms are still crossed. From here, the mover rolls from the fetal crouch all the way to his/her back, while keeping legs and arms crossed.
14. *Rolling to prone*: From back, the mover rolls to belly ending supported by elbows—much like a baby on belly looking up, supported on forearms.
15. *Pull to the elbows*: The mover pulls himself/herself higher onto forearms.
16. *Spiral rolling*: Either alone or with assistance, the mover is encouraged to look over one shoulder so much that he/she ends up rolling to back. Eye tracking is very important in this step.

17. *Ventigrade*: After rolling back to his/her belly, the mover is face down (prone) with arms resting at sides. The mover's vision is no longer stereoscopic but more like a fish—one eye on each side. From here the mover slides arms out to sides and up toward the head all the while moving through alternating pronation/supination of forearms, finishing with arms above the head and back of wrists and hands touching. This is called "fish arms" and echoes the movement of pectoral fins.
18. *Creeping-quadrupedal*: This movement is what most lay people think of as crawling (the accurate developmental term is actually *creeping*. *Crawling* is closer to the floor and at times not yet quadrupedal). The mover is on all fours with opposite upper and lower body limbs propelling him/her through space. The intent is to look for the chair with spatial intent and creep/crawl to it.
19. *Clambering*: Having found the chair, like a toddler pulling to standing from all fours, the mover uses the seat of the chair to pull up back into an inclined squat in this order: hand, hand, foot, foot.
20. *Upright/relevé/on toes*: Pressing off the seat of the chair, the mover swings up to a full standing position. The mover rises on toes once again but this time adding the arms stretched up and overhead. Dart's idea of fully evolved poise is a person balancing on one toe, one leg lifted, spiraled, and arms overhead [1–3].

The Essentials of Performing the Dart Procedures

According to Dart, the fetal curve or what in the procedures is described as the *fetal crouch* is the most important element of the sequence. In an interview for *Dance and the Alexander Technique*, the Murray's recounted that, in his 80s, Dart jumped up on top of a table to demonstrate how it should be done [1]. It bears noting that a paleoanthropologist insisted that this was developmentally the most important and pivotal movement in the sequence [1]. The fetal curve (the rounded prominence of the thoracic and sacral spine) is one of our most formative and primal bodily experiences. In human development, as room in the womb becomes limited by the growing fetus, all late-stage gestational movement pushes away from and returns to this position in preparation for birth [13]. After birth, many cultures traditionally swaddle infants to calm the nervous system and as a gentle transition into the world of larger personal space. Alex Murray surmised that in their initial exchange, Dart had perhaps omitted a description of the fetal curve because to him, it was so obviously ontologically fundamental [2]. Murray classifies fetal, or the *fetal crouch*, as a "total movement" [2, p.170].

From birth, for humans of all ages, the fetal curve is a position with an emphasis toward our original primal spinal flexion that offers rest and relief from habitual muscular pulls (think of *Child's Pose* in yoga practices or curling up on the couch or in bed after a long day). From the "end" of that deep spinal flexion in the sagittal plane, the opposite resultant spinal extension and lengthening are easier and, according to Joan Murray, a logical developmental progression that moves from introversion to connecting to one's environment [1, 15].

In the Dart Procedures, that bodily progression of extension following flexion relates to another important hallmark of Dart's work: his challenge of traditional Western compartmentalization of human anatomy. Of the body's musculature design, he insisted:

> Man suspends the remainder of his body from his head and spine. He swings his body from his head by means of two spirally arranged but interwoven sheets of voluntary musculature in exactly the same manner that his fishy and amphibian forefathers swung their bodies from their heads... [2, p.90].

These interwoven sheets are what he called the *double spiral* musculature and might be less obvious when witnessed in the bilateral symmetry of a position such as the fetal crouch or in what Bonnie Bainbridge Cohen terms *homologous* movement/patterning (e.g., a "frog leap" with both arms reaching out and then both legs following shortly after) [13]. But, when the double spiral musculature is operative in asymmetry—for example, a swimmer reaching forward with the right arm and turning the head left to take a breath—what is characterized as *spiral* movement is at play.

In the Dart Procedures, after the fetal crouch, the transition to spinal extension is through what Alex Murray refers to as "rotational movement" [2]. *Rolling to semi-supine (*and the later *spiral rolling*) is characterized by looking right and left and then rolling to rest on the back. Murray believes that when this *spiraling* movement is performed slowly and purposefully, the mover can notice habits of obvious strain, breath holding, possible fear of falling, etc. and gently work through all possible challenges to ease [2]. This movement also echoes a baby's experience of being born (in a traditional delivery). The legacy of Dart's double spiral musculature (Fig. 15.2) continues to influence ongoing research in myofascial release work [14], Murray's methods of training Alexander Technique teachers, and Rebecca Nettl–Fiol and Luc Vanier's *Framework for Integration* [1, 15].

Framework for Integration

The recent *Framework for Integration* [15] is a particular distillation of overall bodily attitudes and patterning found in the Dart Procedures. This analytical tool considers spinal patterning in various models. The original "simple" model looks at the head and spine in the sagittal plane to see whether the mover/performer prefers an overall pattern of *primary*—Dart's *fetal crouch* (emphasizing an overall pattern of spinal flexion)—or *secondary* (emphasizing an overall pattern of spinal extension/hyperextension) [15]. These patterns can be analyzed in formal physical training but also in the context of daily activities [1, 15]. It is theorized that when balances of these spinal patterns are less than optimal, over time, chronic pain or injury may occur.

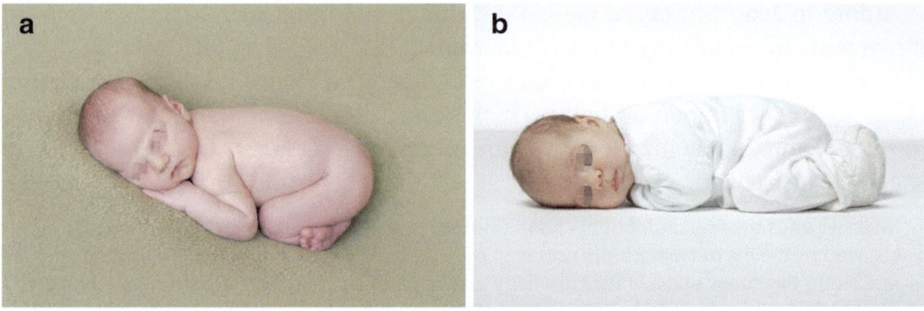

Fig. 15.3 (**a**, **b**) In *primary*, the spinal curves emphasized are the thoracic and sacral. (Source: (**a**) Tatyana Vyc/Shutterstock.com. (**b**) Source: paffy/Shutterstock.com)

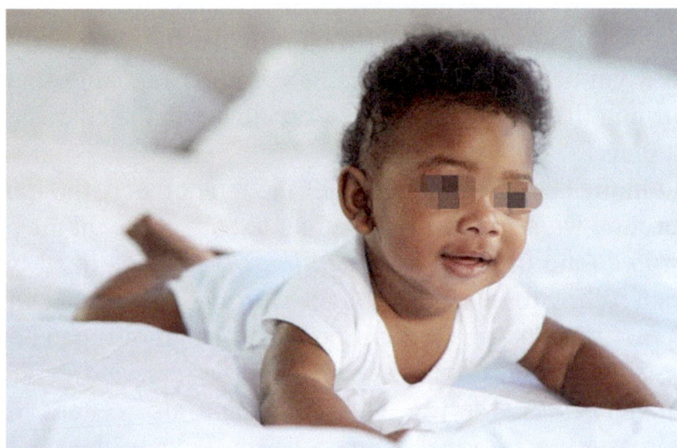

Fig. 15.4 In *secondary*, the spinal curves emphasized are the cervical and lumbar. (Source: Monkey Business Images/Shutterstock.com)

As evident in Fig. 15.3a, b, in *primary*, the whole-body patterning tends toward overall flexion of the spine, softening of the limbs toward the midline, and a general body attitude of rest or introversion [15].

In *secondary*, whole-body patterning tends toward overall spinal extension and hyperextension, with the limbs freeing away from the midline and a general body attitude of engagement with the environment or extroversion [15] (Fig. 15.4).

In the simple model of the *Framework for Integration*, the release of one pattern toward the other encourages a recuperative recalibration of the whole called a *reset* [8]. And, though these two generalized patterns are simple and easy to see, most movement is a more complex spiraling of the two according to the body's double spiral musculature [1, 2] (Fig. 15.5). The sequence of a baby rolling shown in Fig. 15.5 illustrates the baby starting from a general *secondary* pattern (spinal extension/hyperextension), turning the head into a spiral, and then rolling in transition to rest on the back—more toward *primary* but also in a recuperative *reset.*

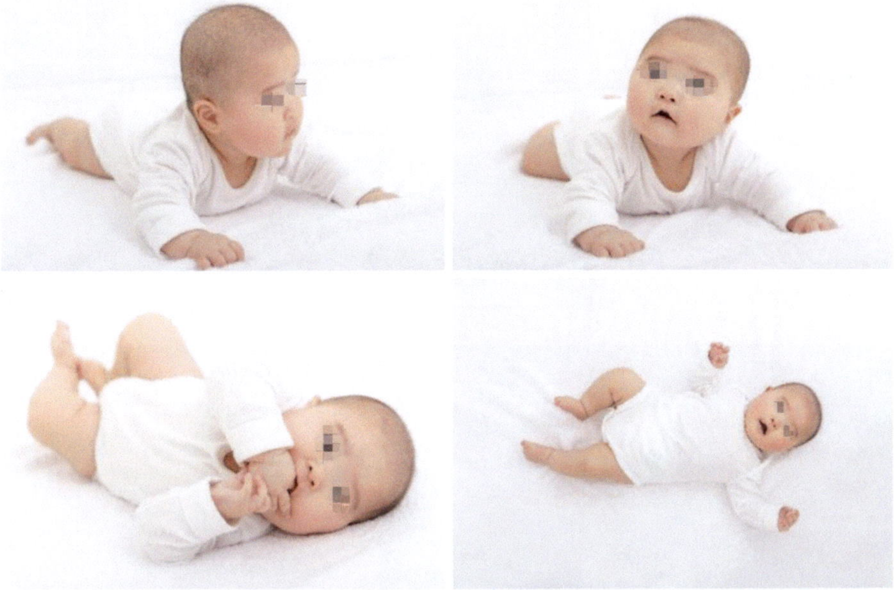

Fig. 15.5 Sequence of a baby rolling. Starting from a general *secondary* pattern (spinal extension/hyperextension), the baby turns the head into a spiral and then rolls in transition to rest on the back—more toward *primary* but also in a recuperative *reset*. (Source: kai keisuke/Shutterstock.com)

Performance Examples

Framework for Integration is, in essence, a movement analysis lens. Because movement is ephemeral and often does not repeat itself identically, practicing seeing the simple model (*primary*, *secondary*, and *spirals*) in still photos develops the confidence needed to recognize the patterns in moving bodies. The patterns are not static shapes but rather point to how the body (or parts of the body) trends toward, away, and through these movement intentions.

In Fig.15.6, each dancer is embodying the oppositional patterning in the simple model of the *Framework for Integration*. The male dancer on the bottom is in a deep, rounded *primary,* while the female dancer on top is in a fully, arched *secondary*.

In Fig. 15.7, from left to right, the dancers are embodying *primary* (toward fetal), *secondary* (full hyperextension), and a *spiral* combination of both (reminiscent of the rolling patterning in Fig. 15.5).

In illustrations less extreme than those of the dancers, the violinist on the left is adopting an overall patterning of *primary*, while the violinist on the right is adopting a patterning that tends more toward *secondary* (Fig. 15.8). In each example, when the performers release their intention of the present activity in which they are pictured, they should, in theory, *reset*. For example, the male dancer in the arched jump in Fig. 15.7 will need to release the extreme arching, so his head and spine can

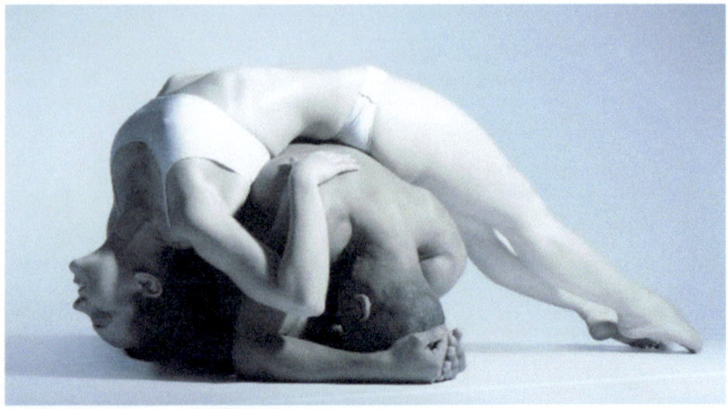

Fig. 15.6 Dancers embodying the ends of the spectrum of *primary* and *secondary*. (Source: sirtravelalot/Shutterstock.com)

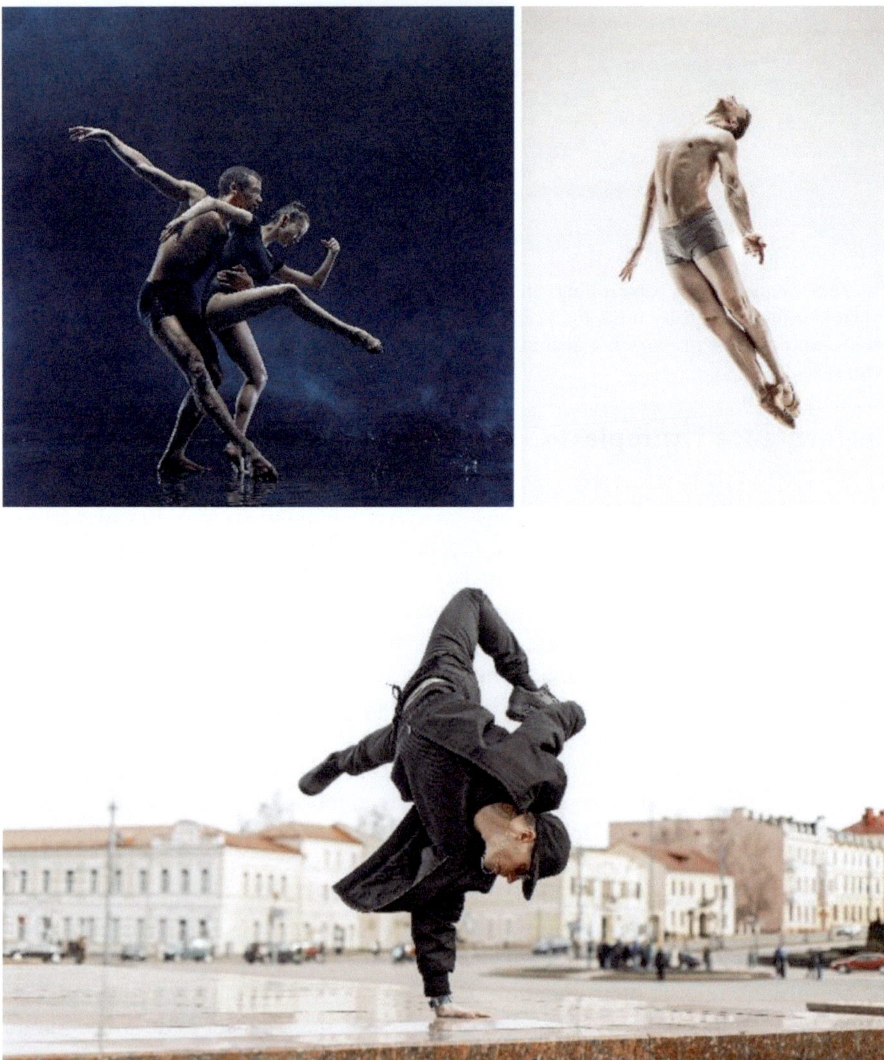

Fig. 15.7 Dancers in clear patterns of Framework for Integration vocabulary: *primary*, *secondary*, and combinations of both in *spirals*. (Source: Master1305/Shutterstock.com; Alones/Shutterstock.com)

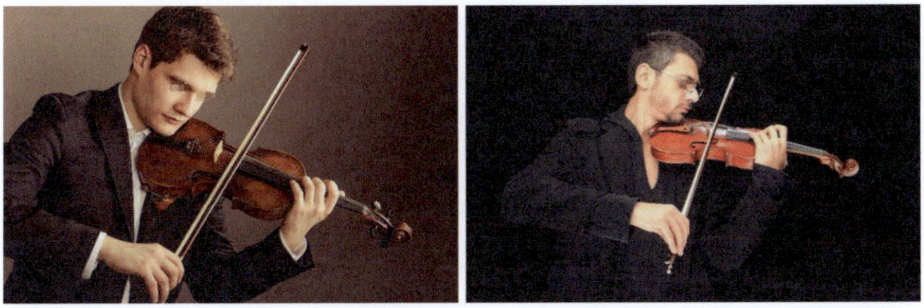

Fig. 15.8 Violinists in subtle but overall *primary* (L) and *secondary* (R) patterning. (Source: Voyagerix/Shutterstock.com; Netfalls Remy Musser/Shutterstock.com)

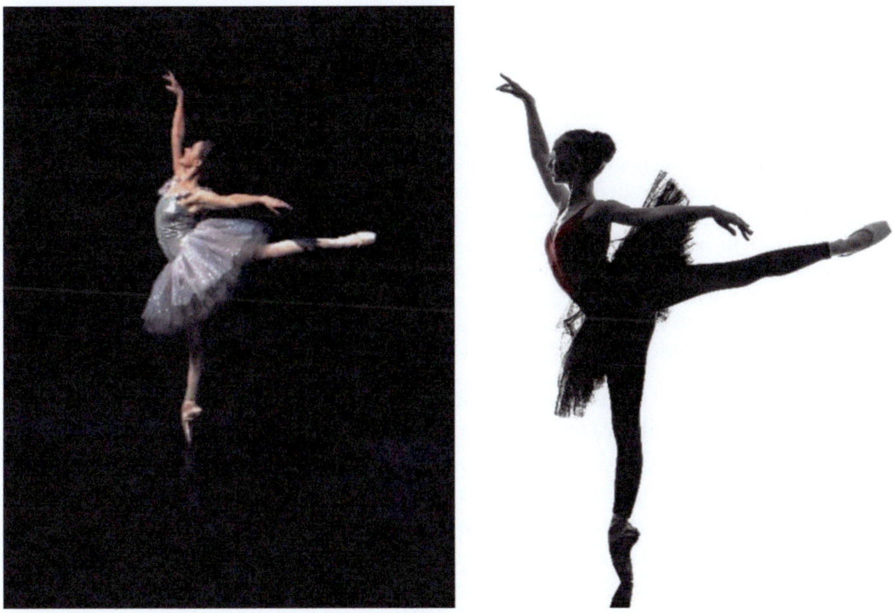

Fig. 15.9 Ballet arabesque with *secondary* patterning. Dancer on left is overly engaged in hyperextension, while dancer on the right has clearer, more efficient *secondary* intention. (Source: Hudson Hintz/unsplash.com; OSTILL is Franck Camhi/Shutterstock.com)

realign vertically, and his feet and legs can reach efficiently toward the floor to land safely. To land well, he must release his *secondary* activity to *reset* more toward *primary*. He will not actively do the opposite of what he is doing in the jump but, rather, will simply let go of the arching to *reset*. All performers in Figs. 15.6, 15.7, and 15.8 are in momentary activities that will change intention and shape according to choreography and composition. If any are caught in one pattern more strongly than the other and are not able to *reset*, unnecessary struggle and muscular tension will hinder efficient and organic movement or playing.

Figure 15.9 is an example of dissonance in patterning. A ballet step called an *arabesque* is an activity that requires extreme range of motion and hyperextension of the spine—the whole body in a *secondary* and lengthened state. Classical Alexander Technique directions for the head are for it to go "forward and up" in length (length at the base of the skull) as opposed to "back and down" (shortening at the base of the skull) [1]. In the *arabesque* on the left, the overarching in the back (too much *secondary*) is causing the head of the dancer to go backward behind verticality and causing extra tension in the musculature of the neck (the sternocleidomastoid specifically). On the right, as in the baby in Fig. 15.5, the *arabesque* balances the use of the body in hyperextension, features clear upward thrust, and reaches into the forward space.

Tools for Teaching

In his 1992 introduction to Dart's *Skill and Poise,*[1] Alex Murray said of the Dart Procedures:

> …these procedures will not teach one the Alexander Technique, but patient and intelligent investigation by one with no Alexander experience may still lead to a certain enlightenment by revealing inefficient patterns of movement and helping to discard them. Undertaken with the guidance of a skilled Alexander teacher, they are a constant source of insight and a point of reference in one's patterns of behavior. One can continually return to these as to Alexander's 'positions of mechanical advantage' in which category they certainly belong. Dart has often said that '*Man can only look ahead as far as he can look back*'. These patterns take us back to the origins of human movement and open up corresponding vistas for our future as mobile human beings. [2, 11 p.10][1]

The Framework for Integration can help those who train and teach performance practices to identify in their students overall bodily patterning that either supports or interferes with successful practice and performance [15]. Practicing parts or all of the Dart Procedures in tandem with Alexander Technique lessons results in greater bodily awareness and capacity for choice and change. Applying the AT principles of *inhibition*—the practice of non-reactivity/non-doing (much like the aforementioned *reset*)—and *faulty sensory awareness*, which is understanding that feedback from the nervous system may be maladapted or too strongly habituated, the mover can learn to approach the Dart work with ongoing process and patience. Integrating these approaches as central tools in training can facilitate greater bodily awareness, increased efficiency and functionality, and improved technical and aesthetic aspects of performance, thus minimizing overuse and chronic injury.

---

[1] This quote was originally in the introduction to the 1992 version of *Skill and Poise* which was a limited, self-published booklet presented at the North American Society of Teachers of the Alexander Technique (NASTAT) Annual General Meeting in Chicago in 1992. The subsequent 1996 STAT Books edition does not include this quote [2].

References

1. Nettl-Fiol R, Vanier L. Dance and the Alexander Technique. Urbana: University of Illinois Press; 2011. p. 23–40, 122–24.
2. Dart RA. Skill and poise: articles of skill, poise and the F.M. Alexander Technique. London: STAT Books; 1996.
3. Murray A, Murray J. Dart procedures (internet video). YouTube. 2010. https://www.youtube.com/watch?v=KnYUvIRZe_o. Accessed 25 Mar 2019.
4. Cacciatore T, Horak F, Henry H. Improvement in automatic postural coordination following Alexander Technique lessons in a person with low back pain. Phys Ther. 2005;85(6):565–78. Available from: https://www.ncbi.nlm.nih.gov/pmc/articles/PMC1351283/pdf/nihms7407.pdf. Accessed 7 June 2019.
5. Klein S, Bayard C, Wolf U. The Alexander Technique and musicians: a systematic review of controlled trials. BMC Complement Altern Med. 2014;14:414. https://doi.org/10.1186/1472-6882-14-414. Accessed 7 June 2019.
6. The Juilliard School: college catalog 2019–2020. DSDAN 100 – Alexander Technique. https://catalog.juilliard.edu/content.php?catoid=36&navoid=3983. Accessed 7 July 2019.
7. The Juilliard School: college catalog 2019–2020. MSMUS 001 – Alexander Technique. https://catalog.juilliard.edu/content.php?catoid=36&catoid=36&navoid=3967&filter%5Bitem_type%5D=3&filter%5Bonly_active%5D=1&filter%5B3%5D=1&filter%5Bcpage%5D=3#acalog_template_course_filter. Accessed 7 July 2019.
8. The Juilliard School: college catalog 2019–2020. Drama 1031-41-Alexander Technique I. https://catalog.juilliard.edu/preview_course_nopop.php?catoid=36&coid=20916. Accessed 7 July 2019.
9. MacPherson H, Tilbrook H, Richmond S, Woodman J, Ballard K, Atkin K, Bland M, et al. Alexander Technique lessons or acupuncture sessions for persons with chronic neck pain: a randomized trial. Ann Intern Med. 2015;163(9):653–62. Available from: https://www.amsatonline.org/aws/AMSAT/asset_manager/get_file/176988?ver=3457. Accessed 7 June 2019.
10. Wheelhouse F. Raymond Arthur Dart: a pictorial profile. Sydney: Transpareon Press; 1983.
11. Bronec R, Carbaugh R. The Dart procedures: history and background. 2011. http://issuu.com/alextechurbana/docs/the_dart_procedures/10?e=0. Accessed 25 Mar 2019.
12. Barnes M. Ernst Haeckel's biogenetic law (1866). In: Embryo project encyclopedia. 2014. https://embryo.asu.edu/pages/ernst-haeckels-biogenetic-law-1866. Accessed 25 Mar 2019.
13. Bainbridge Cohen B. Basic neurocellular patterns: exploring developmental movement. El Sobrante: Burchfield Rose Publishers; 2018. p. 259–82.
14. Myers TW, Chambers G, Maizels D, Wilson P. Anatomy trains: myofascial meridians for manual and movement therapists. Edinburgh: Churchill Livingstone/Elsevier; 2017.
15. Vanier L, Nettl-Fiol R. Developing a framework for integration. AmSAT J. 2016;2016(9):41–5.

Chapter 16
Individualizing Training for Dancers

Tom Welsh, Kaitlin Morgan, and Gabriel Williams

Introduction

For many years, our research group has been advocating the use of small-N, within-subject experiments to study phenomena of interest to performing artists, particularly dancers [1–5]. Readers who are interested in learning more about within-subject experimental methods, also called single-case research methods, may wish to consult the references at the end of the chapter to explore the special features, benefits, and requirements of the within-subject approach to experimental analysis.

The purpose of this chapter is to reflect on what we have been learning about training dancers while conducting within-subject experiments. We begin with a brief description of how dancers have traditionally trained and contrast that approach with how musicians train to reveal an opportunity that some dancers and teachers may find useful. Before reviewing five studies that used within-subject experimental methods to evaluate individualized approaches to training dancers, we describe key features of within-subject experiments. Finally, we identify elements that are common across the studies and suggest training strategies that may permit dancers to engage in more deliberate practice [6] with individually tailored feedback.

Approaches to Training in the Performing Arts

Traditionally, dancers aspiring to a performing career in Western dance forms do most of their training in groups continually integrating their individual technical development and their interactions with other dancers. Dancers usually take a daily technique class in which 15–30 dancers are instructed by a single dance teacher,

T. Welsh (✉) · K. Morgan · G. Williams
Florida State University, Tallahassee, FL, USA
e-mail: twelsh@dance.fsu.edu

S.-H. Lee et al. (eds.), *Perspectives in Performing Arts Medicine Practice*,
https://doi.org/10.1007/978-3-030-37480-8_16

sometimes accompanied by a dance musician. The number of dancers the teacher is responsible for teaching concurrently limits the frequency and intensity of individually tailored cueing and feedback that can be provided to each dancer in the class. It also limits the amount of time the dance teacher can focus on a single skill that a particular dancer needs to improve.

Some dancers engage in individual practice in brief episodes after class when trying to master a movement skill or phrase that challenged them during class. Some dancers review phrases and skills taught in a previous class as part of their warm-up for a new class. In both cases, the individual practice is commonly done with little or no individual attention from their technique teacher.

One exception to this general pattern is when dancers are learning a solo or refining a section of a work that their choreographer is trying to perfect. Another is when dancers are learning and performing a therapeutic exercise under the guidance of a PT or athletic trainer. In these circumstances, dancers receive individualized instruction but it is more often the exception than the rule for training in dance.

Those who have studied music extensively will recognize a different pattern in the training of professional musicians. Musicians normally take a weekly, private lesson with an expert teacher who: (1) assigns etudes tailored to the musician's developing abilities, and (2) provides instructions, cueing, feedback, and reinforcement that match the individual musician's evolving abilities. Between lessons, musicians engage in individual daily practice to maintain and advance the technical skills reflected in the exercises prescribed by their teacher.

As they develop competence with their instrument through individual practice and private lessons, musicians begin to rehearse and perform with ensembles where they can refine their performance skills as they practice working collectively with other musicians to create musical experiences that are interactive, integrated, and whole.

Clearly, neither all dancers nor all musicians train identically and the general patterns of training in both groups evolve. Our purpose in describing the differences in training practices is to reveal an opportunity that some dancers and teachers may wish to pursue when a dancer's technical capabilities are not growing as rapidly or fully as desired when using a traditional approach to dance training.

Individualized Training for Dancers

In this section, we summarize a number of studies that evaluated individualized approaches to building skills and capacities in pre-professional, university dancers. We also introduce one study evaluating an individualized approach to teaching complex dance skills to younger dancers. We will briefly describe the methods, results, and major conclusions for each study. The question we posit is: "What can dancers accomplish by individualizing some of their dance training?" We encourage readers interested in learning additional details about any of these studies to access a copy of the original article. Before describing each study, we will highlight several common features of the research methodology used to conduct the studies.

Common Features of Within-Subject Experiments

All of the studies described in this chapter used small-N, within-subject experimental designs. Within-subject experimentation developed as an elaboration of Interrupted Time-Series designs, which Campbell and Stanley [7] described as a method prevalent in the "more successful sciences." The field of behavior analysis has refined the use of within-subject designs over the past 60 years and this approach to experimentation is becoming increasingly popular in many social sciences that currently rely on large-N, between group experimentation [8, 9].

Two threats to internal validity must be addressed in time-series analyses: instrumentation and history [7]. In the laboratory sciences, they are addressed by (1) establishing thorough control of any variables that might influence the phenomena under study and (2) carefully calibrating the instruments used to measure the dependent variable (DV). In applied studies, within-subject experimenters address the instrumentation threat by assessing inter-observer agreement (IOA) repeatedly throughout a study and requiring high levels of agreement between the independent observers. By doing so, researchers ensure that changes in the outcome measures are not simply reflecting unintended changes in the measurement device or the measurement protocol. IOA is a direct approach to assessing measurement reliability.

Within-subject researchers address the history threat by measuring the dependent variable repeatedly until a stable baseline level of performance is established. The potential influence of coincidental variables is ruled out by offsetting the application of the independent variable (IV) across participants, behaviors, or settings or by reversing the application of the IV. If application of the IV (normally treatment or training) is followed by a sizeable change in the level of performance (DV) each time the IV is systematically changed, researchers suspect a possible causal relationship between the variables. Within-subject researchers require that changes in the DV coincide with changes in the application of the IV several times before they conclude that the IV is causing observed changes in the DV. This amounts to replicating the experimental effect within each experiment. Researchers may repeat the application (or removal) of the IV as many times as needed to produce an unambiguous demonstration of the influence of the IV (or the absence thereof) on the DV.

Additional features of within-subject experiments deserve mention. First, the frequent assessments of the DV reveal patterns of performance over time and across conditions. Second, every participant experiences every experimental condition. This approach allows each participant's performance during treatment or training to be compared with their own performance during baseline, thereby eliminating a major source of variability that has to be addressed statistically in between-group experiments. In within-subject research, each participant serves as their own experimental control.

Within-subject experiments commonly employ a convention used for time-series analyses: displaying repeated measurements of the dependent variable graphically to facilitate the comparison of performances over time and across experimental conditions. For within-subject researchers to conclude that there is a causal relationship between the variables under study, changes in performance must be of a visually detectable magnitude, they must occur relatively soon after a change in experimental conditions, and they must be replicated with each change in experimental conditions.

Within-subject advocates argue that this analytic approach is often more rigorous than group comparison statistical analyses [9, 10]. They also warn researchers that interventions tested in within-subject experiments must be robust enough to produce a clear and consistent change in performance in order to have a chance of offering convincing evidence that an IV is actually responsible for changes observed in a DV. Interventions that have weak or inconsistent effects may not produce a convincing demonstration of experimental control (increasing the likelihood of a Type 2 error). Within-subject pioneers have suggested that the emphasis on robust interventions that this limitation encourages may be pragmatically useful in young, applied fields of research [10].

Finally, within-subject experimenters assess the social validity of the interventions they are testing to sample the perspective of the study participants. At the end of a study, participants (and sometimes teachers or clinicians) judge (1) the importance of the problem addressed; (2) the appropriateness of the treatment or training used; and (3) the value of the benefits received relative to the cost in terms of time and effort by offering written ratings on a 5, 6, or 7-point Likert scale. Treatment or training protocols that receive high social validity ratings may be more likely to be adopted by users [11].

Back Strengthening

In the late 1990s, Welsh, Jones, Lucker, and Weaver [12] evaluated the influences of twice weekly training using MedX and Nautilus equipment on dancers' lumbar extensor strength and related outcomes in pre-professional university dancers. Training lasted for 7–10 weeks as determined appropriate for each dancer by the supervising physician. Training was administered by the clinic staff at an off-campus, back-treatment clinic.

Dancers completed 3 min of training on MedX equipment (MedX Corporation, Ocala, FL) that was engineered to isolate use of the lumbar spine extensors. The supervising physician designed a program for each of the six dancers participating in the study. Training was designed to produce complete fatigue of the lumbar extensors by the end of the 3 min training session. If a dancer could not complete the entire session before fatiguing, the resistance was reduced for the next session. If the dancer did not show signs of fatigue by the end of the 3 min session, the resistance was increased for the next training session. The supervising physician made decisions about adjusting and progressing the resistance. Following each session on the MedX equipment, the dancers completed a 20 min program of complementary exercises on Nautilus equipment housed in the same clinic. All training sessions were directly supervised by the clinic staff. Total training time for each dancer was approximately 5 h.

Back strength increased from 14% to 151% for each of the six dancers when they received training. At the end of the first phase of the study, arabesque height (standing on one leg with the other leg extended behind the body) increased 3.6 degrees for the dancers who had received training and arabesque height decreased 2.6 degrees for the dancers who had not yet received training. The total number of classes and rehearsals missed by all dancers due to low back pain decreased from 25 to 4 per semester following training. Social validity ratings showed that, following training, dancers rated their back strength as greater, its limiting influence on their dance abilities as less, their work on the MedX and Nautilus equipment as the major contributing factor for their improvements, and the investment they made to pursue the training worth the benefits achieved.

Pelvic Alignment

Finding and maintaining good pelvic alignment is challenging for many dancers and their teachers consider good alignment important [13]. We conducted two within-subject experiments to see if a targeted approach to training might help dancers manage this training challenge. Deckert and her colleagues [13] assessed sagittal plane pelvic alignment (see Fig. 16.1) of first-year ballet dancers in a major university dance training program. They found that 12 of the 17 (70%) first-year dancers

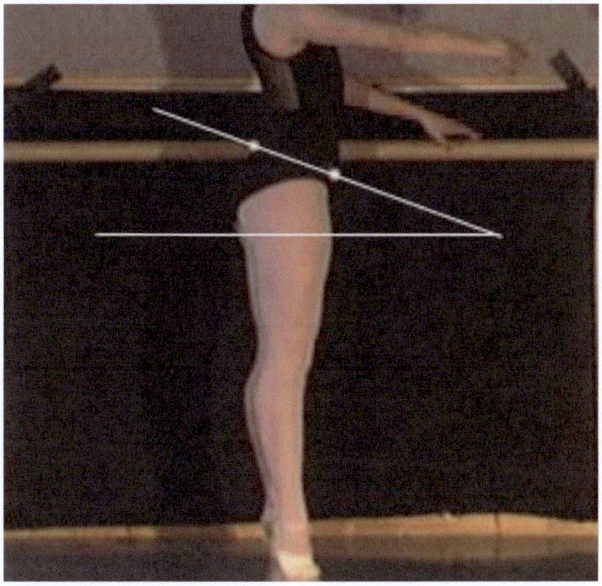

Fig. 16.1 Sample marker placement and measurement of pelvic tilt. (Modified with permission from: Deckert JL, Berry SM, Welsh TM. Analysis of pelvic alignment in university ballet majors. J Dance Med Sci. 2007 Dec;11(4):110–7.)

who volunteered for the study displayed a degree of anterior pelvic tilt that exceeded the amount judged acceptable by their teachers.

Deckert invited three dancers who displayed excessive anterior pelvic tilt during twice weekly baseline measurements, and who expressed an interest in improving their alignment, to participate in an experimental evaluation of an intervention designed to improve pelvic alignment. Deckert implemented a tutoring program that involved brief anatomy lessons, exercises designed to improve pelvic alignment, video feedback, individual coaching, and a home training program that each dancer could perform on their own between training sessions.

She met with each dancer twice weekly for 3 weeks to conduct training one dancer at a time while continuing to measure all three dancers' pelvic alignment each session. When the alignment training was applied individually following four, seven, and ten baseline measurements for Dancers 11, 15, and 16, respectively, pelvic alignment improved 3–4 degrees as each dancer received training (see Fig. 16.2). These improvements were sufficient to move two of the dancers from the unacceptable range (as determined by their teachers in a prior phase of the study) to the acceptable range. Alignment for the third dancer improved from unacceptable to borderline. The end-of-study social validity ratings revealed that the dancers believed good pelvic alignment is important, that tutoring was the major contributor to their improvement, and that participation in tutoring was worth the time and effort they invested.

In a second study of pelvic alignment, Holt and her colleagues [14] used an inexpensive, remote cueing device to remind two dancers in a similar university training program to maintain good pelvic alignment while performing ballet barre warm-up combinations. The researchers refined the measurement protocol used by Deckert and her colleagues to achieve high levels of inter-observer agreement, which is the within-subjects researcher's tool for ensuring measurement reliability and for controlling the instrumentation threat to internal validity. The dancers participated individually in twice weekly 20 min warm-up sessions for eight and a half weeks immediately before their morning technique classes. The first author taught and led the dancers through five typical ballet barre combinations. A more comprehensive sixth combination was video-taped and used for alignment assessments.

Once stable baseline performances were established for each dancer (5 sessions for Dancer 1, and 9 sessions for Dancer 2), remote cueing by an alignment coach was added during practice of the five warm-up combinations. When the alignment coach saw the dancer tilt her pelvis anteriorly (when it might be expected to be neutral), the coach pushed a button on a remote transmitter to activate a cueing device in a pocket on the dancer's abdomen causing it to vibrate four times in quick succession. When the five warm-up combinations were completed, the cueing device was removed and the dancer performed the sixth combination without cueing for the video-taped assessment.

When remote cueing was administered for each dancer individually, pelvic alignment improved 2.3 degrees (17% of baseline) for Dancer 1 and 1 degree (28% of baseline) for Dancer 2. Of the eight movements measured, all but one movement for one of the dancers improved. Social validity ratings by the dancers collected at the

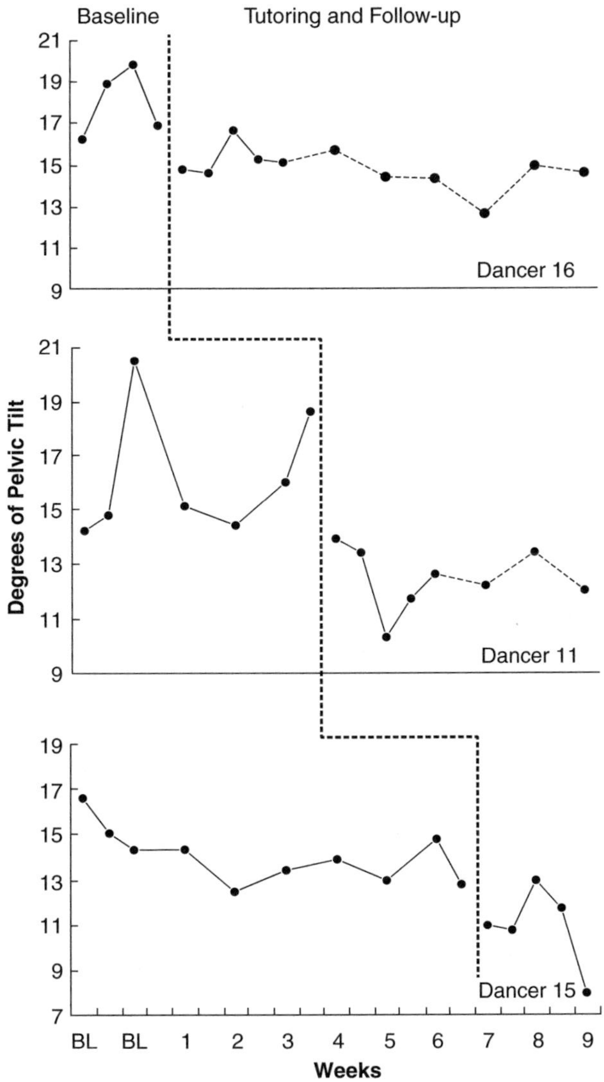

Fig. 16.2 Anterior pelvic title before, during, and following tutoring for all the dancers who received tutoring. Dashed lines show the initiation of tutoring for each dancer. Data points connected with dashed lines were gathered after tutoring was completed for each dancer. (Reprinted with permission from: Deckert JL Berry SM, Welsh TM. Analysis of pelvic alignment in university ballet majors. J Dance Med Sci. 2007 Dec;11(4):110–7.)

end of the study suggested the dancers believed that good pelvic alignment is important, that their alignment had improved, that cue training was an appropriate approach to improving pelvic alignment, and that the benefits of training were worth the time invested. Ratings by the dancers' ballet teacher paralleled the ratings made by the dancers. The teacher also commented on the need for dancers to engage in training beyond technique classes to encourage the maintenance of new movement habits.

One interesting finding from these two studies is that the degree of anterior tilt judged ideal by the dancers' teachers was not zero degrees and the ideal was different for each dancer. Focusing on individual dancer performance was key to calibrating the training and the goals of the training to each dancer's unique dance instrument. It is also interesting that the changes observed in both studies were achieved with approximately 6 h of individualized training per dancer.

We conducted a third study to determine whether improvements in pelvic alignment observed in the training setting were generalizing to the dancers' technique classes. It revealed that consistent improvements in alignment began to appear in technique classes *only* after the researcher added a generalization training component to the training protocol [15]. This finding will not surprise practitioners who have helped clients acquire a new capability in a training setting only to see them fail to use that ability in settings where its use is most important. This study demonstrates a nascent strategy for assessing the generalization of dance skills. It also suggests that principles explored by learning specialists [16] may be useful in addressing some of the challenges faced in training performing artists. Further research will be needed to confirm and extend the findings of this preliminary research.

Turnout

Turnout is a skill that many dancers strive to optimize [17, 18]. Pata and her colleagues conducted a within-subject experiment to evaluate a targeted-training program designed to improve the use of turnout in six, female dancers who were enrolled in a university-based, professional training program [19].

The researchers adapted a protocol developed by their colleagues [20] that was based on recommendations offered by Grossman [21] to measure each dancer's total active turnout [22] after technique classes 4 days per week over a nine-week period (see Fig. 16.3). After daily baseline turnout measurements stabilized for each dancer (5 sessions for Dancers 1 and 6, 13 and 15 sessions for Dancers 3 and 5, and

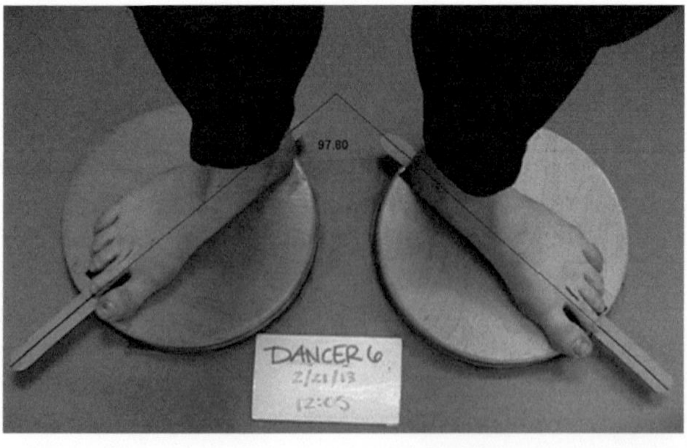

Fig. 16.3 Measurement of Total Active Turnout on modified frictionless rotational disks. (Reprinted with permission from: Pata D, Welsh T, Bailey J, Range V. Improving turnout in university dancers. J Dance Med Sci. 2014 Dec;18(4):169–77.)

25 and 23 sessions for Dancers 2 and 4), the dancers received individualized training designed to improve turnout, two dancers at a time.

Training was conducted twice a week for 45 min before morning technique classes for 5 weeks. Training sessions were designed and led by the first author who was actively training as a dancer herself when the study was conducted. Training focused on creating awareness of the efficient muscles to use to optimize turnout, building strength, improving flexibility, releasing unnecessary tension, and applying these abilities to the performance of dance movements. The trainer taught, cued, provided feedback, and made modifications as needed to tailor the training to each dancer's evolving abilities. She was able to interact intensively with each dancer because training was conducted with two dancers at a time.

Training for a second pair of dancers was initiated when their baseline turnout measurements stabilized and training for the first pair of dancers concluded. Training for the third pair of dancers began as the second pair of dancers completed turnout training. By measuring turnout for each dancer daily and administering training in a staggered fashion across dancers, the influences of turnout training were revealed in the graphic display of the dancers' turnout measurements over time and across conditions for each dancer.

Increases in Total Active Turnout (TAT) ranged from 9 to 20 degrees for each of the six participating dancers. The increases corresponded with the initiation of turnout-training for five of the six dancers. TAT for Dancer 4, one of the last dancers to be trained, began to increase in week 6, before she started turnout training. When training was initiated for this dancer, TAT continued on the same trajectory with no further improvements or decrements associated with training (see Fig. 16.4).

A dance teacher who had substantial experience in the body sciences rated each dancer's before and after training performance of an adagio phrase designed to challenge turnout control. Without knowing which recording was made before and which after training, she identified the after-training video as showing greater control of turnout for all six of the dancers. At the end of the study, the dancers rated the importance of improving turnout, the appropriateness of the training program, and the value of the gains relative to the effort they invested. All ratings were either 6 or 7 on a 7-point scale (7 being the most positive). Training time averaged 7.5 h per dancer over the 10 sessions conducted for each pair of dancer.

In a parallel study of the effects of a training program designed to improve développé performance, Morgan and her colleagues [3] observed développé height improvements of 5–38 degrees for each of the six dancers participating in the study (under review).

Turn, Kick, Leap

Quinn, Miltenberger, and Fogel [23] conducted a within-subject, multiple-baseline-across-behaviors experiment to evaluate the effects of brief supplemental training sessions designed to help four young dancers (6–9 years old) acquire skills they

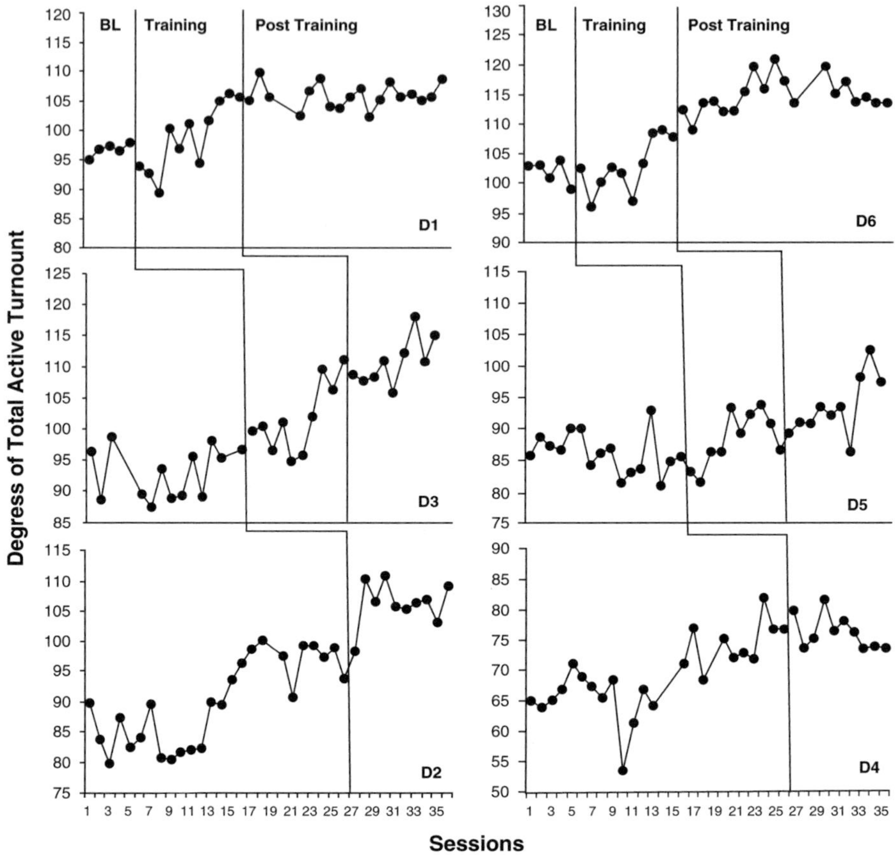

Fig. 16.4 Total Active Turnout measurements for each dancer. The stepped vertical lines mark the beginning and end of training for each dancer. The study concluded when the last two dancers (D2 & D4) finished training. No post training measurements were made for these two dancers. (Reprinted with permission from: Pata D, Welsh T, Bailey J, Range V. Improving turnout in university dancers. J Dance Med Sci. 2014 Dec;18(4):169–77.)

were finding challenging in their dance technique classes. The dance teachers were taught to use a "TAG-Teach" procedure [24] to provide auditory feedback (a click) for correct performance of pre-identified, challenging components of each of three dance skills (Kick, Leap, and Turn). The goals of training were tailored to each dancer's ability.

The researcher worked with each dance teacher to develop a task-analysis of the skills being targeted for each dancer. Each dancer's performance of 8–14 components of each of the targeted dance skills was assessed at least once a week during the 4 months in which the study was conducted. The dependent variable was the percentage of skill components performed correctly for each skill targeted for each dancer.

Training was administered by two dance teachers who met individually for a brief training session with one dancer immediately before or after technique class. Focusing on one component of each skill at a time, the teacher used a clicker to signal to the dancer, "Yes, that is correct" while resisting making "corrections" or offering other verbal feedback. If the dancer was unable to execute the component of the skill correctly after three tries, the teacher used her traditional instructional approach, but she focused on the individual dancer and the skill component being targeted. Once the dancer achieved the targeted component, the teacher moved on to repeat the sequence with the next component of the skill in the task analysis. The weekly investment in supplemental training amounted to 4 min per skill, 12 min per dancer for all three skills. Over the 4 months that the study was conducted, each dancer would have received approximately 3.5 h of individualized training.

When training was applied for each dancer, performance of the targeted skill began to improve promptly, with one exception in which the skill (Kick) took several months to improve for one dancer. As an additional experimental control, one of the skills (Leap) for one dancer never received supplemental training beyond what was offered in the technique classes. It remained unimproved at approximately 60% correct throughout the study. Otherwise, every dancer improved in all skills targeted by the supplemental training. Mean improvements across dance skills ranged from 28% to 44% for the four dancers who participated in the study.

At the end of the study, four dance teachers, including the two involved in TAGteach training, rated video recordings of each dancer's performance of each dance skill before and after TAGteach training without knowing which recording was made before and which was made after training. The combined ratings by the four teachers were consistently higher for the after-training performance of each dance skill.

Social validity ratings of the likeability and feasibility of the training approach by the dancers and teachers were all either 5 or 6 on a 6-point scale, 6 being the most positive rating. Dancers commented that the individualized training approach helped them concentrate, the training was better than their typical class instruction, and they would like to use it more. The teachers said the training approach was more intense and taught them how to break down the skills they were teaching into smaller steps. They also said the dancers were more focused and serious during the one-on-one teaching sessions than they typically were in their technique classes. One teacher commented that the dancers seemed to be having fun and that receiving individualized feedback seemed to make them feel special.

In summary, the handful of studies described in this section show improvements that were judged important by dancers and their teachers and that can be achieved with a modest investment in individualized training for each dancer. In the next two sections, we will highlight common elements of these individualized training approaches and suggest strategies that may allow teachers and dancers to individualize some of the training dancers receive.

Observations and Implications

Common Elements of the Training Approaches

On reviewing this collection of studies, one question that comes to mind is whether there are common elements of these training approaches that may have been instrumental in producing the observed improvements in dancer abilities.

One conspicuous common element is the focus on the individual dancer. Teaching one or two dancers at a time allows teachers to offer lessons based on the skills that each individual dancer is ready to learn. It also allows teachers to design an instructional sequence and use a training approach customized to each dancer's learning abilities. Individualizing training can allow teachers to provide tailored and precisely timed cueing and feedback and to progress through the lesson at a pace that is appropriate for each dancer without concern about leaving other dancers behind or boring advanced dancers. Even when two dancers are taught together [19], teachers are able to give a dancer who is excelling at the current assignment additional work to do on her or his own while momentarily focusing their teaching efforts on a dancer who needs special assistance. Comments by dancers in the Quinn et al. study [23] indicated that they "felt special" when being taught individually by their teacher and the teacher believed her dancers were more "focused" and "serious" in the TAGteach context than during the group technique classes.

Another common element in these studies is the focus on one component, or small collections of integrated components of a dance skill at a time. Focusing training in this way allows both dancer and teacher to be clear about what they are trying to achieve. Clarity of focus creates opportunities for teachers to tailor goals, cues, and feedback to match the skill being addressed as well as the unique abilities of the dancer who is learning to perform it. It also allows the teacher to celebrate each dancer's successes without the complication of creating unintended comparisons with the performance of other dancers who may progress faster or slower than the dancer the teacher is teaching at the moment. The "specialness" of a one-on-one teaching interaction may also motivate a dancer to give full attention to the training challenge.

Each of the speculations we are offering in this section will require further experimental evaluation to better understand the functional relations involved. The use of small-N, within-subject experimental research methods was another common feature in the studies reviewed. It may be that using a research methodology that allows for detailed analysis of individual performance will be necessary to learn whether and how to make the best use of training interventions as intensive and individualized as those described in this chapter. We suspect that greater adoption of within-subject experimental methods will enhance researchers' ability to study individualized treatment and training in the performing arts.

Opportunities to Individualize Training

If dancers and teachers are to try individualized approaches to training, they will need to be able to do so without displacing critical aspects of the training they are already doing. In addition, any investment they make in individualized training will need to return benefits that are valuable to dancers and teachers. Special intervention strategies may be useful in this regard.

One potentially useful strategy may be to individualize only a portion of a dancer's training. The goal should be to supplement, rather than replace the group training that dancers are already using as their primary source of training. The results of the studies reviewed in this chapter show that dancers can make sizeable improvements in capacities that are useful to dancers with as few as 5 h of supplemental training distributed across a few weeks. If individualized training can improve important dance abilities in a modest amount of time, dancers might focus on improving one ability at a time and then change their focus to a new ability when the one they are working on reaches a sustainable level. Future research might be designed to assess this strategy as well as the conditions necessary to make it work.

A second strategy may be to focus individualized training on skills and abilities that are especially important to dancers, either because they are important for all dancers to optimize or because they address a specific limitation for the dancer who is choosing to engage in individualized training. If teachers and dancers use highly efficient training protocols, their investment will be modest and offset by the gains realized. If the dancer feels the investment of their time and energy is worth the improvements they achieve, they may become motivated to try an individualized approach to improving other dance skills. The same probably holds true for teachers; they are more likely to be interested in offering individualized training if they feel their time is being used efficiently and if the gains their dancers are making seem worth the additional effort invested.

A third strategy may be to encourage highly motivated dancers to become early adopters of individualized training approaches and to be sure that any gains achieved by these early adopters are easy for other dancers to see. Other dancers may become interested in trying the training approach if they see dancers they respect benefiting from the practice [25]. It also seems possible that parents of young dancers might seek individualized training for their child if they believe it will allow her or him to excel and remain healthy while doing so. Parental support appears to be a common feature in the backgrounds of individuals who develop high levels of expertise in music, for example [26].

A fourth strategy was exemplified in the studies by Holt and her colleagues [14] and Quinn and her colleagues [23]. Both used simple mechanical devices to make their interventions more focused and easier to apply. Teachers and dancers may want to try devices that show promise in valid empirical research and decide for themselves whether using such devices may be useful in their own training efforts. Video-feedback and modeling is another tool that has been used productively to enhance individualized training in dance and related endeavors [13, 27].

A fifth strategy might be to use partner peers to increase opportunities to individualize cueing, feedback, and reinforcement. In a study subsequent to the one described in the previous section, Quinn and her colleagues [28] showed that dancing peers could be taught to administer TAGteach training to their fellow dancers with experimentally confirmable benefits. Some of the other targeted training approaches described in this chapter also provided opportunities for peer coaching, although those elements were not analyzed separately.

Finally, developers who want to encourage adoption of individualized training approaches may want to allow for some meaningful degree of "re-invention" of their training protocols [25]. If targeted-training procedures can be made robust enough to permit teachers and dancers to modify them modestly without compromising their effectiveness, dancers and teachers may be more willing to use them [25].

Concluding Thoughts

Western concert dance has been taught successfully, and according to tradition, for half a millennium. Many dancers and teachers excel while using a traditional approach to developing expertise in dance. A major change in how dancers train would be ill-advised. However, dancers and teachers who are facing training challenges that are not responding to current training practices may wish to try using an individualized training approach. Future research might be aimed at determining whether a change in a dancer capacity that is initiated with individualized training can be sustained (or further improved) with traditional training approaches.

If dancers who incorporate individualized training into their training practices experience fuller, faster, and safer development of their dance abilities, other dancers may want to try what they are doing. If teachers are able to train a greater number of exceptional dancers, and their dancers remain physically and emotionally healthy as their abilities grow, other teachers may want to try what their colleagues are doing. Dancers and teachers who are achieving their intentions with traditional training methods will continue to be recognized for their successes and may be joined by dancers who overcome a resistant training challenge through individualized training, and thereby, become more capable participants in traditional dance training. Empirical research evaluating individualized training for dancers, like those described in this chapter, may ultimately identify a number of generally functional components of individualized training as well as the conditions under which they can be used to help dancers grow.

We started this chapter by recalling our advocacy of within-subject experiments as a tool for studying skill and capacity development in performing artists. The use of within-subject experimental designs facilitated our ability to study individualized approaches to training dancers. Because within-subject experiments focus on individual performance and permit the study of intensive interventions [29], we, and our colleagues at the University of South Florida, were able to learn a great deal about the influence of targeted training on the development of skills and capacities in the handful of dancers who participated in each study. The repeated measurements and graphic display of dancer performance before, during, and following training revealed nuanced patterns of acquisition over time and across individual dancers while also showing the consistent general influence of the training approaches across dancers.

In group comparison studies, details about individual performance are often hidden within group averages and those averages generally represent assessments made at only one or two points in time. What happens dancer-by-dancer as abilities develop over time is more clearly revealed by within-subject experiments. Researchers interested in better understanding the nuances of individual artistic development may want to consider adding small-N within-subject experimentation to their researcher's tool box.

Acknowledgments This chapter began as a presentation made at the USF-PAMA Conference in Tampa, FL, June 1, 2018 [30]. Jennifer Deckert, Kimberly Holt, Danielle Pata, Sue Carpenter, Alyssa Velazquez, and Veoletta Range contributed to its conceptualization and accuracy. Perceptive editing by Merry Lynn Morris, Santo Nicosia, and Sang-Hie Lee made the chapter better focused and easier to read.

References

1. Welsh TM, Chatfield SC. Within-subject research designs for dance medicine and science research. J Dance Med Sci. 1996;1:16–21.
2. Welsh T, Miller LK, Chatfield SC. Within-subject research with musicians. In: Lee SH, editor. Scholarly research for musicians. New York: Routledge; 2017. p. 125–35.
3. Welsh T, Morgan K, Miller LK, Chatfield S, Mainwaring L, Ambegaonkar J. Within-subject experimental designs: a methodological alternative for dance medicine & science researchers. Presented at the annual meeting of the International Association for Dance Medicine & Science, Houston, TX; 2017.
4. Welsh T. Dance research: facilitating relevance to practice. Presented at the Southeast Regional Performing Arts Medicine Association conference, University of South Florida, Tampa, FL; 2014.
5. Welsh T. Dance medicine & science: a propitious alliance. Presentation at annual meeting of the Performing Arts Medicine Association conference, Snowmass, CO; 2013.
6. Ericsson KA. Deliberate practice and the acquisition of expert performance: an overview. In: Horgensen H, Lehmann AC, editors. Does practice make perfect? Current theory and research on instrument music practice. Oslo: Norges Musikkhogskole; 1997. p. 9–51.
7. Campbell DT, Stanley JC. Experimental and quasi-experimental designs for research. Chicago: Rand McNally; 1963.
8. Bailey JS, Burch MR. Research methods in applied behavior analysis. New York: Taylor & Francis; 2018.
9. Kazdin AE. Single-case research designs: methods of clinical and applied settings. New York: Oxford; 2011.
10. Baer DM. Perhaps it would be better not to know everything. J Appl Behav Anal. 1977;10:167–72.
11. Carter SL. The social validity manual: a guide to subjective evaluation of behavior interventions in applied behavior analysis. Amsterdam: Elsevier; 2010.

12. Welsh TM, Jones GP, Lucker KD, Weaver BC. Back strengthening for dancers: a within-subject experimental analysis. J Dance Med Sci. 1998;2:141–8.
13. Deckert JL, Berry SM, Welsh TM. Analysis of pelvic alignment in university ballet majors. J Dance Med Sci. 2007;11:110–7.
14. Holt KM, Welsh TM, Speights J. A within-subject analysis of the effects of remote cueing on pelvic alignment in dancers. J Dance Med Sci. 2011;15:136–41.
15. Velazquez A, Welsh T. Transferring improved pelvic alignment into ballet technique class. Presented at the Southeast Regional Performing Arts Medicine Association conference, University of South Florida, Tampa, FL; 2018.
16. Stokes TF, Baer DM. An implicit technology of generalization. J Appl Behav Anal. 1977;10:349–67.
17. Clippinger-Robertson K. Biomechanical considerations in turnout. In: Solomon R, Minton S, Solomon J, editors. Preventing dance injuries: an interdisciplinary perspective. 2nd ed. Champaign: Human Kinetics; 2005. p. 135–50.
18. Grossman G, Krasnow D, Welsh T. Effective use of turnout: biomechanical, neuromuscular, and behavioral considerations. J Dance Educ. 2005;5:15–27.
19. Pata D, Welsh T, Bailey J, Range V. Improving turnout in university dancers. J Dance Med Sci. 2014;18:169–77.
20. Welsh TM, Rodriguez M, Beare LW, Barton B, Judge T. Assessing turnout in university dancers. J Dance Med Sci. 2008;12:136–41.
21. Grossman G. Measuring dancer's active and passive turnout. J Dance Med Sci. 2003;7:49–55.
22. Champion LM, Chatfield SJ. Measurement of turnout in dance research: a critical review. J Dance Med Sci. 2008;12:121–35.
23. Quinn MM, Miltenberger RG, Fogel VA. Using TAG-teach to improve the proficiency of dance movements. J Appl Behav Anal. 2015;48:11–24.
24. TAGteach International. http://www.tagteach.com. Accessed 30 Aug 2019.
25. Seekins T, Fawcett SB. Planned diffusion of social technologies for community groups. In: Paine SC, Bellamy GT, Wilcox B, editors. Human services that work: from innovation to standard practice. Baltimore: Brookes; 1984. p. 247–68.
26. Lehmann AC. The acquisition of expertise in music: efficiency of deliberate practice as a moderating variable in accounting for sub-expert performance. In: Deliège I, Sloboda J, editors. Perception and cognition of music. Hove: Psychology Press/Erlbaum (UK) Taylor & Francis; 1997.
27. Kelly H, Miltenberger RG. Using video feedback to improve horseback-riding skills. J Appl Behav Anal. 2016;49:138–47.
28. Quinn M, Miltenberger R, James T, Abreau A. An evaluation of auditory feedback for students of dancers: effects of giving and receiving feedback. Behav Interv. 2017;32:370–8.
29. Hrycaiko D, Martin GL. Applied research studies with single-subject designs: why so few? J Appl Sport Psychol. 1996;8:183–99.
30. Welsh T. Individualizing training for dancers. Presented at the Southeast Regional Performing Arts Medicine Association conference, University of South Florida, Tampa, FL; 2018.

Chapter 17
Creating a Motor Learning Model for Dance Training

Virginia Wilmerding and Donna H. Krasnow

Background

Motor behavior is a general term covering three aspects of human movement: motor development, motor control, and motor learning. Motor development examines changes in movement capabilities through all the stages of life, and they are progressive and irreversible [1]. Motor control describes how the nervous system coordinates muscles and joints to produce movement, using sensory and environmental information [2]. Motor learning examines changes in a person's skill capabilities caused by experience or practice, and these changes can be measured by inferences through observed, relatively permanent alterations in performance [2, 3]. While motor control examines how humans do movement that is already attained, motor learning places an emphasis on acquiring or modifying movement [4].

Over the past 50 years, various theories of how people think and learn have evolved. One well-known theory is *multiple intelligences* by Howard Gardner, which notes eight intelligence types: (1) *linguistic*—ability with words; (2) *logical/mathematical*—ability to reason, consider abstractions, use numerical skills; (3) *spatial*—awareness of space and how objects and the self occupy space; (4) *musical*—a sense of rhythm, pitch, and musical composition; (5) *bodily/kinesthetic*—a sense of the body and movement ability; (6) *interpersonal*—interactions with others; (7) *intrapersonal*—awareness of self and personal goals and standards; and (8) *naturalistic*—relating to the laws of nature and the natural surroundings [5]. This idea has challenged the traditional notion of verbal versus numerical, left versus right brain learning, etc., and offered a new viewpoint about how people think about

V. Wilmerding (✉)
University of New Mexico, Albuquerque, NM, USA
e-mail: pett@unm.edu

D. H. Krasnow
York University, Toronto, ON, Canada

S.-H. Lee et al. (eds.), *Perspectives in Performing Arts Medicine Practice*,
https://doi.org/10.1007/978-3-030-37480-8_17

the world and learn new skills. Gardner's perspective provided the insight to teachers regarding the many ways that students learn and how teachers can develop different approaches to accommodate these variations.

This idea was followed by Bernice McCarthy who described four learning styles in her educational system named 4MAT: (1) dynamic—experimentation and trial-and-error, risk-takers, intuitive; (2) innovative—social interactions and discussion, cooperative; (3) Common sense—hands-on and practical, more cautious; and (4) analytic—logical, seek facts in systematic ways [6, p.187]. These theories are further applied on experiential learning by David Kolb who described a cycle of learning in four stages: (1) concrete experience; (2) reflective observation; (3) abstract conceptualizing based on observing and reflecting; and (4) testing the new ideas through experimentation [7].

Debra Rose and Robert Christina [8] merged these constructs into a single model of learning preferences (see Fig. 17.1). This combined model categorizes learners by personal style and by activity choices for learning. In this construct, a particular dancer might learn best through experimentation (dynamic) with concrete movement experiences while another dancer might prefer logical, analytic descriptions (analytic) and reflecting on what is observed in demonstrations [8].

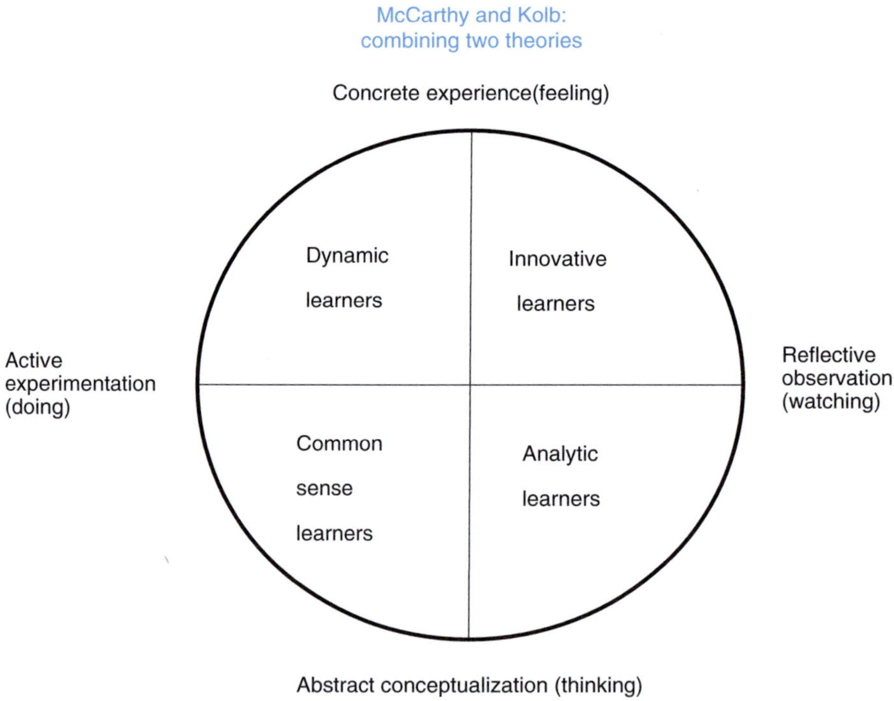

Fig. 17.1 McCarthy's four styles of learning combined with Kolb's cycle of learning. (With permission from Rose and Christina [8], Fig. 6.4, page 188)

The common theme in this line of learning theories is that each student is unique and may have different methods and preferences in the learning process. If teachers only use one teaching strategy, such as the traditional *modeling*, they will only reach some members of the class.

Instructional Strategies: Communicating New Material

Traditionally, the most common dance instructional strategy is demonstration, also known as modeling. It is important for the teacher to understand what the dance students see when they observe a demonstration of new material. Mainly what the dancer perceives deals with the relationships of various body parts to each other, that is, coordination patterns, but not necessarily the effort needed to achieve the movement or what is going on inside the body for stabilization. Timing and frequency of demonstration are key to its usefulness. In terms of timing, dancers should see a demonstration of new material before attempting it. Verbal explanation can be added later. In terms of frequency, unlike what one might think, there is no such thing as too much demonstration, but demonstrations should be mixed with repeated attempts. The concern that students can become dependent on the teacher for demonstrations is not supported by research, and as dancers become more advanced, they will need fewer demonstrations in the learning process [9].

The second teaching strategy upon which teachers rely is verbal instruction. The most important idea to remember, especially with children and beginners, is to not overload them with too much information all at once. A good example of this problem can be seen in Fig. 17.2.

Verbal instructions should be age appropriate [1]. This idea suggests that with children, it is best to keep the information fairly simple and use language with which they are familiar. With older dancers, the teacher can bring in ideas that are more complex and possibly involve conceptual material and anatomy. It is helpful with any age or level or experience to provide information about how to accomplish the movement and not just about what the movement or form is. Additionally, it is crucial to focus on movement outcomes, and not focus on the particular single movements or muscles they are using. In other words, emphasize the use of external rather than internal focus of attention when learning new skills. Internal focus suggests that the dancer is concentrating on the specific components of the movement. External focus suggests that the dancer is concentrating on the effects or the outcome of the movements.

Another teaching modality is the use of verbal cues, which are short phrases, only a few words that suggest movement ideas or approaches. These cues can be introduced during movement demonstration, and then called out as dancers execute the movement. The voice itself can be a powerful tool as a cue, using rhythm, pitch, accent, volume, and tone to affect movement quality and timing.

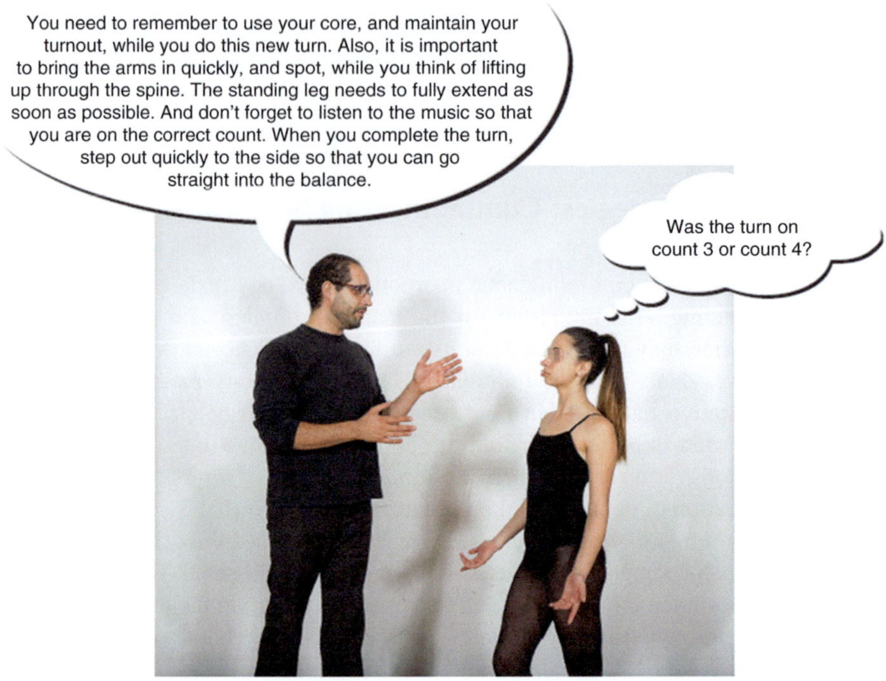
You need to remember to use your core, and maintain your turnout, while you do this new turn. Also, it is important to bring the arms in quickly, and spot, while you think of lifting up through the spine. The standing leg needs to fully extend as soon as possible. And don't forget to listen to the music so that you are on the correct count. When you complete the turn, step out quickly to the side so that you can go straight into the balance.
Was the turn on count 3 or count 4?

Fig. 17.2 The teacher is overloading the dancer with information while she is trying to learn a new movement (Reprinted with permission Krasnow and Wilmerding [9], 247)

Instructional Strategies: Augmented Feedback

During or after dancers have attempted movement, teachers can provide augmented feedback, which gives the dancers information about their relative success at accomplishing the goals. Concurrent feedback is given while the dancers are moving, and terminal feedback is given after the execution is complete. The two types of feedback are: knowledge of results (KR), which is feedback about what has occurred; and knowledge of performance (KP), which is information about the movement features that created what occurred. Often KR is redundant, especially with more advanced dancers, and KP tends to be far more useful in assisting dancers in improving their skills. Table 17.1 shows some examples.

If the teacher is giving concurrent feedback, the emphasis should be on what the dancer is focusing on, as otherwise the feedback can be distracting and have a negative effect. Additional ideas or corrections should occur as terminal feedback. Unlike demonstration, feedback can be overdone, and dancers can become dependent on hearing continuous comments.

Table 17.1 Examples of teacher's feedback to students: Action, Knowledge of Results, and Knowledge of Performance

Action	Knowledge of Results	Knowledge of Performance
Pirouette	You did not complete your triple turn	When you initiate the triple turn, bring the arms in faster
Body roll in standing 2nd position	You lost your balance during the arch	When you arch during the body roll, increase your core support
Jazz layout	You fell backward at the final shape	Keep your body weight forward as the body arches back
Ballroom salsa	You lost contact with your partner on the turning step	As you initiate the turning section, make your steps smaller
Partner lift	You did not get your partner all the way to the intended top of the lift	Use more plié at the onset of the lift, and keep your partner closer to your body on the way up

Reprinted with permission Krasnow and Wilmerding [9], 195

Motivation

Motivating dancers is an important aspect of enhancing motor learning. There are two types of motivation: extrinsic and intrinsic. Examples of extrinsic motivation are praise and social support, while intrinsic motivation refers to self-motivation, often for personal satisfaction. It is important for teachers to realize that younger students rely on extrinsic motivation, but children should be encouraged and guided to develop intrinsic motivation [1].

The teacher can explore various strategies that assist in motivating students. They can set specific short-term and long-term goals, balance praise and criticism, discuss issues of success and failure, use tools such as video to make assessments, and recognize when it is time to move on after a skill has been acquired. The class design can also impact motivation. Class should progress over time in a manner that continues to challenge the dancers but not overwhelm them. Comments can enhance body image rather than seem critical. The class should incorporate safe and sound practices, including pacing and content.

Repetition Versus Variable Material

The question often arises, how much repetition of material is best versus introducing new material to the students. Clearly, a certain amount of repetition is essential. However, unless a skill is going to be executed in the same way in every instance, it is best to vary the skill in a variety of ways, such as timing, dynamics, facings, placement of material before and after the skill, and use of extremities. A good example from sports is the difference between court shots in basketball during play and free throws after fouls. Athletes always practice the free throw from the exact same place on the court, and take some time, as that is how it happens in the game. However, they practice court shots using a variety of timings and placements on the court, and with various players tossing the ball to them, so that this practice is far more random. Additionally, it is better to practice a given skill mixed with practice of other skills (called variable practice), rather than the same movement over and over (constant practice) before moving on to a new idea [9].

Conditions of Practice

Several techniques can be used in teaching motor skills to dancers. The three common ones are segmentation, simplification, and fractionization. With segmentation, the teacher presents only a portion of a movement series, and then continues to add on, for example, teach A, then A + B, then A + B + C, until the entire combination is learned. Simplification involves teaching a foundation of the movement, such as the legs only, and then adding complexity, such as adding arms and then torso. Fractionization is used when different body parts are doing different rhythms, commonly used in music such as drumming. When movement cannot be broken down in any of the above ways, the teacher can use attention as a way of teaching the skill, that is, focusing the dancers' attention on one particular aspect at a time.

Mental Practice and Imagery

Mental practice and imagery are valuable tools in learning and executing dance. Mental practice is rehearsing a skill or sequence of movements using thought, without physical execution. Mental imagery is a psychological activity that calls to mind the characteristics of an absent object or dynamic activity. Mental practice and imagery can be utilized in both the acquisition of new skills and in preparing for performance. Some of the types of imagery include visual, kinesthetic, direct, metaphorical, lines-of-movement, global, and anatomical. Examples include any of the following: "Imagine seeing an expansive ocean in front of you as you dance" (visual). "Imagine feeling sand under your feet as you cross the space" (kinesthetic). "Imagine as you do the movement that you are an arrow flying through space" (direct). "Imagine moving as if you are being pushed by the wind" (metaphorical). "Imagine a string that connects your pubic bone to your navel" (lines-of-movement). "Imagine you are in a sauna and move in a relaxed, fluid way" (global). "Imagine the heads of the femurs or thigh bones as they float inside the hip sockets" (anatomical) [9].

Conclusion

In conclusion, knowledge and application of motor learning principles can support the well-established traditions commonly experienced in dance classes. Teachers can maintain their familiar methods and class content, and enhance their classes with these additional ideas: methods of communicating new material, augmented feedback, motivation, balancing repetition and variable material, conditions of practice, and mental practice and imagery. Drawing from a wide variety of concepts from many sciences, including motor development and learning, dance teachers can help each individual dance student find optimal performance and success.

References

1. Haywood KM, Getchell N. Life span motor development. 5th ed. Champaign: Human Kinetics; 2009.
2. Schmidt RA, Lee TD. Motor control and learning: a behavioral emphasis. 5th ed. Champaign: Human Kinetics; 2011.
3. Magill RA. Motor learning and control. 9th ed. New York: McGraw-Hill; 2011.
4. Shumway-Cook A, Woollacott MH. Motor control: translating research into clinical practice. 4th ed. Philadelphia: Lippincott Williams & Wilkins; 2012.
5. Gardner H. Frames of mind: the theory of multiple intelligences. New York: Basic Books; 1983.
6. McCarthy B. The 4MAT system: teaching to learning styles with right/left mode techniques. Barrington: Excel; 1987.
7. Kolb DA. Learning-style inventory (revised). Boston: McBer and Company; 1985.
8. Rose DJ, Christina RW. A multilevel approach to the study of motor control and learning. 2nd ed. San Francisco: Benjamin Cummings; 2006.
9. Krasnow DH, Wilmerding MV. Motor learning and control for dance: principles and practices for performers and teachers. Champaign: Human Kinetics; 2015.

Chapter 18
Voice and Dance Technique Integration: Triple Threat or Double Trouble?

Jennie Morton

Historical Context and Current Trends in Training

In the modern world of musical theatre, artists are required to sing, dance and act, and have hence become known as "triple threat" performers. However, seamlessly combining challenging vocals while performing a vigorous dance routine can create double trouble! In the early days of musical theatre, these three disciplines were more segregated, with singer/actors typically playing the lead roles and the dance numbers being performed by a troupe of what were known colloquially as "hoofers." As this genre began to develop and musicals began to appear in the world of film, stars such as Gene Kelly became widely known for their ability to perform across all three disciplines—subsequently, the *triple threat performer* began to become a standard requirement in the field. In recent years, there has been an increasing trend toward ever-more spectacular shows as theatres compete with the advent of animation and computer-generated images (CGI) used in the world of film [1]. In order to keep up with audience expectations in the modern world, many shows have attempted to replicate such imagery in their live productions [2]. The result is that the performers are now often required to add skills such as puppetry, aerial and acrobatic work, and the handling of complex props to their repertoires [3]. Examples of this can be seen in shows such as Disney's *The Lion King*, where the costumes themselves have built-in puppetry mechanisms, and *Wicked*, where one of the performers has to operate the large animated Oz head mask. I have personally worked with artists from both these productions who had incurred overuse injuries from the unaccustomed loads these additional skills require. In the Broadway production of *Spider-Man: Turn Off the Dark*, several actors incurred serious injuries when the production attempted to replicate the flying action created by CGI in

J. Morton (✉)
The Colburn School, Los Angeles, California, USA
e-mail: hello@jenniemorton.com

S.-H. Lee et al. (eds.), *Perspectives in Performing Arts Medicine Practice*,
https://doi.org/10.1007/978-3-030-37480-8_18

the movie versions with on-stage flying stunts [4]. To reflect this increased diversity of skills, musical theatre artists are now often referred to as multi-disciplinary performers, as the required skill set now reaches beyond the three prongs of the triple threat. The question then arises as to whether musical theatre training programmes are prepared to facilitate the safe integration of these diverse skills in order to protect the performer from injury and to promote career longevity.

While musical theatre performers are required to integrate all the previously mentioned skills in performance, training programmes still often treat these skills as distinct entities. In fact, there are some musical theatre programmes that focus only on the singing and acting aspects of training, with only one or two dance classes per week. Other performers may attend a pure dance programmes, while taking only occasional private singing lessons. One of the most challenging aspects of performance is to integrate the skills of singing and dancing. For example, how do you maintain a smooth vocal phrase while the choreography requires you to jump up and down? In training, dance classes typically take place in the studio with a dance teacher/choreographer; then vocal work is undertaken with the singing teacher in a room where one is usually sitting or standing still. In the professional world, rehearsals are usually segregated in a similar way as choreography is learned in a dance studio with the choreographer while the vocal work is learned sitting down with the musical director. Usually, around the end of the second week of rehearsal, the performer is asked to put it all together and then may discover that the high B flat note she has to sing occurs choreographically when she is at the height of a leap! It is often left to the performer to find a way to overcome these conflicts so that neither the movement nor the sound is compromised. Sometimes, this may be achievable, but at other times it may not.

Perhaps due to the previously mentioned biases in training, musical theatre performers are often categorized by their dominant skill. Casting calls often state that they are seeking "dancers who sing" or "singers who dance" [5]. Those who fall into the former category will usually have undertaken a high-level dance training programme but may have minimal vocal training. Those in the latter category will usually have a high degree of proficiency in vocal performance but may only have basic dance skills. However, most professional productions require these artists to perform across all skills, and in the context of the usual eight shows per week schedule that may run over weeks, months, or even years, we can begin to see issues arise. Dancers who lack the requisite training to support safe vocalization may experience vocal strain, vocal fatigue and potentially vocal injury [6]. Singers who lack the proficiency and technique training for safe dance practice may experience muscle strains and back problems as the body is pushed beyond its accustomed limits for physical movement [7]. When we take a deeper look at the training protocols for dancing and vocalizing, we begin to see that there are many mutual incompatibilities in terms of body alignment and muscle recruitment patterns that can result in the potential for development of injuries. The following sections highlight these incompatibilities and demonstrate how having a deeper understanding of the underlying anatomical structures can facilitate safer integration of the triple threat skills.

Body Alignment

Dancers

Successful musical theatre productions, as seen on Broadway or in London's West End, usually recruit highly skilled dancers, many of whom have a strong grounding in classical ballet technique [8]. In fact, audition notices often specify "Classically-trained dancers only need apply." Classical ballet is traditionally recognized as the foundational training for many genres of dance; unfortunately, as alluded to earlier, the body alignment and muscle recruitment typically taught in ballet technique are not always compatible with safe vocal production.

Beginning at the feet, ballet training often requires the center of gravity to be shifted toward the forefoot, with the calcaneus (heel bone) barely in contact with the floor in a standing position. This facilitates the seamless shift of body weight required when transitioning to the demi-pointe, full pointe and jump positions (Fig. 18.1). In order for the dancers to be seen to "float" through space, a toe-to-heel gait motion is used, which is in contrast to the usual heel-to-toe pattern seen in

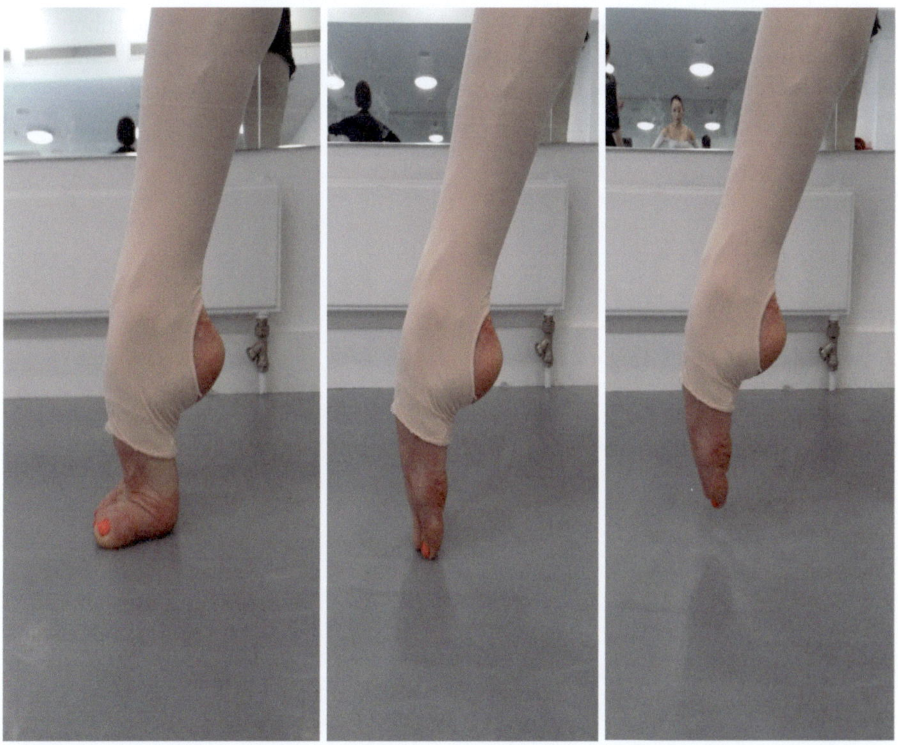

Fig. 18.1 Demi-pointe, full pointe and jump positions. (Photographs courtesy of Claire Calvert and Laura Carter of the Royal Ballet, London)

regular movement. This pattern is also used in jump landings and facilitates improved descent control and shock absorption [9]. However, it can also lead to an increase of loading into the forefoot [10] and therefore good muscle tone and control are required to prevent injury. A high degree of plantar flexion is favored at the foot and ankle, and is often balanced with a hyperextension of the knee joint creating a pleasing line for the gesture leg. However, during weight-bearing this can cause problems as dancers tend to push back into the hyperextended position. This can exacerbate issues of ligament laxity at the knees, leading to joint instability and potentially injury, and impact the generation of optimal breath mechanics when attempting to vocalize from this position.

Another feature of classical ballet training involves the use of extreme external rotation of the hip. This ideally requires the dancer to be able to achieve a 180 degree rotation bilaterally, 90 degrees from each hip. When combined with the aforementioned hyperextension at the knees, this can result in a sway-back posture [11] (Fig. 18.2). This postural combination represents a move away from neutral alignment, which can result in increased spinal and lower limb muscle tension, reflected by increased tone in the muscles of phonation. This can lead to increased phonatory effort and a loss of vocal efficiency [12].

The placement of the pelvis can also present a challenge to optimal vocalizing and this can vary with experience level and training methods. In order to achieve the extremes of hip rotation required, novice dancers often tilt the pelvis anteriorly thereby increasing the lumbar lordosis, while the more experienced dancer tends to

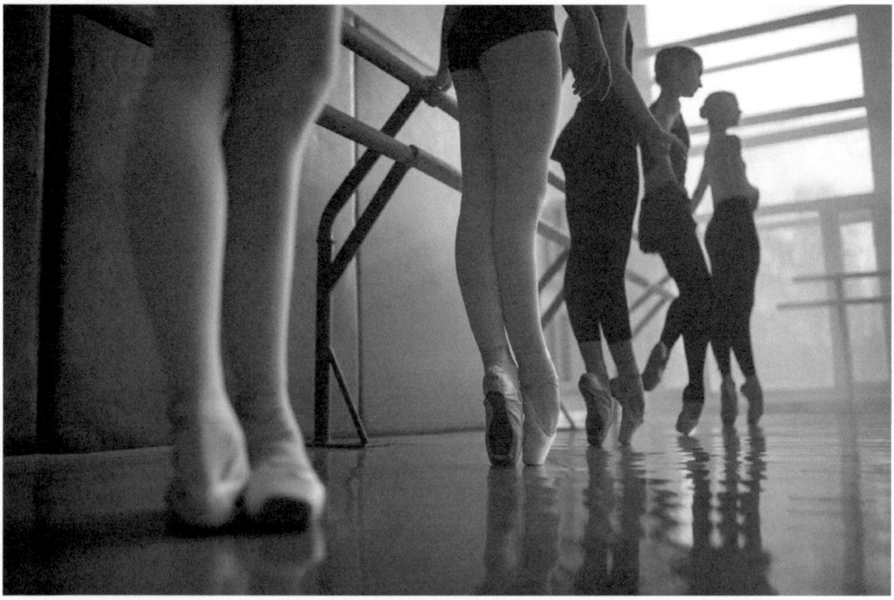

Fig. 18.2 External rotation of the hip with knee hyperextension and foot plantar flexion. (Purchased from Shutterstock.com royalty-free images)

use a posterior tilt of the pelvis to maintain the look of a flattened lumbar spine [13]. Both forms of pelvic tilt may negatively impact effective vocalizing. The posterior tilt of the pelvis, known as "tucking," is taught in some dance training methods to create a straighter look to the spine [14], but it can lead to muscle imbalances between the quadriceps and hamstrings [15] as well as reduce shock absorption for the spine. Similarly, an anterior tilt of the pelvis can produce compensatory actions up the spine, displacing the pelvis to rib cage relationship and altering ideal neck and chin alignment. Therefore, posterior or anterior tilt of the pelvis is currently not recommended in most dance practices—a neutral pelvis is optimal. As will be elucidated in the later section on breath mechanics, a neutral pelvis (and thus neutral spine) is also optimal for safe and effective vocalizing. This can create another area of potential conflict for those dancers who may be using a posterior or anterior pelvic tilt.

Furthermore, in order to support the lengthened spinal alignment, dancers often recruit an inward bracing of the abdominal muscles. This can result in a higher placement of the breath in the upper part of the chest. This can prove challenging to both breath control and efficient vocalizing, and will be discussed later in the chapter.

The final feature of a dancer's typical alignment that can have an effect on vocalizing is the positioning of the neck and chin area. Dancers typically tend to use a high eyeline and this is achieved through a raising of the chin, potentially resulting in increased cervical lordosis. This also creates an upward displacement of the mandible in relation to the sternum that, as described in the later section on vocal anatomy, may have a negative effect on the efficiency of vocal muscle recruitment [12]. This neck and chin alignment can also be a compensation response to the aforementioned hyperextension at the knees and sway-back posture.

Singers

In contrast to the dancers' tendency to place body weight over the forefoot, singers typically use a more normal mid-foot stance that is favorable to neutral placement of the body. Singers also recruit a normal heel-to-toe gait pattern as opposed to the toe-to-heel motion seen in dancers. The knees are held in a more neutral position as well, with some even using a mild flexion of the knees to facilitate a feeling of grounding for some vocal passages. The legs and feet are usually placed in a parallel alignment in contrast to the extreme external rotation seen in dancers. While it is generally accepted that a neutral pelvis is optimal for vocalizing, there are some voice teachers who advocate placing the pelvis into a posterior tilt or "tuck." This is a controversial topic in the realm of vocal pedagogy because of the anatomical challenges that the tucked position can pose [16]. These challenges will be discussed in the following section on anatomy.

With the neutral pelvic placement, the natural curves of the spine are retained, in contrast to either the dancers' flattened spinal alignment (from a posterior pelvic tilt) or the increased lumbar lordosis (often seen in novice dancers) [13]. At the neck and chin area, a neutral relationship between the mandible and sternum is maintained thereby facilitating optimal functioning of the vocal apparatus. Should a singer wish to raise their eyeline, they will tend to do so by initiating the movement from the upper part of the thoracic spine in order to avoid disrupting the chin–sternum relationship. This is in contrast to dancers who tend to displace the chin to raise the eyeline or to perform backward-bending movements of the spine.

The Anatomy of Breathing and Vocalizing

Any form of vocalization, be it for speaking or singing, is a form of controlled exhalation—the voice is being supported upon a column of air. While breathing is a natural and subconscious process for most people, professional vocalizing requires bringing these natural mechanisms under conscious control. In order to do this, it is essential to understand the underlying anatomy of optimal breath patterns. When observing a young infant breathing, it is the abdomen that rises and falls with the breath and not the upper chest or shoulders. However, as infants begin to walk on two feet and the stresses of life begin to take hold, many lose touch with this abdominal connection and resort to a shallower breathing pattern in the chest. Voice training seeks to reconnect performers to the natural breath patterns in order that their conscious choices for breath are in line with the underlying anatomical mechanisms [12].

Many muscles are involved in breath production and all of them have attachment points into the spine, pelvis and rib cage. Muscles are most efficient when they are recruited from a neutral position. Therefore, in the case of the respiratory muscles, this requires a neutral placement of the spine, pelvis and rib cage to which they are attached [17]. That is not to say that these muscles do not function if away from this neutral alignment, but rather that their efficiency would be compromised. Thus, the pelvic and spinal alignment choices made by dancers and singers affect the degree of mechanical advantage of these muscles.

The main muscle of inhalation is the diaphragm. This is a dome-shaped structure that attaches to the lower costal margins, the T12, L1 and L2 vertebrae, the arcuate ligaments posteriorly and the xiphoid process of the sternum anteriorly. Its position in the center of the torso forms the dividing point between the thoracic and abdominal cavities. During inhalation, the diaphragm contracts and the upper portion of the muscle flattens in an inferior direction as the attachment at the lower costal margins moves outwards. This outward movement is a result of the rib cage expanding under the influence of the external intercostal muscles [6]. Beneath the diaphragm lie all the abdominal and pelvic organs and these must move downward and outward in order for the diaphragm to make its full excursion. While most of this outward motion occurs anteriorly via the abdominal wall (as observed in infants), it is also occurring inferiorly (via the pelvic floor) and postero-laterally (although this movement is not as obvious due to fewer elastic structures found around the spine and pelvic rim). In concert with the muscles of the rib cage, the contraction of the diaphragm results in an increase in thoracic cavity volume and a decrease in lung pressure that facilitates the drawing of air into the lungs.

Exhalation results from the release of the diaphragm and its return to the original domed position under elastic recoil. This is further facilitated by the contraction of the internal intercostal muscles returning the rib cage to neutral, and the contraction of the transversus abdominis, the oblique muscles and the muscles of the pelvic floor that assist in the return of the organs to their original position [6]. This motion reverses the pressure gradient in the lungs, resulting in an expulsion of the air. Just like a set of bellows, expansion of the rib cage and abdominal cavity is required to draw air in and contraction of these spaces is required to expel the air outward. When the anatomical information is overlaid with dancers' and singers' alignment and movement choices (see prior sections), the integration of voice and dance technique can be compromised by several factors:

- A posterior tilt of the pelvis, with the resultant flattening of the lumbar spine curve, reduces the efficiency of the respiratory, abdominal, pelvic and spinal musculature in both stabilizing and dynamic functions.
- Posterior pelvic tilt may also affect pelvic and hip stabilization during dance movements due to shortened hamstrings, lengthened psoas and weakness in the gluteus maximus muscle.
- The inward bracing of the abdominal wall seen in dancers can reduce sub-glottal pressure availability and result in an increased tendency for constriction of the vocal muscles that may cause fatigue or damage to the vocal structures.
- Tension in the upper back, neck and shoulders accompanied by an upper chest or clavicular breathing pattern that is sometimes seen in dancers may increase the level of tension in the vocal musculature.
- The placing of the center of gravity over the forefoot, often seen in dancers, can create postural demands on the respiratory and abdominal muscles that may compromise optimal breath mechanics.
- The displacement of the chin–sternum relationship may affect the tracking and glide of the vocal apparatus by compromising the alignment of the vocal muscles.
- For singers undertaking choreographic work, the typical heel-to-toe gait pattern can increase ground reaction forces when landing from jumps possibly leading to lower limb injures [9].

Details of these concerns are addressed in the next sections. Specifically, I will focus upon the breathing complexities associated with inward bracing of the abdominals in dancers; the pelvic alignment concerns for both dancers and vocalists; and the chin–sternum relationship as it relates to optimal breath mechanics.

Issues of Concern for Dancers and Singers

Inward Bracing of the Abdominals in Dancers Impacting Breath Mechanics

As alluded to earlier, several facets of dance training incur challenges for optimal breath patterns. In classical ballet training, *breath* is not often mentioned by teachers. Classically trained ballet dancers actually tend to hold their breath during movements and tend to recruit only upper-chest or clavicular breathing [14]. In modern/contemporary dance, the *breath* is emphasized in some movements; even so, this is often done with swift, audible exhales. Neither of these breath choices lends itself well to the controlled, non-audible exhalation required for safe vocalizing, and this can prove to be challenging for dancers when they are required to sing.

The optimal breathing is especially challenging as most dancers are typically trained to brace the abdominal muscles inward and upward. This was traditionally thought to provide the requisite core stability for strenuous dance movements, while at the same time, lending itself to the aesthetic of the slim body shape that the profession has historically encouraged. This inward bracing necessarily limits the downward excursion of the diaphragm as the internal organs have nowhere to go [6]. The result will be a lower air intake that leads to the over-recruitment of the accessory muscles of respiration and to upper-chest or clavicular breathing. This will be particularly apparent when oxygen demands are high during strenuous dance routines. The accessory muscles include the scalenes and sternocleidomastoid (that attach to the first and second ribs, and the sternum, respectively) and these muscles are also recruited for neck and head movements. Over-recruitment here can lead to neck tension and compromised vocal mechanics [12]. Further, the main issue arising from the inward bracing of the abdominal muscles is that this results in low sub-glottal pressure, a critical element in vocalization.

Sub-Glottal Pressure

When vocalizing, the ability to control volume (loudness) and pitch (higher notes) is a function of sub-glottal pressure. To understand this concept, one must first understand the mechanisms underlying the production of sound, or phonation. Housed within the larynx, or voice box, are the vocal cords. The vocal cords act as a sphincter that, when closed, will protect the airway and prevent the aspiration of food or other foreign objects into the lungs. As air escapes from the lungs during exhalation and passes through the vocal cords, they oscillate, much like splitting a blade of grass and blowing through it to create a buzz-like sound. Thus, at the laryngeal level, the voice is just a reed instrument only capable of producing a "buzz." It is only when this column of air passes through the funnel of our pharynx and oral cavity that each person's distinct vocal "fingerprint" is shaped and produced. The sphincter created by the meeting of the vocal cords is known as the glottis, and the level of air pressure beneath the glottis is referred to as sub-glottal pressure. Sufficient sub-glottal pressure is required to sustain volume over distances and for loudness control [18]. When the available air pressure is insufficient, increases in loudness can only be achieved through an escalation of local muscle activity creating pressing or squeezing of the vocal cords. This is much like the function of a garden hose where a greater stream of water can be created either by turning up the pressure from the faucet (increased sub-glottal pressure) or by placing a thumb over the lumen of the pipe (squeezing the muscles around the vocal cord sphincter). Both mechanisms operate under the physiological principle, pressure = flow × resistance.

When a dancer is physically restricting the downward excursion of the diaphragm by bracing the abdominal muscles inward, he or she is necessarily reducing the amount of available sub-glottal pressure. Therefore, when the dancer is required to sustain vocal volume, particularly at high pitches, the vocal muscles will be constricted. This constriction can significantly increase the risk of injury to the vocal mucosa (the delicate surface of the vocal folds) leading to edema and tissue damage, and may produce hoarseness, vocal fatigue, and pain on vocalizing [6].

Effects of Pelvic Alignment on Vocalizing

The vocal apparatus is located in the most mobile portion of the spine, the anterior region of the neck, the supporting structures of which include the larynx (housing the vocal cords), associated cartilages, and the hyoid bone. This small horseshoe-shaped bone does not articulate with any other bone, but is suspended in space by a sling of muscles (Fig. 18.3) that attach to various locations including the sternum, mandible, temporal bone of the skull, and the scapula (omohyoid muscle). Due to its suspended nature within this highly mobile body area, the neutral placement of the vocal apparatus is dependent upon optimal alignment of the entire musculoskeletal framework above and below. Direct fascial connections that link the plantar surface of the foot to the pelvic floor, diaphragm, hyoid muscles, scalene muscles, and the occipital bone of the skull dictate that the concept of safe and effective vocalizing must be viewed through the lens of whole-body alignment [19, 20].

Considering the aforementioned issues of pelvic alignment in dancers and singers, an overview of the muscular and fascial interconnections involved will demonstrate how pelvic placement choices can affect respiratory mechanics and therefore vocalizing. One of the muscles that influence pelvic positioning is the psoas muscle. This muscle has both superficial and deep layers that originate from the T12 to L5 vertebrae and intervertebral discs, and runs down to the lesser trochanter on the inner portion of the upper femur. This distal attachment is shared by the iliacus muscle that arises from the inner surface of the pelvis and thus these muscles are often referred to conjointly as the iliopsoas (Fig. 18.4). While the psoas is often referred to as a hip flexor, due to the role it plays in bringing the femur towards the torso, its primary role is in stabilization of the lumbar spine. Contraction of the

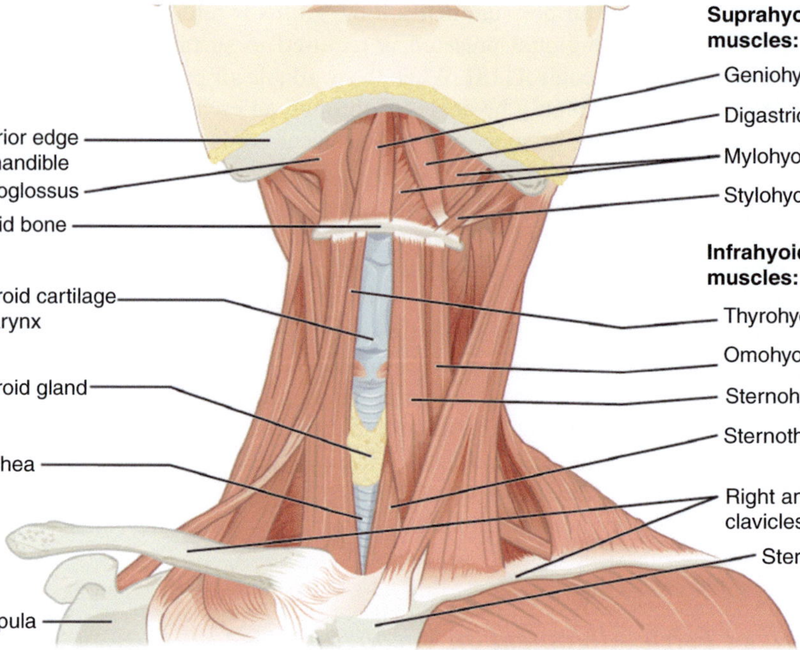

Fig. 18.3 Anatomy of the anterior neck. (From OpenStax College, 23 May 2013, Wikipedia)

psoas muscle bilaterally results in an anterior tilt of the pelvis, and conversely a posterior tilt of the pelvis would indicate slackening of the psoas muscles. Any movement of the pelvis necessarily affects the curvature of the spine, particularly at the T12/L1 junction where the diaphragm has its attachments. The psoas has a direct fascial connection with the diaphragm superiorly and with the pelvic floor muscles inferiorly [21]. Therefore, alterations in pelvic positioning can affect neutral placement and efficient action of the diaphragm.

It is important to note that the diaphragm is not only a muscle of respiration, but also supports lumbar-pelvic stabilization [22]. During normal breathing, the diaphragm works as part of an antagonist pair with the transversus abdominis (TA)—when the diaphragm contracts the TA releases and vice versa. However, when the body is moved away from a neutral alignment, the diaphragm and TA (along with the pelvic floor muscles) co-contract to provide lumbar-pelvic stability [23]. When respiratory demands increase, such as in vigorous dance movements and during vocalizing, the stabilization capacity of the diaphragm is decreased [24]. This can leave performers vulnerable to lower back injury if other core stabilizing muscles are not trained to compensate.

The pelvic floor is comprised of a sling of muscles that span the inferior pelvic outlet. Attachment points arise from the ischial tuberosities laterally, the coccyx bone posteriorly, and the pubic bone anteriorly. While they play a role in pelvic stability and provide the requisite sphincters for excretion, they are also involved in

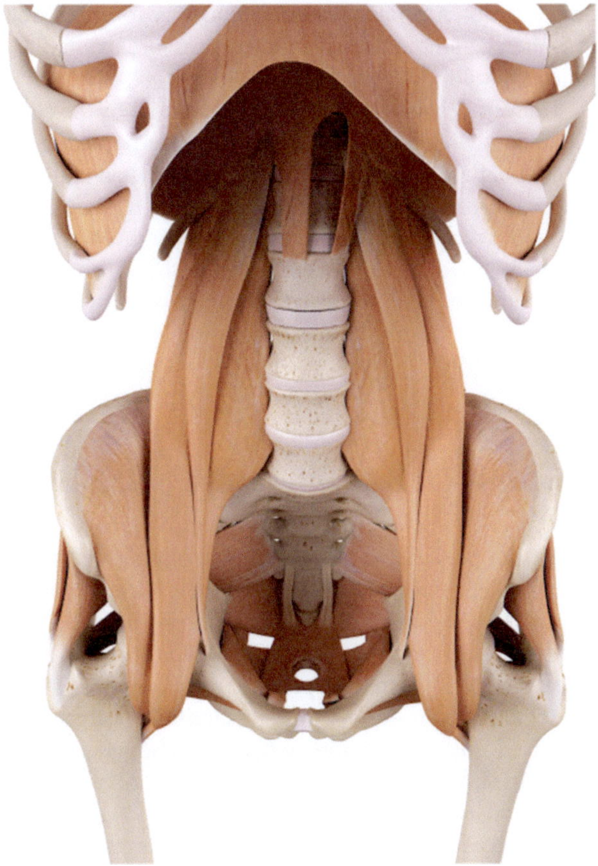

Fig. 18.4 The psoas, iliacus and diaphragm. (Purchased from Shutterstock.com royalty-free images)

respiration. During inhalation, they must release to allow for the downward motion of the pelvic viscera. During exhalation, they contract to assist with the return of the organs and the resultant recoil of the diaphragm. It has been demonstrated that these muscles co-contract with the TA and the internal oblique muscles of the abdomen during breathing [25].

Effects of Chin–Sternum Displacement in Dancers

The hyoid bone is suspended in the anterior neck by the supra-hyoid muscles above and the infra-hyoid muscles below. It is also connected to the larynx inferiorly by the thyrohyoid membrane. The supporting muscles can move the whole vocal apparatus superiorly and inferiorly to achieve changes in vocal pitch. With the chin raised, these muscles will be moved from their neutral position and placed under a stretch. While still able to function from this compromised position, their power will be diminished resulting in increased phonatory effort [12]. The high chin position may also lead to a tendency for high breath placement that may compromise the amount of sub-glottal pressure available—a requirement for safe volume and loudness control [18].

Therefore, the issue of the displacement of the chin—sternum relationship seen in dancers who use a high eyeline during performance will have an effect on efficient vocalizing. The extension in the cervical spine that this alignment will create places increased forces on the muscles of the neck that are involved in breath control and vocal production. When this high chin position accompanies a choreographed movement into a backward bend, then the airway may also become compromised, leading to a constricted sound when vocalizing. This situation will also likely result in increased tension in the jaw muscles, which will also affect phonation [6].

Strategies for Safe Integration of Dance and Voice Technique

While the previous anatomy section highlighted the ideals of neutral body alignment for safe and effective vocalizing, it is clearly unrealistic to think that such ideal posture is consistently achievable during the dynamic choreography of a musical theatre performance. What is essential is that performers have a strong kinesthetic sense of that ideal neutral placement in order for the body to make a connection to a grounded "home base." With this ingrained sense of neutral, the body can develop a form of "auto-correction" where it can always seek to balance itself. Without this sense, the body would be in a perpetual state of controlled falling that may result in excess muscle tension. With the high cardiovascular demands of performance, it is key not to waste precious energy through extraneous and unnecessary muscle activity. Every time the body passes through this neutral placement (if the choreography permits) it will be afforded a moment of respite, and can provide an ideal opportunity to inhale without resistance (if the vocal phrase allows). Therefore, alignment training that helps the dancer to find a neutral pelvic and spinal position, as well as an optimal relationship of the chin to the sternum should be a key component of education programmes.

To overcome the tendency for dancers to inwardly brace the abdominal muscles requires a re-thinking of the underlying reasons for choosing this strategy. Traditionally in dance training it was thought that "pulling in" the abdominal muscles was a key part of stabilizing the core. However, this notion is being challenged by recent research [26]. Simply bracing the abdominal muscles and holding the breath will tend to create rigidity rather than stability. Rigidity can be likened to a high-rise structure that is not designed to flex in the wind—under stormy conditions it is likely to topple! However, a more flexible structure has dynamic stability and can therefore adapt to environmental conditions. If a dancer creates a balanced pose through rigidity, one nudge could knock them over. A dancer who uses dynamic stability will be able to "auto-correct" for any disturbances to balance. The body is instinctively pre-programmed to dynamically activate numerous muscles in order to achieve spinal stability. When we attempt to override this innate system, this can result in imbalances in muscle activation patterns and a decrease in stability [26]. An increase in spinal compression has also been shown to result from inward bracing of the abdominal muscles [27], and sustained tension in the muscles of the trunk can potentially cause spinal damage [28]. In light of this information, it is apparent that the concept of abdominal muscle bracing needs to be revisited. Allowing for abdominal expansion in dance movements would allow for a full excursion of the diaphragm during inhalation with a subsequent increase in sub-glottal pressure to facilitate safe vocalizing, a reduction in potentially damaging spinal compression without compromising core stability, and an increased capacity to meet the cardiorespiratory demands of performance.

There will still be times, particularly in very "off-centre" poses or movements, when extra recruitment of abdominal muscles will be necessary to provide the requisite stability in these challenging positions. Here it is key to teach the dancers to use postero-lateral or circumferential rib cage motion during inhalation [29]. Expanding the lower portions of the rib cage in this manner can compensate for the reduced capacity for abdominal expansion without resorting to the upper chest or clavicular breathing patterns.

Introducing the concept of "breath choreography" into the dance class is a key factor in facilitating the safe addition of vocalizing to movement. There are many dance movements that can be greatly improved if performed using controlled exhalation rather than breath-holding. As previously noted, the transversus abdominis is one of the muscles that controls the rate of exhalation and it is also a key stabilizer of the lumbar spine. Performing movements such as a *pirouette* (when a dancer spins on one leg) using an exhale rather than the typical inhale serves to lower the center of gravity (by reducing shoulder and neck tension) and stabilizes the spine via the cylindrical support of the TA. The result is a calm, stable turn. Should the dancer then be required to sing during this motion, the fact that he or she is already exhaling can allow the transition to be seamless. Strategies for inhalation should also be examined as many dancers tend to actively gasp for air when initiating a vocal or movement phrase (a process that can lead to vocal dryness).

Inhalation occurs naturally as a result of releasing the abdominal muscles at the end of an exhale. Practising a long, slow exhale at the end of which one just allows the abdomen to release will result in a natural, effortless intake of breath. This exercise can put dancers back in touch with natural breathing patterns that will translate easily to voicing. Incorporating breath choices into dance training not only creates a more seamless transition to vocalizing but can actually enhance many dance movements.

In essence, performers need to be taught a wide range of muscle recruitment options for both stability and breath management from which they can create a "recipe" for the various choreographic movements required. There is no single solution that will be applicable to every voice and dance movement combination, so performers need to be given the information from which they can construct (often through trial and error) an optimal strategy for each given situation. A good grounding in the essential anatomy of respiratory, vocal, and core stabilization will be key to building optimal strategies. Therefore, this should ideally be incorporated into musical theatre training.

Proprioceptive training should also be considered in the development of a musical theatre artist. Performance can create very high cognitive and perceptual demands that may not be apparent to the observer. Artists may have to simultaneously recall detailed choreography and complex floor patterns involving other artists, the melody, harmony, and lyrics of the vocal work, handle props, and navigate around the movements of scenery and stage furniture. This may all occur under the blinding stage lights while wearing unwieldy costumes, precarious head-dresses, or masks that restrict vision. Combining all these skills requires a high level of cognitive and proprioceptive ability. Training exercises such as singing a song while performing a basic choreographic phrase, and simultaneously throwing and catching a ball with a partner, are some ways to sharpen the psycho-physical and proprioceptive skills necessary for performance.

Cardiovascular fitness should also be considered in the training of musical theatre performers. Dance class is predominantly an anaerobic form of exercise due to its intermittent nature. Classes tend to be comprised of a sequence of short combinations with dancers waiting and resting while they take their turn. However, performance is more of an endurance activity requiring aerobic fitness [30]. It has been shown that, despite appearances, dancers perform no better than healthy sedentary individuals when assessed in key fitness tests [31]. Performers should therefore include supplemental cardiovascular training into their regime. Wyon recommends 20 min of continuous moderate- to high-impact cardiovascular activity at approximately 70–80% of the maximal heart rate to be repeated two to three times per week [32]. Performers could include vocalizing during this activity by doing vocal exercises or singing a favorite song to enhance their triple threat training.

The role of the production team in both professional and training environments is one final area that needs to be addressed to ensure that musical theatre artists are fully supported. The collaboration between the musical director and choreographer at the early stage is crucial to avoid possible conflicts between the choreography and the vocal lines. If an artist is required to hit a particularly challenging high note, the choreographer could create a movement sequence that is sympathetic to the anatomical requirements for this vocal moment. Similarly, if a challenging piece of choreography is required, the musical director could assist by offering alternative choices for breath phrasing. In collaboration, they could agree to use off-stage or pre-recorded vocals to supplement the vocal line—a strategy that is sometimes used in theatres. Costume design should be sympathetic to the movement needs of the performer. Costumes that restrict abdominal expansion, such as heavy corsets, can create increases in intra-abdominal pressure that are potentially harmful. If the wearing of high heels is required, this can alter neutral pelvic and spinal alignment, shifting the kinetic chain away from neutral and interfering with optimal breath mechanics. Artists should be trained in how to compensate for these types of restrictions by softening at the knee joints and transferring the weight towards the heel rather than toe. Many of these issues are beyond the control of the performer; rather they are in the hands of the production team. Artists should therefore learn to advocate for themselves in these situations in order to pre-empt potentially challenging issues.

Conclusion

In summary, the world of the "triple threat," or multi-disciplinary performer, is a complex and challenging one. As productions become increasingly demanding of artists, it is imperative that training is fit for purpose, in order to prepare them for the profession and its many challenging conditions. A career in musical theatre can be highly rewarding, but clearly it carries many potential risks for injury. It is incumbent upon those who provide care for the artists, as well as those who train them, to ensure successful preparation. For the artists, through having a deep knowledge of the physical requirements for safe performance and the confidence to advocate for themselves, they can enjoy long and healthy careers as "triple threat" performers.

References

1. Marks P. If it's a musical, it was probably a movie. NY Times. [online]. 2002. Available at: https://www.nytimes.com/2002/04/14/movies/if-it-s-a-musical-it-was-probably-a-movie.html. Accessed 5 Jun 2019.
2. Adler S. On broadway: art and commerce on the great white way. Carbondale: Southern Illinois University Press; 2004.
3. Morton J. Musical theatre: the hazards of the performer's workplace. Med Probl Perform Art. 2015;30(1):1–7.
4. Zhang H. Top eight woes of spider-man turn off the dark. [online]. 2011. Available at: https://abcnews.go.com/Entertainment/spider-man-turn-off-dark-top-woes/story?id=13837622. Accessed 5 Jun 2019.
5. Morton J. The integration of voice and dance techniques in musical theatre: anatomical considerations. Med Probl Perform Art. 2015;30(2):71–7.
6. Melton J, Tom K. One voice, integrating singing and theatre voice techniques. Long Grove: Waveland; 2012.
7. Russell JA. Preventing dance injuries: current perspectives. J Sports Med. 2013;4:199–210.
8. Malkogeorgos A, Mavrovouniotis F, Zaggelidis G, Ciucurel C. Common dance related musculoskeletal injuries. J Phys Educ Sport. 2011;11(3):259–66.
9. Volkerding KE, Ketcham CJ. Biomechanics and proprioceptive differences during drop landings between dancers and non-dancers. Int J Exerc Sci. 2013;6(4):289–99.
10. Prochazkova M, Tepla L, Svoboda Z, Janura M, Cieslarová M. Analysis of foot load during ballet dancers' gait. Acta Bioeng Biomech. 2014;16(2):41–5.
11. Trepman E, Gellman R, Solomon R, Murthy K, Micheli L, De Luca C. Electromyographic analysis of standing posture and demi-plie in ballet and modern dancers. Med Sci Sports Exerc. 1994;26(6):771–82.
12. Garfield Davies D, Jahn A. Care of the professional voice. Oxford: Butterworth-Heinemann; 2000.

13. Liederbach M, Richardson M, Dougherty J, Dilgen F. Anterior hip pain in dancers. Clinical observation and literature review. Proceedings of the International Association for Dance Medicine and Science annual meeting, New York; 2002.
14. Melton J. Dancing with voice: a collaborative journey across disciplines. New York: Voice Theatre Solutions; 2015.
15. Fischer Gam C, Urmston E. Dancing with the pelvis: alignment, deviations, and mobility. International Association for Dance Medicine & Science. 2015. https://www.iadms.org/blog-post/1177934/214940/Dancing-with-the-pelvis-Alignment-deviations-and-mobility. Accessed 13 Jan 2019.
16. Melton J. Tucking the pelvis: actual and perceived outcomes. 2011. http://www.joanmelton.com/tucking-pelvis-actual-and-perceived-outcomes-0. Accessed 13 Jan 2019.
17. Hixon TJ. Respiratory function in singing: a primer for singers and singing teachers. Tucson: Reddington Brown; 2006.
18. Sundberg J, Titze I, Scherer R. Phonatory control in male singing: a study of the effects of subglottal pressure, fundamental frequency, and mode of phonation on the voice source. J Voice. 1993;7(1):15–29.
19. Myers T. Anatomy trains: myofascial meridians for manual and movement therapists. 3rd ed. London: Churchill Livingstone; 2014.
20. Bordoni B, Zanier E. Anatomic connections of the diaphragm: influence of respiration on the body system. J Multidiscip Healthc. 2013;6:281–91.
21. Sajko S, Stuber K. Psoas major: a case report and review of its anatomy, biomechanics, and clinical implications. J Can Chiropr Assoc. 2009;53(4):311–8.
22. Hodges PW, Butler JE, McKenzie DK, et al. Contraction of the human diaphragm during rapid postural adjustments. J Physiol. 1997;505(2):539–48.
23. Boyle KL, Olinick J, Lewis C. The value of blowing up a balloon. N Am J Sports Phys Ther. 2010;5(3):179–88.
24. Hodges PW, Heijnen I, Gandevia SC. Postural activity of the diaphragm is reduced in humans when respiratory demand increases. J Physiol. 2001;537(3):999–1008.
25. Neumann P, Gill V. Pelvic floor and abdominal muscle interaction: EMG activity and intra-abdominal pressure. Int Urogynecol J Pelvic Floor Dysfunct. 2002;13(2):125–32.
26. Brown SH, Vera-Garcia FJ, McGill SM. Effects of abdominal muscle coactivation on the externally preloaded trunk: variations in motor control and its effect on spine stability. Spine (Phila Pa 1976). 2006;31(13):E387–93.
27. Vera-Garcia FJ, Elvira JL, Brown SH, McGill SM. Effects of abdominal stabilization maneuvers on the control of spine motion and stability against sudden trunk perturbations. J Electromyogr Kinesiol. 2007;17(5):555–67.
28. Lederman E. The myth of core stability. J Bodyw Mov Ther. 2010;14(1):84–98.
29. Sweigard LE. Human movement potential: its ideokinetic facilitation. New York: Harper & Row; 1974.
30. Rodrigues-Krause J, Krause M, Reischak-Oliveira A. Cardiorespiratory considerations in dance: from classes to performances. J Dance Med Sci. 2015;19(3):91–102.
31. Koutedakis Y, Jamurtas A. The dancer as a performing athlete. Sports Med. 2004;34(10):651–61.
32. Wyon M. Cardiorespiratory training for dancers. J Dance Med Sci. 2005;9:7–12.

Chapter 19
The Role of Nutrition in Injury Prevention Among Ballet Dancers

Lauri Wright and Casey Colin

General Role of Nutrition

Professional and pre-professional ballet is an athletic art; and as such, it creates a unique set of nutrition requirements for optimal performance. Both male and female ballet dancers tend to be more at risk for nutritional disparities in terms of overall health, and more particularly bone health, than their non-athlete counterparts. Athletic performance is enhanced with proper nutritional considerations, but can be weakened without adequate nourishment [1, 2]. The risks associated with nutritional deficiencies are especially concerning with regard to very young ballet dancers who are still growing and developing [2–4]. With careful attention to the risks associated with nutrition in ballet dancers, prevention of adverse short- and long-term health issues can be achieved.

Nutritional Status of Ballet Dancers

Despite the increased needs required for ballet and the important role of nutrition in performance, assessment of the nutritional status of pre-professional and professional ballet dancers has shown multiple nutritional issues. The most prevalent nutritional issues found in pre-professional and professional ballet dancers include low body weight, low energy intake, and delayed puberty and amenorrhea. The following section details these common nutritional problems.

L. Wright (✉) · C. Colin
Department of Nutrition & Dietetics, University of North Florida, Jacksonville, FL, USA
e-mail: l.wright@unf.edu; n01405331@unf.edu

S.-H. Lee et al. (eds.), *Perspectives in Performing Arts Medicine Practice*,
https://doi.org/10.1007/978-3-030-37480-8_19

Low Body Weight

Because of the high demand for an aesthetically appropriate physique, dancers often strive for a much lower body weight than is recommended [2, 5–9]. Further, ballet dancers may have a higher propensity to achieve a body weight that is far too low for stature as a result of distorted body image [2], and without regard to long-term consequences of the pathway toward achieving this suboptimal weight. Freitas and colleagues compared 40 professional dancers with 40 controls who were not athletes and found that body weight and body fat percentages were considerably reduced in the ballet dancers [5]. Frusztajer and colleagues examined 50 ballet dancers compared to 59 "non-dancers" and found that 80% of the ballet dancers were underweight [10]. The degree to which many ballet dancers are underweight has been quantified as less than 10–12% ideal body weight [8]. Ballet dancers may consider having a low body weight to enhance performance more so than having a nutrient-rich diet [2], therefore they must be educated on the impact of nutrition optimization not only for performance, but also for proper growth and development in these adolescent years. Additionally, nutrient deficiencies are likely to occur as a result of the energy restrictions required to achieve a low body weight [7].

Low Energy Intake

In an effort to reduce body weight and maintain a lower body weight, ballet dancers often consume an overall energy intake below that of recommendations [4, 6, 7]. In 2015, Hewett and Tufano emphasized from their findings that inadequate energy intake may be the single most important factor implicated in the female athlete triad [6]. The Female Athlete Triad is a collective term that captures three major disparities that impact female ballet dancers: low energy availability and/or disordered eating; amenorrhea; and low bone mineral density [3, 6, 8–10]. In 1985, Braisted and colleagues found that about 50% of the 45 ballet dancers they surveyed restricted intake compared to about 30% of non-dancer controls [2]. Energy restrictions nearly always come with a sacrifice in terms of overall nutrient status. Nutrition status can be further compromised in the setting of a vegetarian or vegan eating style, especially in terms of iron, calcium, and protein intake [1]. Some data actually suggest that vegetarianism is chosen by some dancers simply as a strategy to reduce weight [1, 10]. In fact, one study by Frusztajer and colleagues in 1990 noted that of the ballet dancers in the group they studied, 60% were vegetarian as compared to only 20% of non-dancer subjects being vegetarian [10]. However, a diet of any kind, including vegetarian and vegan diets, can be nutritionally sufficient for the ballet dancer if it is well-designed [1]. It is important to note that increasing overall energy intake without regard to appropriate nutrient value may not be adequate in terms of improving dance performance [11]. Interestingly, in 2011, Doyle-Lucas and Davy interviewed 39 ballet dancers and found that 100% of them desired nutrition education for better "performance and overall health" if such an option was available at their facilities [8]. Nutrition education and monitoring by a dietitian plays a key role in the assurance of a nutritionally sound diet for ballet dancers, and the registered dietitian nutritionist (RDN) is uniquely qualified to provide this evidence-based guidance [2, 6, 8, 11].

Delayed Puberty and Amenorrhea

The number of female athletes diagnosed with hypothalamic-pituitary menstrual disorders, such as amenorrhea or delayed menarche, is estimated to be as high as 61% [12]. Freitas and colleagues considered amenorrhea as "the absence of menses for three consecutive months," while Lagowska and colleagues considered an amenorrhea diagnosis to include 6 months without menses [5, 13]. Lagowska and colleagues further delineate amenorrhea into two different categories, *primary amenorrhea* and *secondary amenorrhea* [13]. Primary amenorrhea is synonymous with delayed menarche, while secondary amenorrhea is the absence of menses in a female who had previously menstruated [13]. Some consider delayed menarche if the female reaches age 14 without having started menses [6], while some regard age 15 as the standard cutoff [13]. Females were considered to have *oligomenorrhea* if they experienced a long duration (>35 days) between periods, but not as long as that which is considered complete amenorrhea (3–6 months) [12]. Ballet dancers also tend to have a later menarche than their non-athlete peers [12], and the delayed menarche seems to be closely associated with nutritional habits [2, 4–7, 13]. Low bone mineral density is also highly correlated with the presence of amenorrhea in female athletes [5, 6], which may increase the risk of injury in female ballet dancers. Interventions that target increased energy intake and balanced body fat percentage have been directly correlated with reestablishing normal menstruation cycles in female ballet dancers [13].

Nutrition Risk for Injuries

The professional ballet world is plagued by high injury rates that negatively impact both the ballet company and its dancers. Female dancers are particularly prone to stress fractures of the lower extremities. Current research suggests that the incidence of dance injuries in women correlates with the symptoms of the Female Athlete Triad. As previously defined, the Female Athlete Triad is a collective term that captures three major disparities that impact female ballet dancers: low energy availability and/or disordered eating; amenorrhea; and low bone mineral density [3, 6, 8, 9, 11, 13, 14]. The aesthetic nature of ballet and the desire to remain thin may lead many dancers to display the symptoms of the triad, ultimately making them more prone to injury. Researchers emphasize that the low energy availability factor is the cornerstone of the Female Athlete Triad, as the lack of available energy substrate is what leads to delayed or absent menarche and low bone mineral density [6]. The following sections detail the most common nutritional risks associated with injuries in ballet dancers.

Amenorrhea

Estrogen is a hormone well-known for its role in female reproduction. Estrogen also plays a pivotal role in bone mineralization [4, 7]. Braisted and colleagues noted that low body fat percentage in ballet dancers was directly associated with suboptimal estrogen levels [2]. Grochowska-Niedworok and colleagues described the link between body fat's role in hormone production (such as estrogen) and amenorrhea in ballet dancers [3]. Warren and colleagues noted that estrogen levels plummeted during the duration of amenorrhea as well as a positive correlation with occurrence of stress fractures and cases of scoliosis with delayed menarche [4]. Hewett and Tufano found a positive correlation with amenorrhea and suboptimal lumbar spine bone density [6]. Kadel et al. found that incidence of stress fractures was positively associated with longer-lasting amenorrhea [15]. In 2011, Burckhardt and colleagues noted that the earlier menarche started, the better bone density was, which emphasized the role of estrogen in bone mineralization [7]; in 2015, Hewett and Tufano noted the same link [6]. Additionally, many studies have found that amenorrhea is related not only to decreased overall bone density [6], but perhaps and more importantly also with reduced bone-mineral content [7, 10, 15]. However, bone density may not be a useful measurement in young subjects who are still growing [7]. Hewett and Tufano noted that resolution of amenorrhea increased bone density in the wrist and spine of dancers, but resuming what would be "normal" bone density was not achieved [6]. It is worth noting that delayed menses and/or amenorrhea have multiple connected etiologies, and cannot be attributed to either energy intake, body fat, nor physical exertion independently, although all factors may contribute [7, 15].

Low Body Weight

Injury risk is increased in ballet dancers who have a below-average body weight, and the connection is complex and indirect in many ways. Ballet dancers who strive for low body weight are often consuming too few micronutrients, especially calcium and vitamin D [5, 7], which can put the dancer at increased risk for bone fractures. Low body weight in dancers is also highly correlated with low body fat percentage [5], which in turn can compromise estrogen production, and thus further impacts bone mineralization and bone fracture risk. However, Freitas and colleagues found that the weight-bearing nature of ballet seems to offer a significant protection in terms of improving bone density despite the negative impact of low body weight and energy intake [5, 6, 15]. Hewett and colleagues also support the notion that weight-bearing exercise is a significant factor in increasing bone density in ballet dancers as indicated by Wolff's law [6].

Body Composition

Body fat percentages of total body composition tend to be much lower in ballet dancers than in their non-dancer peers and are often below recommended values for age and gender [3, 5, 9]. Sousa and colleagues suggest that the lowest body fat percentages recommended for females and males are 12% and 5%, respectively [11]. Grochowska-Niedworok and colleagues studied 150 pre-professional ballet dancers in Poland and found that 54% had a body fat percentage below average [3]. Kay-yun Yau's dissertation on ballet dancers and risk of injury found that many dancers seem to strive for a lower body fat percentage in an effort toward improved physique and performance without regard to the increased risk for injuries [9].

Disordered Eating

As a group, ballet dancers tend to show higher rates of various eating disorders [7, 11], including (but not limited to) anorexia, binge eating, and bulimia [7]. Eating disorders appear to be far more prevalent in ballet dancers than in non-dancers [2]. One notable observation from Frusztajer et al. was that significant weight gain during competitive off-seasons can be a major indicator of an eating disorder in ballet dancers [10]. Similarly, Burckhardt and colleagues noted that a significant variance in a ballet dancer's weight when compared to standardized recommendations for growth should trigger concern with regard to a possible eating disorder [7]. In 1986, Warren and colleagues reported the rate of eating disorders in ballet dancers to be estimated between 5% and 22% [4]. Not surprisingly, survey data suggest a significant correlation between poor body image and prevalence of eating disorders [2, 7, 16].

Restricted Diet

Even in the absence of a true eating disorder diagnosis, many ballet dancers practice some form of energy restriction to control body weight [2, 4, 8, 16]. As with any restrictive eating pattern, nutritional insufficiency, or even deficiencies, can contribute to increased risk of injury [11]. In the case of ballet dancers, the impact of nutritional insufficiency on performance is often the most evident [8]. In many individuals, obtaining adequate iron, calcium, and vitamin D is difficult; this is especially true when overall energy intake is restricted [2, 11]. Frusztajer and colleagues found that 70% of the ballet dancers who had experienced stress fractures were consuming less than 85% of their estimated energy needs [10]. Sousa and colleagues and Doyle-Lucas and Davy both found that most female ballet dancers are consuming far less than 80% of their estimated energy needs [8–11]. These, along with other observations in this population, indicated that incidence of injuries, such as stress fractures, are positively associated with restrictive eating [10]. Warren and colleagues noted that 24% of the 75 ballet dancers they studied had scoliosis; and those who had scoliosis also "were found to have more deviant eating behavior than the dancers without scoliosis" [4].

Nutrition Prescription

Nutrition recommendations for ballet dancers are not outside the typical parameters that exist in sports nutrition. Ballet dancers are athletes, after all, and exhibit a higher energy expenditure than non-athletes due to high energy demands of training and competition [12]. However, the nutrition professional must take care to provide advice that is realistic and sustainable in the context of the inherent need for the ballet dancer to maintain the physique and body fat standards specific to the industry [1, 11]. Efforts must also consider the nutrient density of the diet, not just the total caloric load [11].

Most available evidence for estimating overall energy needs for ballet dancers center around fat-free mass (FFM) [11]. Estimated energy needs for ballet dancers range from 30 to 45 kcal/kg FFM/day, adjustable for individual training demands, gender, and age [11]. Studies have shown that less than 30 kcal/kg FFM/day appears to be a significant mark between adequate energy versus a negative energy balance [8, 11, 12]. Little evidence exists for a macronutrient breakdown specifically for ballet dancers [11]. However, it seems the most accepted recommendation for protein, fat, and carbohydrates (CHO) is as follows:

- Protein: 1.2–1.7 g/kg/day [1, 11] or 12–15% of total kcal/day [1]
- Fat: 20–35% of total kcal/day [1, 11]
- Carbohydrate: 3–5 g/kg/day [11] or 55–60% of total kcal/day [1]

Efforts should be made to choose good-quality, whole-food sources of all nutrients to ensure a nutrient-dense diet rich in fiber and omega-3 fatty acids [1]. Recommendations for nourishment and hydration before, during, and after exercise for ballet dancers along with specific examples of implementation can be found in Table 19.1.

Risk for inadequate micronutrients is high in ballet dancers, especially when energy restrictions are present. The most significant micronutrients in question for ballet dancers are iron, calcium, and vitamin D [11]. In addition to iron, calcium,

Table 19.1 Nutrition specifics for ballet dancers Before, During, and After Training

Before exercise	1–4 g CHO/kg eaten 1–4 h before exercise 5–7 mL/kg of fluid 4 h before exercise If under-hydrated: additional 3–4 mL/kg 2 h before exercise	Snacks providing 50 g of CHO: 600 mL of sports drink with 6% CHO 2–3 cereal/muesli bar 2 medium bananas or 3 pieces other fruit 80 g of dried fruit 2 slices of bread with jam
During exercise (>1 h)	30–60 g CHO/h 150–350 mL of fluid every 20 min	Dancers should weigh themselves before and after training to adjust the amount of fluid intake. The weight difference must not be >2%
After exercise	0.8 g CHO/kg/h 0.2–0.4 g protein/kg/h (The first meal should be taken during the first 30 min and again every 2 h for 4–6 h) 1500 mL of fluids for each kg lost	Snacks providing 50 g CHO and 10 g Protein: 500 mL of chocolate low-fat milk 2 cups of low-fat breakfast cereal with 1 cup of low-fat milk 2 slices of bread with cheese/ham/meat/chicken and 1 large piece of fruit 250–350 mL of milkshake or fruit smoothie

Modified from Sousa et al. [11]

Table 19.2 Micronutrients at risk, recommended intake, food sources

Micronutrient at risk	Recommended intake	Food sources
Iron	Females (14–18 years) 15 mg Females (19–50 years) 18 mg Males (14–18 years) 11 mg Males (19–50 years) 8 mg	Fortified breakfast cereals, beans, beef, sardines and oysters, nuts, tofu
Calcium	Females (14–18 years) 1300 mg Females (19–50 years) 1000 mg Males (14–18 years) 1300 mg Males (19–50 years) 1000 mg	Yogurt, cheese, milk, tofu, sardines, salmon, calcium-fortified orange juice, greens
Vitamin D	Females (14–50 years) 600 IU Males (14–50 years) 600 IU	Salmon, tuna, vitamin-D orange juice, vitamin-D fortified milk, liver, eggs, vitamin-D fortified breakfast cereals
Vitamin B12	Females (14+ years) 2.4 mcg Males (14+ years) 2.4 mcg	Clams, salmon, tuna, beef, fortified breakfast cereal, milk, yogurt, eggs

and vitamin D, vegetarian and vegan ballet dancers may also have some difficulty achieving adequate intake of vitamin B12, although a well-planned diet can provide sufficient amounts of vitamin B12 [11]. Although the primary emphasis for obtaining micronutrients is from food sources, and sun exposure in the case of vitamin D, some ballet dancers may require supplementation to meet their recommended micronutrient needs [11]. Lagowska et al. suggest that supplemental vitamin D be considered as a protocol for female athletes who are the most vulnerable to the Female Athlete Triad [12]. Table 19.2 details the micronutrients at risk, recommended intake, and food sources of the micronutrient.

Nutrition Education and Monitoring

Ballet dancers have increased nutritional requirements to support the physical demands of training and performance. However, a high prevalence of nutritional issues including low body weight, low calorie intake, nutrient deficiencies, disordered eating, reduced bone density, delayed menarche, and amenorrhea has been demonstrated. These nutritional issues, in turn, increase the risk of performance injuries and delayed recovering when injuries do include. To prevent this downward spiral and improve nutritional health and performance, nutrition education should be incorporated into ballet training programs and ballet companies. Doyle-Lucas et al. found that a nutrition education series of three lectures to pre-professional adolescent ballet dancers significantly increased nutrition knowledge, perceived susceptibility to the Female Athlete Triad, and self-efficacy [3]. Improvements in dietary intake were also observed. Summer program workshops and company professional series would be ideal to provide nutrition education. Nutrition education should be scientifically based as athletes are often susceptible to fad diets and nutrition information that is unsound and potentially dangerous. Further, the nutrition education should be tailored to the needs and concerns of the dancers such as injury prevention rather than simply generalized healthy eating guidelines.

Pre-professional and professional ballet dancers' nutritional status should be monitored closely. Nutritional screening should include weight status, changes in weight, body composition, bone density, nutritional intake, and disordered eating behaviors. Dancers found at risk should be referred to a registered dietitian nutritionist for comprehensive nutritional counseling and medical nutrition therapy.

References

1. Brown DD. Nutritional considerations for the vegetarian and vegan dancer. J Dance Med Sci. 2018;22(1):44–53.
2. Braisted JR, Mellin L, Gong EJ, Irwin CE. The adolescent ballet dancer. J Adolesc Health. 1985;6(5):365–71.
3. Grochowska-Niedworok E, Kardas M, Fatyga E, Piorkowska-Staniek K, Muc-Wierzgon M, Kokot T. Study of top ballet school students revealed large deficiencies in their body weight and body fat. Acta Paediatr. 2018;107(6):1077–82.
4. Warren MP, Gunn JB, Hamilton LH, Warren F, Hamilton WG. Scoliosis and fractures in young ballet dancers. NEJM. 1986;314(21):1348–53.
5. Freitas L, Amorim T, Humbert L, et al. Cortical and trabecular bone analysis of professional dancers using 3D-DXA: a case-control study. J Sports Sci. 2019;37:82–9.
6. Hewett EM, et al. Bone health in female ballet dancers: a review. EJSS. 3(2). ISSN 2282–5673.
7. Burckhardt P, Wynn E, Krieg MA, Bagutti C, Faouzi M. The effects of nutrition, puberty, and dancing on bone density in adolescent ballet dancers. JDMS. 2011;15:51–60.
8. Doyle-Lucas AF, Davy B. Development and evaluation of an educational intervention program for pre-professional adolescent ballet dancers nutrition for optimal performance. JDMS. 2011;15:65–75.

9. Yau RKY. Injuries and possible disordered eating among elite pre-professional ballet and contemporary cancers: department of epidemiology. Chapel Hill: University of North Carolina; 2016.
10. Frusztajer NT, Dhuper S, Warren MP, Brooks-Gunn J, Fox RP. Nutrition and the incidence of stress fractures in ballet dancers. Am J Clin Nutr. 1990;51:779–83.
11. Sousa M, Carvalho P, Moreira P, Teixeira VH. Nutrition and nutritional issues for dancers. Med Probl Perform Art. 2013;28:119–23.
12. Lagowska K, Kapczuk K. Testosterone concentrations in female athletes and ballet dancers with menstrual disorders. Eur J Sport Sci. 2016;16(4):490–7.
13. Lagowska K, Kapczuk K, Jeszka J. Nine-month nutritional intervention improves restoration of menses in young female athletes and ballet dancers. J Int Soc Sports Nutr. 2014;11(1):52.
14. Williams NI, Statuta SM, Austin A. Female athlete triad: future directions for energy availability and eating disorder research and practice. Clin Sports Med. 2017;36(4):671–86.
15. Kadel NJ, Teitz C, Kronmal RA. Stress fractures in ballet dancers. Orthop J Sports Med. 1992;20(4):445–9.
16. Jauregui Lobera I, Bolanos-Rios P, Valero-Blanco E, Ortega-de-la-Torre A. Eating attitudes, body image and risk for eating disorders in a group of Spanish dancers. Nutr Hosp. 2016;33(5):588.

Chapter 20
When Prevention Makes Good Music

Carina Joly

Introduction

Research data from the past four decades report the prevalence of performing-related physical problems ranging from 55% to 81.3% among orchestra musicians [1–5] and from 13% to 89% among music students [6–14]. With the establishment of the first medical clinics designed to provide musician-tailored treatment in the 1980s, music medicine specialists started to advocate the idea of preventive education as a promising strategy to help to decrease the high incidence of injury in musicians [15]. In 1988, Alice Brandfonbrener, the founding editor of the journal *Medical Problems of Performing Artists*, affirmed that among the most effective strategies to reduce the risk of injury among musicians "early training grounded in scientifically as well as musically sound principles" and "committed partnership of musicians, physicians and other concerned parties," are both essential [16, p., 0].

Other health practitioners joined the mission and developed programs that included regular practice of physical exercises and/or sports and measured the effects of such programs after a period of time. Some projects directed to music students offered lectures on health and prevention, basic knowledge of functional anatomy, psychological aspects of performance and stress coping strategies, relaxation techniques and physical exercises [17–20]; others focused on pre- and post-measurements after exposing orchestral musicians to an exercise program [21, 22]. Although the outcomes pointed to a potential for preventing performing-related health problems among musicians, varying standards of prevalence and the generally small sample sizes of these studies have failed to provide statistically significant results [23].

The original version of this chapter was revised. The correction to this chapter can be found at https://doi.org/10.1007/978-3-030-37480-8_26

C. Joly (✉)
Music Department, Universidade Federal de São João del-Rei, São João del-Rei, MG, Brazil

S.-H. Lee et al. (eds.), *Perspectives in Performing Arts Medicine Practice*,
https://doi.org/10.1007/978-3-030-37480-8_20

A systematic review of 15 research papers rigorously selected for methodological quality dealing with risk factors of musculoskeletal disorders in musicians by Baadjou et al. [23] reported neither positive nor negative association between sports or exercise behavior and injuries. However, the three best-rated papers in Baadjou's review supported the effectiveness of preventive programs [24–26]. Zaza et al. reiterated the need for further examination on the impact of prevention programs [24]; Kenny and Ackermann confirmed the positive impact of physical exercises tailored to musicians [25]; and Leaver et al. emphasized the importance of generic advice considering different instruments and their relation to posture, seating/standing, warm-up practices, the use of adjustable stands and chairs as well as chin rests, among other ergonomic considerations [26]. Chan et al., on the other hand, suggested that generic exercise may target neither muscles directly involved in the performance nor muscles that would compensate for strength imbalance caused by awkward postures and typical maladaptive movement patterns, and suggested instrument-tailored exercise programs [22]. Lee et al. [27] developed an integrative program that included yoga, physical therapy exercises, mental training (i.e., imagery, mental rehearsal, and mind clearing) and improvisational practices to college students attaining an improvement in overall physical and musical efficacy as well as posture, muscle strength, aerobic endurance, and freedom of movement during the performance.

The Workshop

Aiming to contribute to the prevention of performing-related injury, the author of this chapter developed a workshop specially designed to improve musicians' body awareness and overall posture, as well as to target typical strength imbalances in key muscle groups. The uniqueness of the proposed approach lies in the awareness gained from the exercises, which may be practiced in either standing or seated positions, during breaks and while performing.

Participating volunteer musicians performed short musical excerpts before and after a session mobilizing their bodies for 45 min using selected physical exercises. The mobilization sessions could be extended to 3–4 h. Audience members, who practiced the exercises without the performances, commented observing postural and musical changes in the pre- and post-performances of the volunteer musicians.

The workshop exercises are selected from courses and literature studied during a music physiology specialization curriculum at the Zurich University of the Arts, Zurich, Switzerland [28–32]. In this three-year program, music educators are introduced to the physiological aspects and psychological processes involved in music performance, acquiring basic knowledge of anatomy, biomechanics, and performance training. The curriculum also introduces a variety of principles from physical therapy and body therapies such as Alexander Technique, Feldenkreis, *Spiraldynamik*, *Dispokinesis*, and other contemplative practices, such as Tai chi, Qigong, and Yoga, all believed to have potential for significantly improving musicians' physical and psychological conditions.

The Exercises

As different instruments and performing situations may affect whether musicians perform seated or standing, the exercises were selected considering aspects of postural stabilization in both situations [32]. Participants mobilize the whole body, starting with a sensitization drill followed by exercises targeting the stimulation of the supporting musculature of the lower back, the pelvic area, the shoulder, and the neck, as recommended by physical therapists [33]. Due to its relevance to musicians who use the hands to perform (e.g., pianists, clarinetists, guitar players), one exercise for the strengthening of intrinsic muscles of the hand was also included [25].

Screening Your Body

Higher awareness (sensitization) may be stimulated by observing the reactions after a full body tap. The participants are invited to stand up, vigorously tap their whole body with their hands, traveling from head to toes, stop tapping, relaxing and feeling the bodily responses. If group members are familiar with each other, they may be encouraged to tap their neighbors' back and shoulders. This exercise works well in classroom settings, helping students of all ages to release tension and preparing them for more concentrated activities. It also works well as a final activity before group dismissal.

Pelvis

As the pelvis affects the whole body alignment, it deserves special attention during the performance in both seated and standing positions. In cases where individuals encounter difficulties holding the pelvis into a neutral position, it would be beneficial to seek professional help to find out what is preventing the appropriate alignment. Once the alignment is no longer an issue, the next step is to learn to keep a minimal level of stable muscle tonus in the pelvic area while performing.

Two exercises may be used to mobilize the pelvis and to bring more awareness towards the relevance this area assigns to the overall posture. In a seated position and imagining that the sit bones (ischial tuberosities) represent the feet, participants are asked to "walk with the sit bones" over the surface of their flat chair, moving forward and backwards (Fig. 20.1). One should be careful not to slide with their sit bones over the surface, correctly executing the stepping movement, lifting each "foot" for the "step."

A second exercise includes circular pelvic movements, imagining that the pelvis is a bowl full of honey, participants draw a circle with the bottom of the bowl over

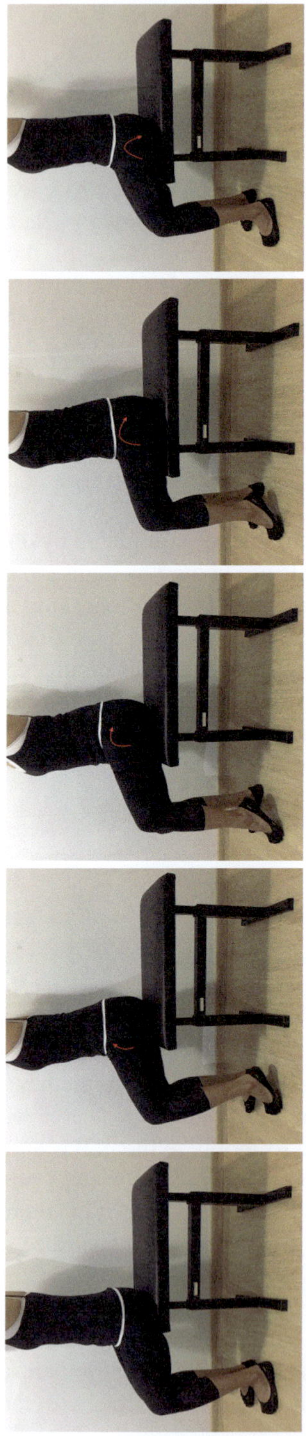

Fig. 20.1 Walking over the chair sequence of the left side moving backwards. The arms are up to facilitate movement observation

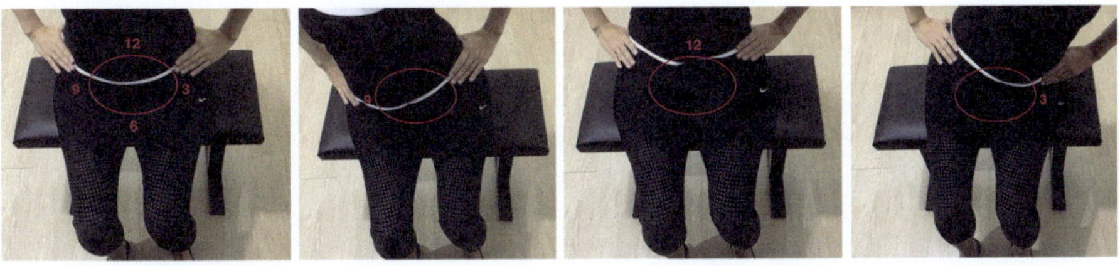

Fig. 20.2 Pelvic clockwise rotation

the chair's surface, making the honey perform vortex-like movements, clockwise and counterclockwise in variable diameters and speeds (Fig. 20.2).

While practicing these two exercises, one should observe how the pelvic mobilization affects the overall alignment of the upper body, especially the position of the head, neck, and shoulders. To avoid compensatory movements in the upper body, it is essential for musicians who usually play in seated positions to seek a neutral pelvic alignment whenever possible.

Feet/Standing

In a standing position, the ideal tonus is achieved through a raised awareness of the foot contact with the floor and a supporting muscle action in the pelvic area, which can be stimulated while standing on one foot. The muscular engagement necessary to stand on one foot should be reproduced with both feet on the ground. In a seated position, the same idea applies by seeking quality contact of the sit bones on the chair and proper engagement of the pelvic muscles as if one would be ready to stand up if necessary. It is essential to point out that in this process, simultaneously to the proposed sustained muscle tonus, the breathing movements of the lower abdominal area should occur naturally. In spite of the initial required concentration, with time, as these muscles learn to actively hold a minimal amount of tonus, this practice becomes effortless.

In a standing position, the pelvis also plays an important role as it directly affects the upper body alignment. While standing up, through the practice of a sequence of alternating anterior and posterior pelvic tilts, participants are able to identify their pelvic postural habit. Due to long hours of activities in seated position, the *iliopsoas* muscle group may be shortened in certain individuals who have the tendency to stand throwing the weight toward the front (Fig. 20.3a). In these cases, *iliopsoas* stretches are highly recommended in order to enrich the amplitude of the pelvic movements and to bring more comfort when these individuals seek the neutral pelvic position.

In most cases, the recruitment of the pelvic muscles in either seated or standing positions results in an overall improvement of the alignment in the upper body. When necessary, depending on the performer's postural behavior, the alignment of the shoulders, neck, and head may achieve optimal levels through simply remembering the feeling achieved after the practice of the exercises taught in the workshop. These interventions, after a full body mobilization during the workshop, are in most cases enough to bring the positive performance results observed by the participants.

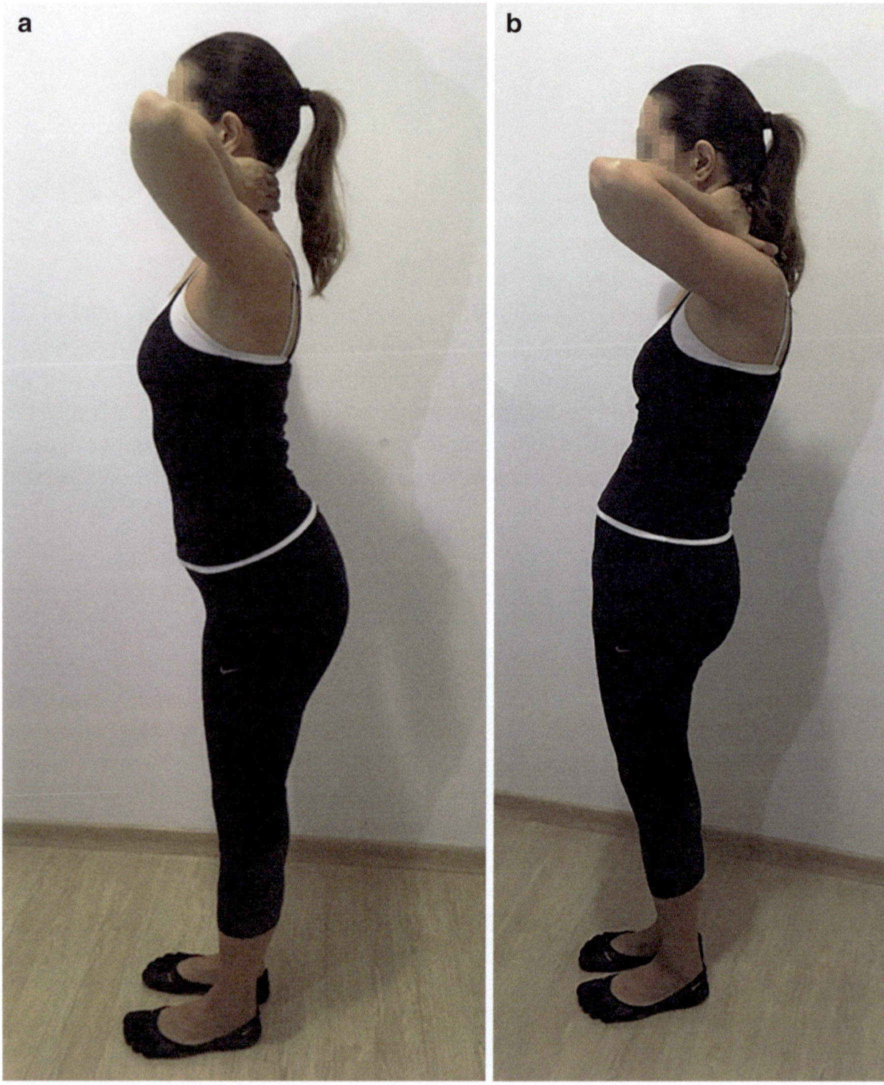

Fig. 20.3 (**a**) Anterior pelvic tilt. (**b**) Posterior pelvic tilt

The Shoulders

As the shoulders present high variability of movement, it is common, after a long period of nonaligned postural behavior, to observe compensatory behavior that usually results in discomfort and pain. Shoulders are directly affected by the stabilization of the pelvis and tend to react when the pelvis is not in neutral position. For

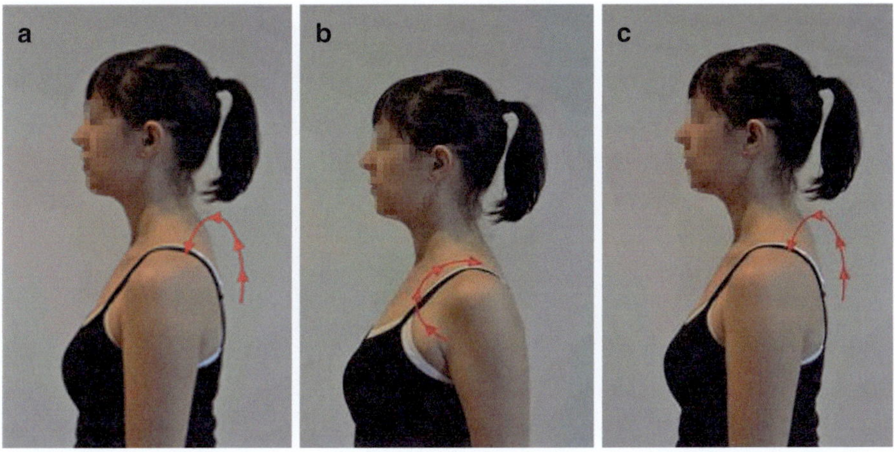

Fig. 20.4 (**a–c**) Finding the correct shoulder position. Positions are shown as incorrect (**a**, **b**) and correct (**c**)

Fig. 20.5 Shoulder and back stretch

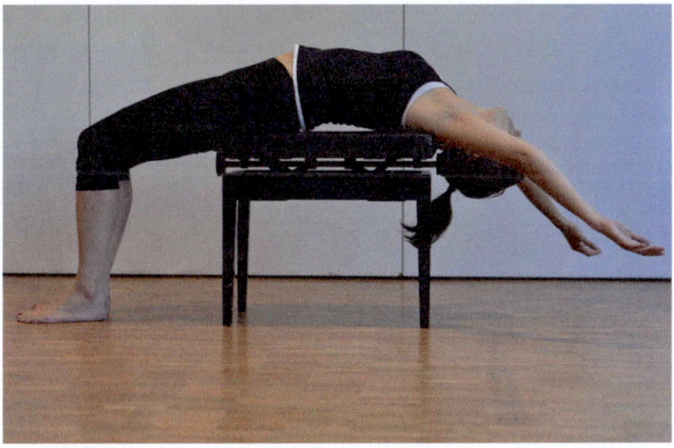

this reason, the participants are encouraged to seek an aligned pelvis while trying to find the correct position of the shoulders. Step-by-step rotating movements, shown by the red arrows in Fig. 20.4a–c, may help to easily find the final correct position.

As humans execute most of the shoulder-engaging arm movements toward the front, it is essential to stretch the shoulders in the opposite direction as often as possible (Fig. 20.5).

Sporadic easier variations of arm push-ups (i.e., against the wall, in standing position) can be effective to strengthen and to reset the placement of the shoulder muscles (Fig. 20.6).

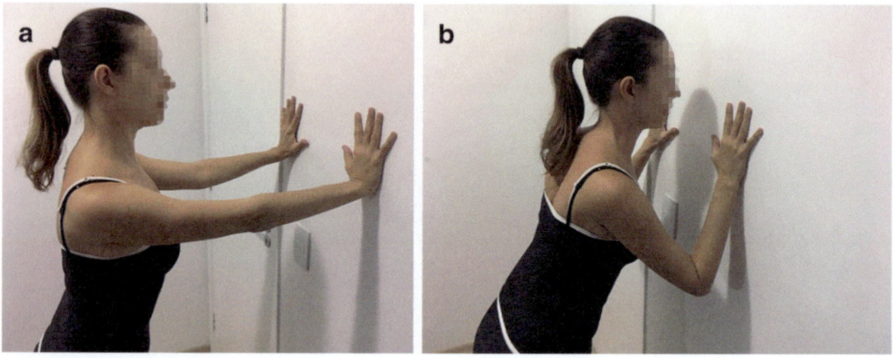

Fig. 20.6 Standing arm push up

The Head and the Neck

Similar to the shoulders, both head and neck tend to react to the postural behavior of the whole body. A simple forward movement of the head, emphasizing the awareness of the incorrect position followed by a slow return to the neutral position may encourage the more comfortable position (sensitization). During this exercise, participants are reminded to seek a more aligned pelvis. Other highly recommended neck mobilizations include self-massage using the hands or using medium-sized balls (placing them in the back of the neck and performing head movements leaning against the wall or laying on the floor), as well as neck stretches.

Hands

For musicians who produce sound through finger action, strengthening the intrinsic muscles of the hand (i.e., the *interossei* and the *lumbricals*) is an essential preventive measure against playing-related injuries. Workshop participants are invited to search for a flat surface where they can lean their whole lower arm and observe the alignment of the hand (Fig. 20.7a–c).

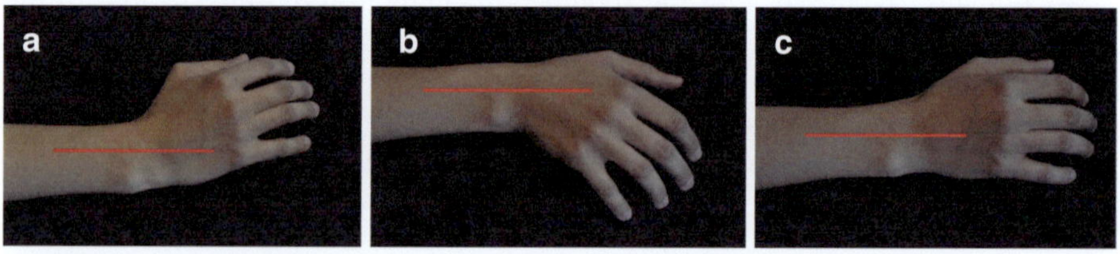

Fig. 20.7 Hand alignment shown as incorrect (**a**, **b**) and correct (**c**)

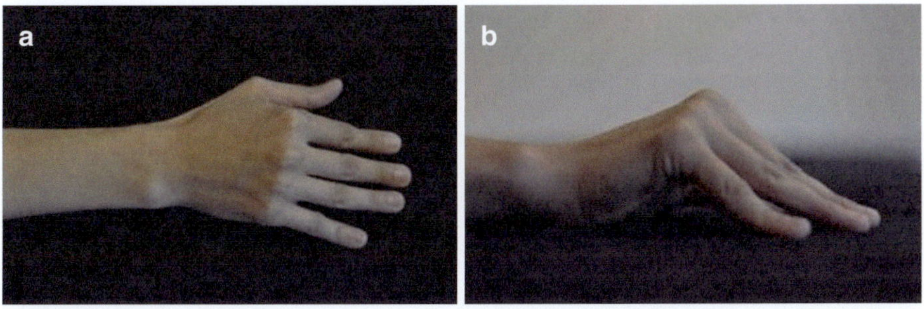

Fig. 20.8 Hand strengthening exercise

Once the correct hand alignment and full elbow and wrist contact with the surface are achieved, in an overstretched position, each fingertip should press against the surface until the third knuckles (*metacarpophalangeal joints*, known as the bridge of the hand) of all fingers except the thumb start to raise (Fig. 20.8a, b). It is recommended up to ten repetitions daily, holding the bridge for 3–10 seconds (depending on hand strength) and then relaxing.

Application Into Performance

Workshop Volunteers

Standing and sitting positions require concentration on the part of the participants to align the structures optimally (see section "Feet/Standing"). Three examples of pre- and post-workshop postural behavior of volunteers show visually recognizable changes.

Pianist

In her pre-workshop performance, Volunteer 1 presented a collapsed chest, slightly rounded shoulders (i.e., protracted shoulders) and a forwardly positioned head, all reinforced by a low tonus level in the pelvic area. The low pelvic muscles' tonus associated to the use of the right foot pedal rooted her tendency to lean toward the left.

In her post-workshop performance, Volunteer 1 was instructed to adjust the bench height. As there was no adjustable bench available, some stacks of paper were used to raise her seating position. The recruitment of the pelvic muscles was enough to raise the chest and a light hair band positioned on top of her head was used to remind her of the correct head positioning (Fig. 20.9).

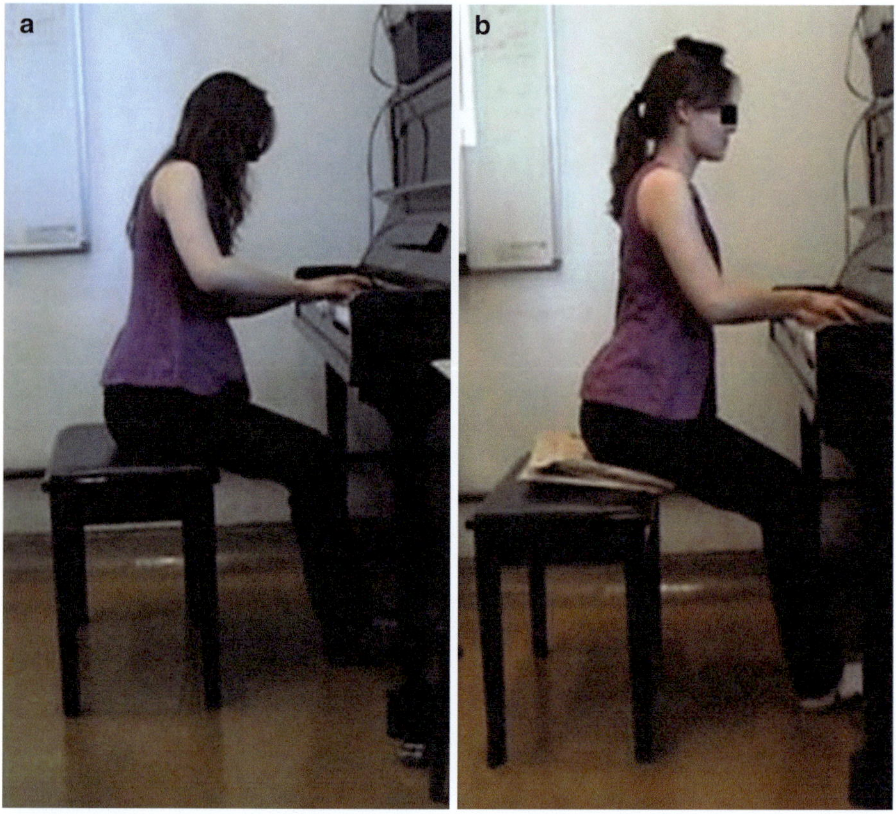

Fig. 20.9 Pianist performing before (**a**) and after (**b**) workshop

Trombonist

In his pre-workshop performance, Volunteer 2 presented a tendency to lean his full body weight over both outer laterals of his feet (i.e., supination), a more prominent lower back curvature caused by the positioning of his pelvis (anterior pelvic tilt), rounded shoulders (i.e., protracted), forwardly positioned head, and elevated elbow (Fig. 20.10).

In his post-workshop performance, Volunteer 2 improved the contact of the inner lateral of the foot with the floor by first stepping on a slightly inclined wooden platform and then standing on the flat surface reproducing the same muscle tonus level achieved over the platform. Special attention was given to the alignment of his

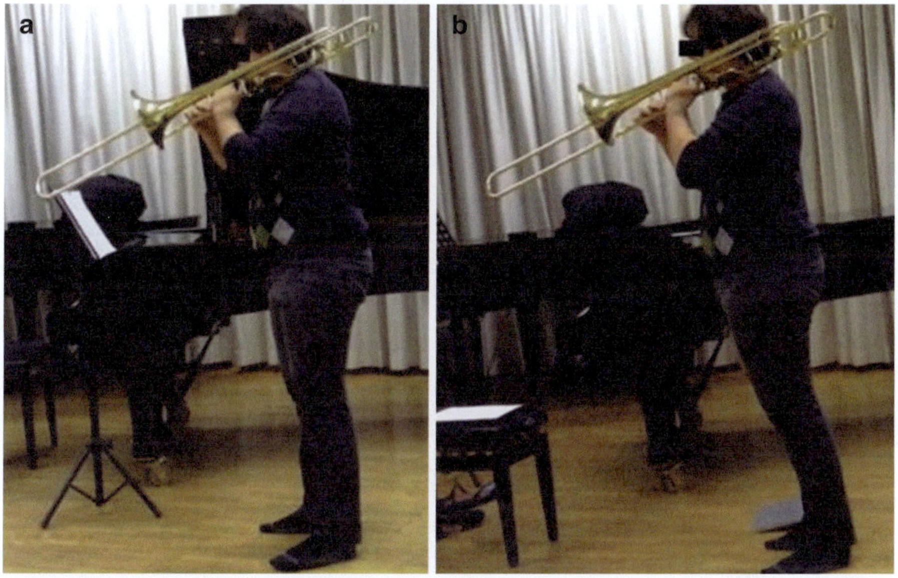

Fig. 20.10 Trombonist performing before (**a**) and after (**b**) workshop

pelvis, which was accomplished by a short repetition of the pelvis exercises. Through this intervention, the lower back curvature minimized, the shoulders, neck, and head found their correct position and the arms relaxed.

Violist

In her pre-workshop performance, Volunteer 3 presented great postural instability by constantly alternating the weight of her body between feet, allowing for pelvic reactions such as lateral flexion and rotation. This instability reflected in typical upper body responses, such as collapsed chest, rounded shoulders (i.e., protraction) and forwardly positioned head (Fig. 20.11).

In her post-workshop performance, Volunteer 3 sought for an improvement of the floor contact by focusing on directing her body weight over the balls of each foot. This mobilization was sufficient to positively engage the upper body in a more aligned posture.

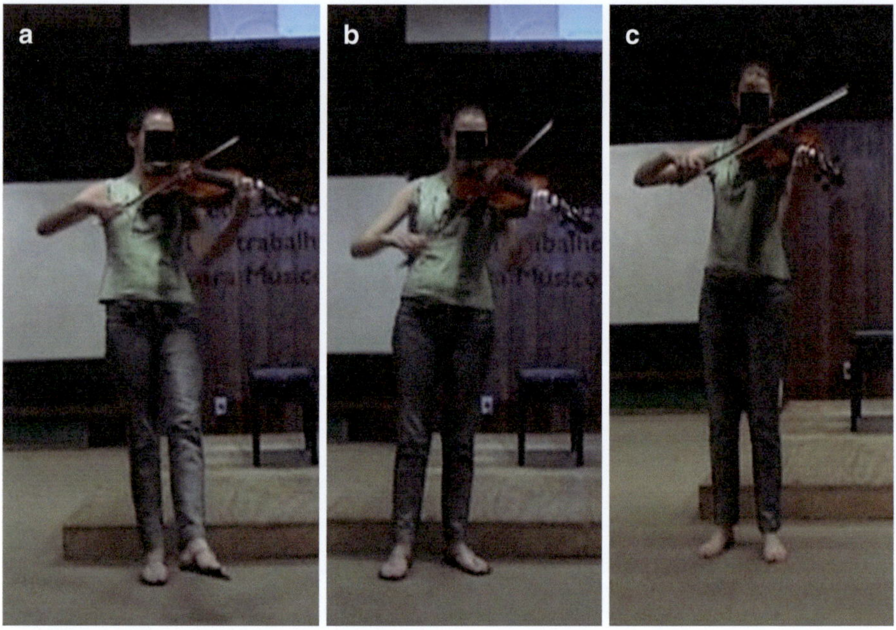

Fig. 20.11 Violinist performing before (**a**, **b**) and after (**c**) workshop

Final Considerations

Workshop Participants

In over 50 PRMDs workshops that I conducted in Europe, North and South Americas, and the Middle East, the participating groups often comprised musicians who had suffered some sort of performance-related physical discomfort or injury. Although also present in the workshops, musicians who had never dealt with such impairing conditions and/or who, during their early music education, had never been encouraged to become aware of their bodies while performing showed lower interest in changing their performing mode solely for preventive reasons. The "no pain, no gain" mentality described in 1995 by Shoup still prevails in music educational institutions and orchestras, as musicians continue to share high motivation to find ways to sound better, gladly choosing to endure painful physical behavior and neglecting preventive measures [9, 34]. Although workshop participants reported to be aware of the benefits of cardiovascular and muscular exercises for the overall health, it was rare to find musicians who practiced them regularly [35].

During the workshops, participants were encouraged to experience a new way of perceiving their bodies and to apply this new perception directly into performance. When a few volunteers performed before and after the body mobilization, other participants, in most cases, witnessed positive musical results. Through this experience, they seemed more enthusiastic to incorporate a preventive approach into their practicing/playing routines.

While many preventive programs in universities and conservatoires tend to direct students into sports or physical activity to be developed in parallel to the musical performance, the current workshop focuses on strategies to be directly applied during the performance. The empowering character of the proposed approach may justify the observed high acceptance of these workshops. The prospect of possibly enhancing technical and sound control through the engagement of the whole body seems to be far more appealing to musicians than the preventive undertaking.

Further Research

These workshops have produced an array of anecdotal observations and outcome feedback. For future study, the establishment of consistent standards of prevalence is essential for quality assessment of the incidence, causation, and risk factors of PRMDs in musicians. The influence of the most common individual variables, such as gender, age, experience, health history, and anthropometric features on the overall postural behavior in playing their instrument should be considered. Specifically based on the reactions of the workshop participants, a thorough investigation on the correlation between body behavior and performance quality could bring new insights to music performance pedagogy and to the mentality of the musicians of the future.

References

1. Fry Hunter JH. Incidence of overuse syndrome in the symphony orchestra. Med Probl Perform Art. 1986;1(2):51–5.
2. Fishbein M, Middlestadt SE, Ottati V, Straus S, Ellis A. Medical problems among ICSOM musicians: overview of a national survey. Med Probl Perform Art. 1988;3(1):1–8.
3. Middlestadt SE, Fishbein M. The prevalence of severe musculoskeletal problems among male and female symphony orchestra string players. Med Probl Perform Art. 1989;4(1):41–8.
4. Abréu-Ramos AM, Micheo WF. Lifetime prevalence of upper-body musculoskeletal problems in a professional-level symphony orchestra. Med Probl Perform Art. 2007;22(3):97–104.
5. Gembris H, Heye A, Seifert A. Health problems of orchestral musicians from a life-span perspective: results of a large-scale study. Music Sci. 2018;1:1–20.
6. Fry HJH. Prevalence of overuse (injury) syndrome in Australian music schools. Br J Ind Med. 1987;44(1):35–40.
7. Lockwood A. Medical problems in secondary school-aged musicians. Med Probl Perform Art. 1988;3(4):129–32.
8. Zaza C. Playing-related health problems at a Canadian music school. Med Probl Perform Art. 1992;2:48–51.
9. Shoup D. Survey of performance-related problems among high school and junior high school musicians. Med Probl Perform Art. 1995;10(3):100–5.
10. Zetterberg C, Backlund H, Karlsson J, Werner H, Olsson L. Musculoskeletal problems among male and female music students. Med Probl Perform Art. 1998;13(1):160–6.
11. Spahn C, Strukely S, Lehmann A. Health conditions, attitudes toward study, and attitudes toward health at the beginning of university study: music students in comparison with other student populations. Med Probl Perform Art. 2004;19(1):26–33.

12. Spahn C, Nusseck M, Zander M. Long-term analysis of health status and preventive behavior in music students across an entire university program. Med Probl Perform Art. 2014;29(1):8–15.
13. Arnason K, Árnason Á, Briem K. Playing-related musculoskeletal disorders among Icelandic music students: differences between students playing classical vs rhythmic music. Med Probl Perform Art. 2014;29(2):74–9.
14. Ioannou CI, Hafer J, Lee A, Altenmüller E. Epidemiology, treatment efficacy, and anxiety aspects of music students affected by playing-related pain: a retrospective evaluation with follow-up. Med Probl Perform Art. 2018;33(1):26–38.
15. Brandfonbrener AG. Performing arts medicine: a Checkup. Med Probl Perform Art. 1988;20(2):101–2.
16. Brandfonbrener AG. Medical problems and the young music student. Med Probl Perform Art. 1988;20(2), Editorial.
17. Spahn C, Hildebrandt H, Seidenglanz K. Effectiveness of a prophylactic course to prevent playing-related health problems of music students. Med Probl Perform Art. 2001;16(1):24–31.
18. Barton R, Feinberg JR. Effectiveness of an educational program in health promotion and injury prevention for freshman music majors. Med Probl Perform Art. 2008;23(2):47–53.
19. Zander MF, Voltmer E, Spahn C. Health promotion and prevention in higher music education: results of a longitudinal study. Med Probl Perform Art. 2010;25(2):54–65.
20. López TM, Martínez JF. Strategies to promote health and prevent musculoskeletal injuries in students from the high conservatory of music of Salamanca, Spain. Med Probl Perform Art. 2013;28(2):100–6.
21. Brandfonbrener AG. Orchestral injury prevention: intervention study. Med Probl Perform Art. 1997;12(1):9–14.
22. Chan C, Driscoll T, Ackermann BJ. Effect of a musicians' exercise intervention on performance-related musculoskeletal disorders. Med Probl Perform Art. 2014;29(4):81–188.
23. Baadjou VAE, Roussel NA, Verbunt JA, Smeets RJ, de Bie RA. Systematic review on risk factors for musculoskeletal disorders in musicians. Occup Med. 2016;66(8):614–22.
24. Zaza C, Farewell VT. Musicians' playing-related musculo-skeletal disorders: an examination of risk factors. Am J Ind Med. 1997;32:292–300.
25. Kenny D, Ackermann B. Performance-related musculoskeletal pain, depression and music performance anxiety in professional orchestral musicians: a population study. Psychol Music. 2015;43:43–60.
26. Leaver R, Clare Harris E, Palmer KT. Musculoskeletal pain in elite professional musicians from British symphony orchestras. Occup Med. 2011;61:549–55.
27. Lee SH, Carey S, Lazinski M, Kim KS. An integrative intervention program for college musicians and kinematics in cello playing. Eur J Intern Med. 2019;25:34–40.
28. Gutzwiller J. Körperklang – Klangkörper: ein Arbeitsbuch über Körperarbeit für Chorleiter, Sänger und Instrumentalisten. Basel: Hbs Nepomuk; 1997.
29. Klein-Vogelbach S, Lahme A, Spirgi-Gantert I. Interpretación musical y postura corporal madrid. Madrid: Ediciones Akal S.A; 2010.
30. Larsen C, Larsen C, Hartelt O. Körperhaltungen: analysieren und verbessern. Stuttgart: Trias Verlag; 2008.
31. Mätzener H, Gutzwiller J, Sick B, Maier HC, Tomatis L. Klarinettenklang: Versuch einer physiologischen Analyse. http://www.dissonance.ch/en/archive/main_articles/360/abstract/en. Accessed 15 Jan 2019.
32. Spirgi-Gantert I, Gutzwiller J. Kleines Kompendium der Bewegung. Zürcher Hochschule der Künste. Zurich: Sihldruck AG; 2015.
33. Chan CL, Driscoll T, Ackermann B. Development of a specific exercise programme for professional orchestral musicians. Inj Prev. 2013;19:257–63.
34. Ioannou CI, Altenmüller E. Approaches to and treatment strategies for playing-related pain problems among Czech instrumental music students: an epidemiological study. Med Probl Perform Art. 2015;30(3):135–42.
35. Chan CL, Ackermann B. Evidence-informed physical therapy management of performance-related musculoskeletal disorders in musicians. Front Psychol. 2014;5:1–14.

Part IV
Program Implementation

Chapter 21
Exploring Traditional Chinese Medicine in Musician Health

Stephanie L. Mayer-Sattin and David B. Kaplan

Introduction

Research suggests that over 50% of musicians have chronic pain from injuries sustained while making music, and that the level of pain that musicians suffer is twice that of the general population [1–6]. Common physical health concerns may be grouped into three categories: playing-related musculoskeletal disorders (PRMD); task-specific focal dystonias; and nerve entrapments. The reader is referred to Chaps. 11 and 13 where these conditions are described extensively.

Causes for the high injury rate include postural asymmetries, instrument designs and demands, contact pressure and compression, flaws in musician technique, muscle tension, and overuse [7]. Gross and Musgrave commented that musicians' lifestyle and work environment further exacerbate musicians' mental health [8]. As a result of these injuries and other job-related factors, musicians experience psychological disorders, fatigue, and stress that negatively impact their general physical health [1, 8]. In addition, lack of sleep places musicians at risk for obesity and chronic diseases including diabetes, cardiovascular disorders (such as coronary heart disease, hypertension, peripheral vascular disease, and stroke), dementia, Alzheimer's disease, Parkinson's disease, memory loss, and psychiatric disorders [9].

Musicians with performance-related sleep loss also have a 95% risk for Major Depressive Disorders [9]. Mental health in the professional music community continues to be reported as a serious problem [1]. In a study of 1227 musicians conducted by the

S. L. Mayer-Sattin (✉)
Instrumental Music Department, Bullis School, Potomac, MD, USA

Wudang Wellness, Rockville, MD, USA
e-mail: stephanie_mayer@bullis.org

D. B. Kaplan (✉)
Wudang Wellness, Rockville, MD, USA

Edgewood Surgical Hospital, Transfer, PA, USA

S.-H. Lee et al. (eds.), *Perspectives in Performing Arts Medicine Practice*,
https://doi.org/10.1007/978-3-030-37480-8_21

Music Industry Research Association (MIRA), almost 12% of respondents reported suicidal thoughts in the preceding two-week period [2]. This statistic ranks musicians four times more likely to have suicidal thoughts than the general population, yet research and effective interventions designed for musicians with mental illness remain limited [2]. Further, substance abuse continues to be a concern within the music community. Over 30% of musicians report frequent drinking in contrast to over 15% in the general population [2]. Reports of overall drug use in musicians are documented at over 5%, while average drug use in the general public is less than 2% [2]. Musicians' use of opium and heroin is almost three times that of the general population [2]. Self-medication of prescribed or illegal substances both creates and worsens musician mental health and constitutes a serious impediment to a musician's career [2]. In light of such evidence, it is clear that there is a need for continued research in musician wellness and in intervention resources designed to improve musicians' physical and mental health. Therefore, to address these significant and prevalent issues, we created a mindfulness intervention program for use in music practice, rehearsal, and performance employing traditional Chinese physical and mental techniques.

Traditional Chinese Medical Practice as a Health Intervention for Musicians

Traditional Chinese Medicine (TCM), martial arts, and meditation methodology can be traced in print to the *Mawangdui silk texts* of 168 BC in Changsha, Hunan, China and has been used to treat and prevent physical and mental health disease since its inception [10]. Among the vast array of TCM methods and treatments, mindfulness interventions such as taichi, qigong, meditation, and acupressure massage, when regularly executed, have shown promise in safely addressing a variety of conditions in Western medical clinical trials and studies. Some of the most compelling study results support that *taichi, qigong*, and acupressure massage alleviate symptoms of depression [11], improve sleep [12], reduce anxiety [13], increase stamina [14], reduce stress [15], and reduce musculoskeletal pain [16]. As musicians are at increased risk for all of these conditions, there is a demonstrated need for early prevention, sound pedagogy in the music classroom, and effective interventions such as found in traditional Chinese methods that prevent disease, treat the symptoms of disease, and reduce a musician's need for medication [2].

Wudang Daoist Sanfeng Pai *Methods*

Music is hardwired in human physiology and it stands to reason that music educators must concern themselves with all biological matters involved in music-making [17]. With this concept in mind, we selected physical warm-up techniques of acupressure massage, *qigong, taichi*, and meditation to help instrumental musicians play with efficacy, relaxation, and mindfulness. This intervention employed the practices and

Fig. 21.1 Wudang Five Animal Qigong Snake (David Kaplan, MD Yuxu Palace, Wudangshan, China)

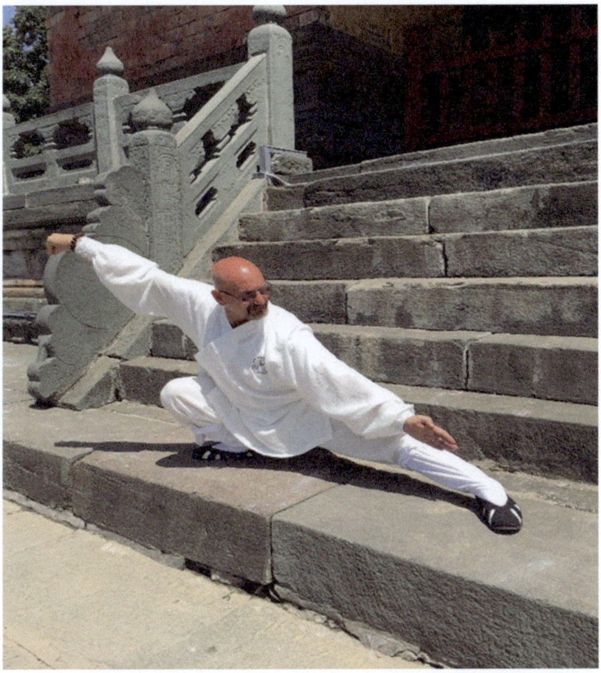

principles of the Wudang Daoist Sanfeng Pai lineage of Wudangshan, China in Hubei Province, China with a documented lineage of active disciples to the present day. *Wudang Sanfeng Pai* takes its name from the legendary inventor of *taichi, Zhang Sanfeng*, and has preserved an oral tradition lineage of martial artists for nearly 800 years [18]. The practices and martial arts of *Wudang Sanfeng Pai* are designated and protected by the Chinese government as intangible heritage, and the numerous temples of Wudangshan, China have been declared official UNESCO world heritage sites [19].

Specific methods used in the intervention from the *Wudang Daoist Sanfeng Pai* tradition included acupressure self-massage of the well, spring, stream, river, and sea acupuncture points [20], *Wudang Five Animal Qigong* [21] (Fig. 21.1), *Wudang Taichi* [22], and *meditation* (Fig. 21.2). These methods were taught to the authors of this chapter over 9 years by *Wudang Daoist Sanfeng Pai* Chinese martial arts master, *Yuan Xiu Gang* and his *kungfu* brothers, *Zhong Xue Chao* and *Zhou Xuan Yun*. As a result, Stephanie Mayer-Sattin, coauthor, became the first American woman to be chosen as an official disciple of the *Wudang Daoist Sanfeng Pai lineage.*

Curriculum Enhancement Program

From 2009 through 2018, approximately 100 third through twelfth grade students took part in the intervention each year at the Bullis School, a suburban private school in Potomac, Maryland. Students were taught *acupressure massage*, *qigong, taichi*, and a meditation moving-mindfulness warm-up sequence during instrumental music

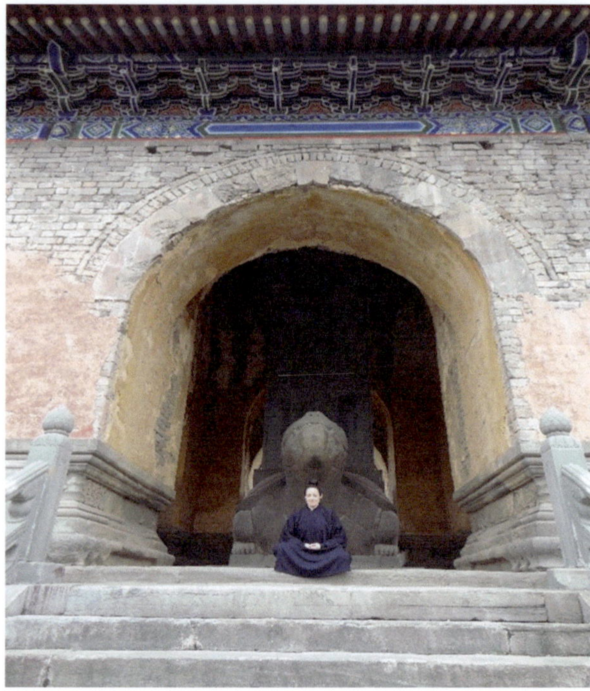

Fig. 21.2 Wudang Sanfeng Pai Meditation (Stephanie Mayer-Sattin, Yuxu Palace, Wudangshan, China)

rehearsals as an enhancement to the curriculum. With generous funding provided by the school, faculty was sent to Wudangshan, China for training. The school also provided funding for *Daoist Master Yuan Xiu Gang* to travel to the United States to launch the initial efforts through a two-week residency teaching *Wudang Sanfeng Pai* methods to all music students at the school. In addition, financial support was given by the school for faculty and Master *Yuan Xiu Gang* to report the intervention pedagogy and initial results of the intervention at the International Society for Music Education (ISME) World Conference in Beijing, China in 2010. These methods continued to be incorporated into the music curriculum as an educational enhancement to music rehearsals at the school over a nine-year period. Final refinements to the *acupressure massage, qigong, taichi*, and the *meditation* intervention warm-up protocol sequence used in the curriculum were made in the 2017–2018 school year. Thus, we will primarily report on the intervention process and observations for the year 2017–2018. The majority of the students who participated in the orchestral and concert bands were high school age and 60% were male.

Moving-Mindfulness Intervention Process 2017–2018

Students engaged in a three-step intervention sequence process based on the *Wudang Daoist Sanfeng Pai* tradition. Third through eighth-grade students were led by the instructor, while ninth through twelfth-grade students were led by the instructor or by an instructor-trained student. Class sizes in this school year contained 52 students in concert band, 20 students in each chamber orchestra, and 10 students in each beginning instrumental class. During each rehearsal session of 70 min in length, students performed the 20 min *moving-mindfulness intervention* warm-up sequence at the beginning of class. Students massaged acupressure points, then proceeded with the intervention *qigong* and *taichi* sequences. Each *qigong* exercise and *taichi* sequence was followed by silent *meditation* of 1–2 min in length. Students then played a developmentally appropriate piece of music that they had prepared for 3 months. Finally, students self-reflected through in-class surveys and ePortfolio essays at home on whether or not they had improvement in physical and mental well-being, mental focus, finger speed, and breath-support while playing the piece of music after the intervention. Students also considered whether or not existing pain and stiffness prior to the sequence was improved after the intervention warm-up sequence. Throughout the remainder of the rehearsal, students also used *acupressure massage* every 15 min to reduce static load. Pedagogical rationale for the implementation of these warm-up techniques mirrors the educational theory of Estelle Jorgensen in support of mind–body integration of the whole musician [23]. By focusing the mind and body with these specialized Chinese martial arts warm-ups, it was hypothesized that music students would improve physical and mental health outcomes and be better able to connect with themselves and with others in the ensemble. Informal and casual testimonies were collected through teacher observation, student reflective essays on course materials, informal conversations, and course surveys.

Program Observations and Results

We observed students demonstrating intrinsic motivation to incorporate the intervention into their everyday lives, both in music and in other high-stress events such as athletic contests and academic testing, to alleviate performance anxiety. This is especially surprising given that adolescents often express reluctance to participate in unusual activities out of fear that they will be judged by their peers due to a heightened level of Intolerance of Uncertainty (IU) [24]. Contrary to the common developmental IU in adolescence [24], students expressed that they enjoyed the intervention and volunteered to lead the instrumental ensembles through the intervention at the beginning of rehearsals. When altered school schedules shortened the rehearsal and there was not enough time to perform the intervention, students expressed disappointment. Their continued interest in eagerly participating and leading the intervention in each rehearsal without instructor prompting suggests an individual investment of value into the intervention itself.

Students also perceived receiving benefit from the intervention. All students participated in the acupressure self-massage, *qigong*, and *taichi*. One student asked to be excused from the meditation portion because meditating in a large group setting was too distracting with so many people present. In the 2017–2018 school year, students reflected in the Part III Course Surveys (see Appendix) and ePortfolio essays that they felt more relaxed, experienced less preexisting stiffness with more flexibility and experienced less pain after the intervention at the rate of 77%, 87%, and 56%, respectively. The teacher and students observed several qualitative benefits as well, which included: relaxed bow holds for string instruments, relaxed shoulder position for all instrumentalists, better focus, flow, and mental agility in rehearsal, and less in-class disruption.

Short answer responses from the yearly Part II Course Survey question "What did you enjoy about this class?" include the following responses: Student #1 "I also like how she incorporates health tips to make sure we aren't hurting ourselves when playing. For example: the practice of *qigong*." Student #2, "Highlight of my day. *Qigong* was great!" Student #3, "*Qigong* was definitely the best part." Student #4, "We don't only play music but we do exercise to prepare ourselves to play music."

Student benefits from the intervention spanning an entire year was also documented in student ePortfolios. In a reflective essay for his ePortfolio, one student noted, "*Qigong* is the highlight of my work [in band]. It is so relaxing while also helping me to focus. Because of that, I try to meditate once a week." Another band student remarked, "I started using *qigong* before my track meets and every time I do, I get a faster time." Additionally, one orchestra student reported, "At the school concert, I was comfortable because I was in a familiar place. On the other hand, at the honors recital, at the Strathmore Mansion, I was in an unfamiliar place and the stage was small and the audience felt like they were really close to where I was performing. I felt my knees shake while I was playing at the Strathmore Mansion. It is probable that some people thought I looked nervous. I, in fact, played nervously. I never practiced playing nervously. I was not able to control my nerves in the moment." The student then documented the desire to "meditate and stretch more" with *qigong* as part of the ePortfolio school year goals. Subsequently, in the end of year ePortfolio reflection, the student reported that, "Because of *qigong* and meditation, my sanity and health was preserved. I had a great year [in orchestra] internally and externally."

Discussion

The outcomes of a *moving-mindfulness intervention* integrated into an instrumental music program were informally observed as part of a music curriculum over a nine-year period. Multiple benefits were noted by both students and teachers involved in the experience, indicating the need for systematic collection and analysis of the data for future research directions. Key benefits included improvements in focus, levels of body tension, and reported reductions in pain and stiffness. The next step would be to address the need for randomized trials and more formal study to assess causal benefit. Consideration of age differences and how formalized study of this intervention can accurately be measured across the developmental expanse of third through twelfth-grade students need to be taken into account. In addition, the logical path for studying the effects of the intervention on the reduction of repetitive use syndromes would include a separate study that examines the intervention in light of music practice norms at teaching institutions. With some of these ideas in mind, a formal study of this *moving-mindfulness intervention* with university music student participants was completed in February 2019. Early survey results from the study reveal that 93% of participants reported feeling more relaxed after the *moving-mindfulness intervention*. While these results are promising, it is important to note that the majority of respondents were 18–22 years of age. It needs to be seen if these findings would yield similar results from a more diverse group of participants. A complete reporting with metrics of this study's findings will be released later in 2020.

Appendix

Course Survey Part III (Mindfulness Warm-Up)

Month

❑ January	❑ March	❑ May	❑ July	❑ September	❑ November
❑ February	❑ April	❑ June	❑ August	❑ October	❑ December

Day

❑ 1	❑ 4	❑ 7	❑ 10	❑ 13	❑ 16	❑ 19	❑ 22	❑ 25	❑ 28	❑ 31
❑ 2	❑ 5	❑ 8	❑ 11	❑ 14	❑ 17	❑ 20	❑ 23	❑ 26	❑ 29	
❑ 3	❑ 6	❑ 9	❑ 12	❑ 15	❑ 18	❑ 21	❑ 24	❑ 27	❑ 30	

Year

❑ 2018 ❑ 2019

I am (gender):

❑ Female ❑ Male

I am (age):

❑ 1	❑ 3	❑ 5	❑ 7	❑ 9	❑ 11	❑ 13	❑ 15	❑ 17	❑ 19
❑ 2	❑ 4	❑ 6	❑ 8	❑ 10	❑ 12	❑ 14	❑ 16	❑ 18	❑ 20

What instrument do you play?

❑ Violin	❑ Piano	❑ Soprano Saxophone	❑ Trombome
❑ Viola	❑ Flute	❑ Alto Saxophone	❑ Baritone Horn
❑ Cello	❑ Oboe	❑ Tenor Saxophone	❑ Tuba
❑ String Bass	❑ Clarinet	❑ Baritone Saxophone	❑ Percussion
❑ Electric Bass	❑ Bass Clarinet	❑ Trumpet	
❑ Guitar	❑ Bassoon	❑ French Horn	

List other instruments here:

How many year(s) have you played your primary instrument?

❑ 1	❑ 3	❑ 5	❑ 7	❑ 9	❑ 11	❑ 13	❑ 15
❑ 2	❑ 4	❑ 6	❑ 8	❑ 10	❑ 12	❑ 14	

Did you notice any of the following before or during the qigong and meditation?

❑ Pain	❑ Weakness	❑ Fatique
❑ Soreness	❑ Numbness	❑ I did not experience any of these conditions or discomforts
❑ Uncomfortable Tingling	❑ Loss of Physical Control	
❑ Stiffness	❑ Physical Hypersensitivity	

If you experienced physical discomfort before or during qigong, please identify the location(s) of your discomfort:

- ❑ Head
- ❑ Eyes
- ❑ Jaw
- ❑ Neck (Front)
- ❑ Neck (Back)
- ❑ Shoulder (Front)
- ❑ Shoulder (Back)
- ❑ Chest
- ❑ Upper Back
- ❑ Middle Back
- ❑ Lower Back
- ❑ Upper Arm
- ❑ Lower Arm
- ❑ Wrist
- ❑ Thumb
- ❑ Fingers
- ❑ Buttocks
- ❑ Upper Leg
- ❑ Lower Leg
- ❑ I did not experience any discomfort

Did you feel discomfort/pain before qigong?

❑ No ❑ Yes

If yes above, rate the level of discomfort you felt before qigong. (1 - low degree of physical discomfort, 10 - high degree of physical discomfort)

- ❑ 1 - Low degree of pain or discomfort
- ❑ 2
- ❑ 3
- ❑ 4
- ❑ 5
- ❑ 6
- ❑ 7
- ❑ 8
- ❑ 9
- ❑ 10 - High degree of pain or discomfort

Did you feel discomfort/pain during qigong?

❑ No ❑ Yes

If yes above, rate the level of discomfort you felt during qigong. (1 - low degree of physical discomfort, 10 - high degree of physical discomfort)

- ❑ 1 - Low degree of pain or discomfort
- ❑ 2
- ❑ 3
- ❑ 4
- ❑ 5
- ❑ 6
- ❑ 7
- ❑ 8
- ❑ 9
- ❑ 10 - High degree of pain or discomfort

After completing qigong exercises and meditation, did you feel pain:

❑ No ❑ Yes

If yes above, after completing qigong exercises and meditation, did you feel pain:

❑ Less pain ❑ I did not notice a diference ❑ More pain

After completing qigong exercises and meditation, did you feel stiffness:

❑ No ❑ Yes

If yes above, after completing qigong exercises and meditation, did you feel stiffness:

❑ Less stiff ❑ I did not notice a diference ❑ More stiff

After completing qigong exercises and meditation, did you feel relaxed:

❑ Less ❑ Same ❑ More

After completing qigong exercises and meditation, did you feel mentally focused:

❑ Less mentally focused ❑ I did not notice a difference in mental focus ❑ More mentally focused

After completing qigong exercises and meditation, did awakeness change:

❑ Less awake ❑ I did not notice a difference ❑ More awake

After completing qigong exercises and meditation, did finger speed change:

❑ Less finger speed ❑ I did not notice a difference ❑ More finger speed

After completing qigong exercises and meditation, did your sense of physical well-being change:

❑ Less sense of physical well-being ❑ I did not notice of difference in my physical well-being ❑ More sense of physical well-being

After completing qigong exercises and meditation, did your sense of mental well-being change:

❑ Less sense of mental well-being ❑ I did not notice a difference in my mental well-being ❑ More sense of mental well-being

After completing qigong exercises and meditation, did your sense of physical energy change:

❑ Less physical energy ❑ I did not notice a diference in physical energy ❑ More physical energy

After completing qigong exercises and meditation, did your sense of energized breath control change

❑ Less energized breath support ❑ I did not notice a change in my energized breath support ❑ More energized breath support

Pain

❑ Less ❑ Same ❑ More

Stiffness

❑ Less ❑ Same ❑ More

Relaxed

❑ Less ❑ Same ❑ More

Mentally focused

❑ Less ❑ Same ❑ More

Awakeness

❑ Less ❑ Same ❑ More

Finger speed

❑ Less ❑ Same ❑ More

Physical well-being

❑ Less ❑ Same ❑ More

Mental well-being

❑ Less ❑ Same ❑ More

Physical energy

❑ Less ❑ Same ❑ More

Energized breath control

❑ Less ❑ Same ❑ More

References

1. Voltmer E, Zander M, Fischer JE, Kudielka BM, Richter B, Spahn C. Physical and mental health of different types of orchestra musicians compared to other professions. Med Probl Perform Art. 2012;27(1):9–14.
2. Krueger AB, Zhen Y. Inaugural Music Industry Research Association (MIRA) survey of musicians. Music Industry Research Association. 2018. https://img1.wsimg.com/blobby/go/53aaa2d4-793a-4400b6c995d6618809f9/downloads/1cgjrbs3b_761615.pdf. Accessed 21 Oct 2018.
3. Fishbein M, Middlestadt SE, Ottati V, Straus S, Ellis A. Medical problems among ICSOM musicians: overview of a national survey. Med Probl Perform Art. 1988;3(1):1–8.
4. Fry HJH, Ross P, Rutherford M. Medical problems in secondary school-aged musicians. Med Probl Perform Art. 1988;3(4):133–4.
5. Lockwood A. Medical problems in secondary school-aged musicians. Med Probl Perform Art. 1988;3(4):129–32.

6. Lockwood A. Medical problems of musicians. NEJM. 1989;320(4):221–7. https://doi.org/10.1056/NEJM198901263200405.
7. Dommerholt J. Performing arts medicine – instrumentalist musicians, part II – examination. J Bodyw Mov Ther. 2010;14:65–72. https://doi.org/10.1016/j.jbmt.2009.02.004.
8. Gross SA, Musgrave G. (2016, November). Can music make you sick? Music and depression: a study into the incidence of musicians' mental health (Report No. 1). MusicTank Publishing. 2016. https://issuu.com/helpmusiciansuk/doc/can_music_make_you_sick_part_1_pil. Accessed 24 Nov 2018.
9. Colten HR, Altevogt BM. Sleep disorders and sleep deprivation: an unmet public health problem. Washington DC: National Academic Press; 2006. https://doi.org/10.17226/11617.
10. Xia A. (Presenter). Introduction to acupuncture. Speech presented at The National Institute of Health, Bethesda, MD/USA; 1 Feb 2016.
11. Zou L, Yeung A, Li C, Wei GX, Chen KW, Kinser PA, et al. Effects of meditative movements on major depressive disorder: a systematic review and meta-analysis of randomized controlled trials. J Clin Med. 2018;7(8):195. https://doi.org/10.3390/jcm7080195.
12. Du S, Dong J, Zhang H, Jin S, Xu G, Liu Z, et al. Taichi exercise for self-rated sleep quality in older people: a systematic review and meta-analysis. Int J Nurs Stud. 2015;52(1):368–79. https://doi.org/10.1016/j.ijnurstu.2014.05.009.
13. McClure M. Use of Tai Chi to treat mental health disorders in Veterans, ProQuest Dissertations and Theses. 2017. https://search-proquestcom.ezproxy.bu.edu/docview/1964397920?pq-origsite=primo. Accessed 12 Jan 2019.
14. Johansson M, Hassmén P, Jouper J. Acute effects of qigong exercise on mood and anxiety. Sport Exerc Perform Psychol. 2011;1:60–5. https://doi.org/10.1037/21573905.1.S.60.
15. Wang C. Improving health among elementary school children: a comparison of aerobic and mind-body exercise, ProQuest Dissertations and Theses. 2012. https://search-proquest-com.ezproxy.bu.edu/docview/1176549271/?pq-origsite=primo. Accessed 10 Jan 2019.
16. Sousa CM, Moreira L, Coimbra D, Machado J, Greten HJ. Immediate effects of Tuina techniques on working-related musculoskeletal disorder of professional orchestra musicians. J Integr Med. 2015;13(4):257–61. https://doi.org/10.1016/S2095-4964(15)60181-9.
17. Elliot DJ, Silverman M. Music matters: a philosophy of music education. 2nd ed. New York: Oxford University Press; 2015. p. 180–5.
18. Yang LZ. (Presenter). A brief history of Wudang Mountain Daoism. Speech presented at Daoist Studies Institute, Danjiangkou, Hubei, China; 18 Jul 2010.
19. Ancient Building Complex in the Wudang Mountains, Danjiangkou City, Hubei Province, N32 28 0.012E11100, date of inscription: 1994, criteria: (i), (ii), (vi), Ref: 705. https://whc.unesco.org/en/list/705. Accessed 5 Jan 2019.
20. Keown D. The spark in the machine. Singing Dragon: London; 2014.
21. Yuan XG. Wudang five animal Qigong [Video file]. 16 Jan 2010. https://www.youtube.com/watch?v=8Up2Mnq7JSM. Accessed 20 Nov 2018.
22. Yuan XG. Wudang Taiji 28 quan [Video file]. 23 Jul 2007. https://www.youtube.com/watch?v=j1DM1M3Tsds. Accessed 20 Nov 2018.
23. Jorgensen E. The aims of music education: a preliminary excursion. JAE. 2002;36(1):31–49. https://doi.org/10.2307/3333624.
24. Dekkers L, Jansen B, Salemink E, Huizenga H. Intolerance of uncertainty scale: measurement invariance among adolescent boys and girls and relationships with anxiety and risk taking. J Behav Ther Exp Psychiatry. 2017;55:57–65. https://doi.org/10.1016/j.jbtep.2016.11.009.

Chapter 22
Youth Dance Fundamental Movement Skills and Assessment

Juanita Patterson-Price

Introduction: Footprints Dance Project and Program Rationale

Footprints Dance Project is a nonprofit organization providing free, high-quality dance and arts programs to children and youth ages 3–18 years throughout Calgary, Alberta, Canada. The mission ensures that children and youth facing economic, physical, and social barriers have an opportunity to experience and enjoy the performing arts [1]. The organization has served over 2000 children and youth primarily through its summer camp programs in the City of Calgary since it was founded in 1999. In 2005, Footprints received grant support through RBC Learn to Play and Canadian Tire Jumpstart, and mentorship by Canadian Sport for Life to develop a dance teaching resource for children and youth. The aim of this teaching resource was to help other individuals and organizations elevate their teaching practice by incorporating fundamental movement skill instruction. The resource that was consequently developed is called the **Footprints Dance Project - Movement Tool** (FMT) [2].

Dance teachers at Footprints Dance Project noticed that an increasing number of their students struggled with movements that should be appropriate for their age level. The same issue has been observed in other athletic and health organizations, prompting new physical activity initiatives in Canada. These initiatives include a push to add physical activity counseling within the Canadian primary care network [3], Alberta's "Prescription To Get Active" program [4], and other initiatives through "Canadian Sport For Life" [5]. Physical Education is mandatory in schools up to the ninth grade throughout Canada, and there has also been an effort in Canada to

J. Patterson-Price (✉)
Department of Mental Health Law and Policy, College of Behavioral and Community Sciences, University of South Florida, Tampa, FL, USA
e-mail: juanitap@mail.usf.edu

S.-H. Lee et al. (eds.), *Perspectives in Performing Arts Medicine Practice*,
https://doi.org/10.1007/978-3-030-37480-8_22

increase physical activity outside of the classroom in community settings. Many unique and creative short-term interventions, such as free archery for underprivileged youth and a variety of dance and sport programs, have been used in a large variety of settings, often in conjunction with Canada Sport for Life [5]. The ideology grounding many of these initiatives is that kids just need to be doing *something* active, as opposed to finding what the *best* activity would be.

Some initiatives have taken a more rigorous research-based approach in developing program theory and outcome monitoring and assessment, such as Julie Beaulac's initiative at the University of Ottawa. While searching for types of physical activities to use to implement a community-based physical activity program for disadvantaged youth, Julie Beaulac—using qualitative methodology, consultation, and focus groups—discovered that hip hop dance had the most popular support in that community and would provide the maximum benefits [6]. Due to the combination of its ease of implementation and cultural acceptance, hip hop dance became the most ideal intervention for this population, and results indicated improvement in multiple facets of life, including physical health [7].

There are also efforts to teach educators and coaches about fundamental skills and their impacts in order to improve skills in students [8]. For instance, Thomas van Rossum and David Morley's work, developed at Sheffield Hallam University in the UK, is an easy-to-use computer application program for school teachers that teaches them fundamental skills and provides assessments that can be used during class time [9]. Another example of fundamental skills teaching guidance is Kamla and Freeman's activities and guidance for early childhood physical education teachers and programmers, published in the USA [10]. The work of Kamla and Freeman specifically supports Standard 1 of the National Association for Sport and Physical Education (NASPE) National Standards for Physical Education, which is that "the physically literate individual demonstrates competency in a variety of motor skills and movement patterns" [11]. Beurden et al. conducted a quasi-experimental evaluation of the "Move It Groove It" primary school intervention in New South Wales, Australia, which confirmed the effectiveness of including fundamental skill development in a school setting. They noted improvements in all tested skills ranging from 7.2% to 25.7% [12]. These examples comprise a pool of both research and pilot programs indicating that when the awareness of fundamental movement skills is incorporated in physical education and activity programs, there is significant improvement in children's skill development [8–10, 12].

Fundamental Movement Skills

Fundamental movement skills are "basic observable patterns of behaviour present from childhood to adulthood" [13]. The Victoria Fundamental Motor Skills Manual for Teachers, practiced in Australia, lists 11 specific skills considered to be fundamental: the ability to catch, kick, run, vertical jump, overhand throw, ball bounce, leap, dodge, punt, forehand strike, and two-hand sidearm strike [14]. Similarly,

Canadian Sport for Life identified 12 skills as essential: dodge, hop, skip, log roll, stork stand, jump, kick, dribble, overarm throw, catch, run, and sidearm strike [15]. These specific skills, while varied depending on the country or region, share significant consistencies. Firstly, they are expected to be mastered before the age of 9 years (see Fig. 22.1). Each skill has a critical window of development where it is best learned. Missing a critical window of development results in permanent difficulty and limits future abilities even with intense training [16]. Secondly, all the skills are sports-based and generally measured by simple metrics of relative success or failure, generally categorized as emerging, developing, or established competence [5, 9]. Lastly, the skills and skill development discussed in these works all reference typically abled bodies, and do not account for the full range of physical capabilities, such as including children with disabilities.

Fundamental Movement Skills are understood as building blocks for producing efficient movement. Without them, it is not possible to proceed to the next step of more complicated movement or activities [10, 13]. Therefore, it is crucial to teach these fundamental movement skills at an early age. If a child cannot walk, they will not be able to move to the next step of running or playing conventional sports. In sports fundamentals, if a child cannot catch or throw a ball, they will be unable to play any sport activity that involves those skills. In our Footprints dance classes, we often notice the younger participants demonstrating an easier time mastering the movement skills as compared to the teenaged participants. This supports the theory

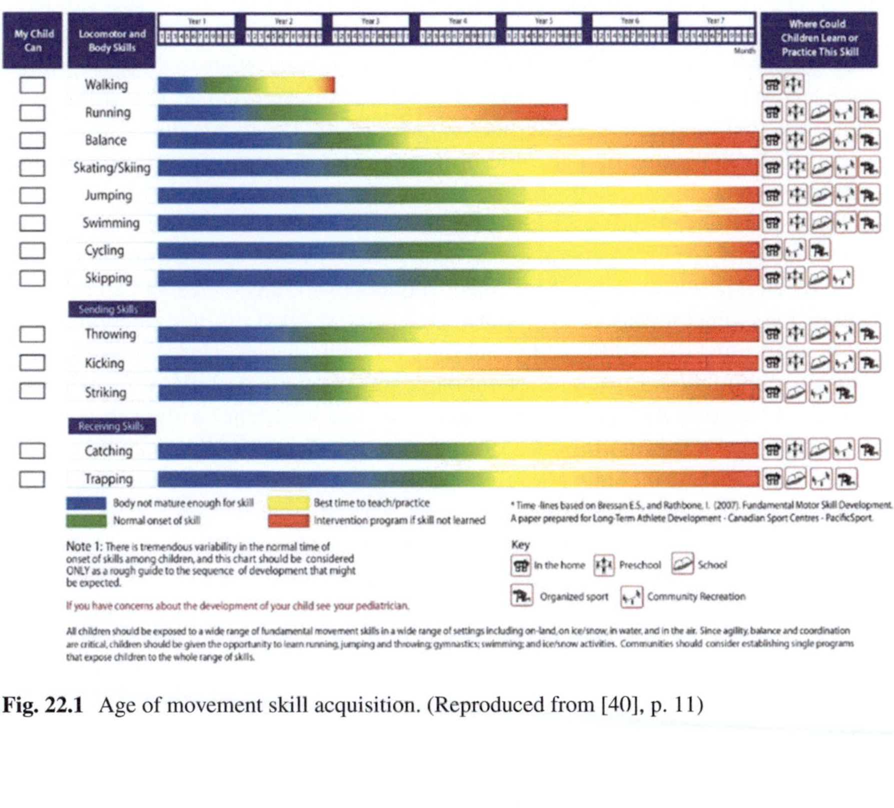

Fig. 22.1 Age of movement skill acquisition. (Reproduced from [40], p. 11)

of early developmental windows, and highlights both the critical issue of addressing skill development at a young age, and the difficulty of correcting issues at an older age. Therefore, for practitioners treating injuries in adults resulting from problems in these developmental skills, it is important to note that fixing the underlying issue will require substantial time and effort. For practitioners treating the same issues in young children, directing them to appropriate activities will be essential. For dancers, this may require involving the dance instructor in the treatment plan.

Using Dance for Teaching Fundamental Movement Skills

While lack of physical skills is an established issue, there is no consensus on how best to address it. Dance may be an ideal context in which to address these fundamental physical skills. Chatzihidiroglou, Chatzopoulos, Lykesas, and Doganis demonstrated that dance improves sensorimotor synchronization and balance in pre-schoolers and recommended dance be included in standard physical education for young children [17]. Additionally, dance can be a convenient place to teach fundamental movement skills because, unlike sports, it does not have limitations regarding activity boundary—such as a narrow (although challenging) goal of moving a ball from one place to another. The dance goal of artistic expression may provide more expansive opportunities to explore fundamental movement skills. Even highly structured genres, such as traditional ballet or highland dance, still have some flexibility and areas where instructors can creatively adapt and incorporate novel concepts. For example, while a soccer coach may wish to improve spinal awareness with their player to support healthy back development, it is difficult to incorporate that fundamental skill into the game itself. The coach may use a warm-up or cool-down routine or a specific drill; however, that requires time allotments away from game time. Contrastingly, a dance instructor could simply decide to highlight spinal awareness as a key element of a choreographed dance routine or add it as an activity in the general dance class, thereby never taking time away from the designated activity, dance. Movement sequences in dance classes can often be manipulated to encompass all the fundamental movement skills, and finely focus on specific skill sets [18]. Additionally, not only do many dance classes offer the flexibility to accommodate teaching of fundamental movement skills, it is generally understood that it is desirable for instructors to equip students with high levels of physical movement skills. Because of the movement proficiency goals that dance educators often have, including developing body awareness and addressing foundational skills in their students, dance educators may be a particularly receptive audience for adding the teaching of these skills to their practice [19].

Another reason we believe dance is an optimal tool for teaching fundamental movement skills is that dance can be easily adapted to different individual needs and interests [18]. Even something as simple as line dancing in the Dance for Health program—a community-based participatory research initiative evaluated by Schroeder et al. from 2012 to 2016—was effective and enjoyed by participants aged 2–79 years [20]. The choice of music, cultural elements, theme, and presentation are key factors to making a dance program successful across multiple interests and demographics [18], and can entice even reluctant participants (see Case Example 1). A well-trained dance instructor will be able to tailor these choices for their participants and their audience; a teaching practice that is highlighted in the FMT. Due to the capacity for versatility, dance programs have been successfully used as therapeutic tools in diverse environments such as prisons [21, 22], nursing homes [23] and youth programs [6] across the globe. Additionally, over the past four decades, dance programs and companies have increasingly included individuals with disabilities. Examples include MOMO Movement (formerly MOMO Mixed Ability Dance Theatre) in Calgary, Alberta, Canada [24]; AXIS Dance Company in Oakland, California, USA [25]; REVolutions Dance Inc. in Tampa, Florida USA [26, 27]; and the international breakdance crew ILL-ABILITIES™ [28], based in Montreal, Canada.

In the interest of versatility, FDP incorporates multiple dance genres in their programs. The range of dance forms includes hip hop, ballet, jazz, tap, contemporary, African and Latin dance. The variety of genres not only broadens artistic exposure, but it provides a larger range in which to capture each student's passion and develop their full abilities. While hip hop may be a popular choice in modern North America, as seen in Case Example 1, under the right conditions even often stigmatized genres, such as ballet, can be appealing. The diversity of genres and variety in approaches supports the notion that dance can be a highly accessible tool for teaching fundamental movement skills and addressing the prevailing issue of poor motor development and its co-occurring negative social and cognitive repercussions.

Case Example 1

'Abdul' arrived at a community demonstration for dance program highly skeptical of his peers participating in ballet. He and his friends had mocked and teased them after learning from the neighborhood girls that the boys were involved in ballet. The participants became self-conscious and considered leaving the dance program. On the day of the demonstration, Abdul and his friends watched with the expectation that they would ridicule the performers. However, when he saw the grace strength and physical agility, he became silent. At one point, a performer leapt and performed a split jump high in the air and Abdul recognized how the skill could transfer to his own athletic sports endeavors. Instead of mocking the performers, he quietly watched and later confessed he was impressed by the physical and mental determination of his peers. The next time the community program ran, he immersed himself in it and today he champions dance. Today, as a youth leader he encourages others to get involved and support each other to build strength and cooperation in the community.

Many of the issues within our society come from our biases and lack of understanding and perspective. Dance provides the opportunity for building understanding and perspective. Helping us bridge the gap between us and them.

Andrea Pass, Artistic Director of Footprints Dance Project, Calgary, Canada.

Practical Issues in the School and Community Setting

Previous explorations of the effectiveness of dance interventions have focused on well-trained instructors delivering semi-structured dance programs. However, professionally trained dance instructors are not always available in a school or community setting. An ideal scenario would involve dance teachers who are not only well trained in their genre(s) and dance pedagogy, but who also possess an in-depth knowledge of anatomy, biomechanics, and human development [29]. This is an unrealistic expectation in actual practice [30]. While a holistic program with a well-trained and experienced dance instructor is ideal, even someone with a minimal dance background can successfully create a *very basic* dance program if given the right resources. It is this latter group, in particular, which is the focus of the FMT. Education and local government systems increasingly ask untrained or inexperienced individuals to provide dance programs as part of their daily work. For example, "dance" is a required component of the provincial curriculum for physical education in Alberta, Canada, for kindergarten through grade 12 [31]. Some schools may hire a dance consultant to deliver this section of program, some may have a physical education specialist, and many expect the general classroom teacher to provide it. Therefore, in developing the FMT, we wanted to be sure that it could be useful for a variety of levels of teachers, from inexperienced dance teachers to experienced practitioners looking for intervention-style tools.

Dance Fundamental Movement Skills (DFMS)

While the aforementioned sports fundamental movement skills are tied to success in athletics [13], in Footprints Dance Project, we noticed that the proficiency in the standard sport fundamental movement skills was not necessarily an indicator of success in dance. In day camps at the City of Calgary recreation, where several of the Footprints staff also worked, children had access to playground equipment during breaks and could demonstrate proficiencies with ball play, skipping, and running. However, instructors commented that children who excelled at these traditional sports activities could still struggle with dancing, or vice versa. It was clear that these published skill sets were not good indicators of general physical competency in a dance class.

The fundamental movement concepts frequently applied in dance, originate from the Bartenieff Fundamentals (BF) and the Laban Movement Analysis (LMA) framework. These differ from the basic human motor skills and sports-oriented development concepts discussed previously [32, 33]. While these movements have been established as useful in the dance education community, there is a lack of scientific evidence demonstrating any relationship of the LMA/BF concepts to a dancer's successful progress or injury prevention. These concepts are particularly common in the contemporary dance genre.

Other genres of dance, such as Highland or Ballet, have foundational movements such as specific named positions of the arms and feet, as well as an established pattern of pedagogy in which certain movements are learned before others [34]. In Highland, that could be learning shedding before a crossover, and in ballet, learning a plié before a pirouette. In ballet, basic movements and dance concepts were historically established in a manual by E.A Théleur in 1831. For instance, Théleur established seven basic movements of dancing, which are: plier—to bend; etendre—to stretch; relever—to rise; glisser—to slide; sauter—to jump; elancer—to dart; and tourner—to turn [35]. These are all essential skills for a dancer; however, we believe that, like the sports fundamentals, they can be broken down into further components. Some of these components are discussed in the BF and LMA frameworks.

Laban Movement theory focuses on the concepts of Effort, Space, Shape, and Body,[1] and how they can be applied by performing artists to enhance their work. The Body principle of Laban Movement, which focuses on connectedness and physical organization, formed the cornerstone of Bartenieff Fundamentals. Bartenieff, a physical therapist, described movement patterns based on neurological development. For example, the neurological development of contralateral movement (as seen in crawling or walking) formed the theoretical basis for cross- lateral connections. "When using Cross-Laterality we can come to clear connection from fingertips of one hand through the core and to toes of the opposite foot. Such a clear connection may be seen in a beautiful soaring leap of ballet's *grand jeté* [32]. Bartenieff Fundamentals also address breath, core–distal connectivity, head–tail connectivity, upper–lower connectivity, body-half connectivity, and integration. Each component relates to a neurological developmental stage, such as when first learning to stand, and is subsequently extended to the practice of dance [32].

In the development of our tool, we drew from these fundamental movement concepts because they are applied frequently in dance education. There are parallel relationships between many of our skill parameters identified in the FMT and the BF/LMA framework. For instance, in DFMS and DFMS-A, we discuss the release and absorption of force, extension and retraction of the limbs, general flow, spinal awareness, and balance and weight transfer. The use of force is expressed in the BF/LMA framework as a combination of Weight and Time factors. Extension and retraction of the limbs is based on the BF concept of core–distal body connectivity, which is not only essential for aesthetics of the desired movements, but also for injury prevention. Flow is one of Laban's four primary Effort components of human movement, and it relates to how one approaches the regulation of control in the body [33]. When we analyze general flow in the DFMS-A, we directly examine this idea. Spinal awareness discussed in the FMT mirrors the BF premise of head–tail connectivity, and the different balance and weight transfer categories reflect use of Weight Factor in the LMA framework. Our goal was to simplify the concepts as much as possible for ease of implementation by teachers, while bridging the gap between dance and medical terminology.

[1] The terms "Effort," "Space," "Shape," and "Body" are specific terms used in LMA and are thus capitalized.

Breaking Down Fundamental Movement

We intended to address the gap between dance and sports movement fundamentals by developing a dance-specific framework for basic skill development: the *Dance Fundamental Movement Skills (DFMS)*. Figure 22.2 (and Appendix 1) shows the

General

- **Confidence:** Is the participant approaching the activity with confidence or trepidation?
- **Motivation:** Is the participant demonstrating motivation to do their best, or are they simply marking places until the activity is over?
- **Comprehension:** Does the participant understand the direction and follow along with the video?
- **Awareness:** Is the participant aware of their body in space? Example, in a growth spurt this score will drop.
- **Fitness:** Subjective measure in place to allow for reasonable doubt if lack of fitness affects ability to perform.

Balance:

- **Simple Balance (static) one foot:** Static balance while on one foot only
- **Simple Balance (dynamic) two feet:** Dynamic balance with both feet, for example walking.
- **Complex Balance (static) combination:** Static balance while holding a complex pose, such as breakdance freeze.
- **Complex balance, dynamic:** Dynamic balance during more complex movements, such as a grapevine.

Weight Transfer

- **Front/Back weight transfer:** Shifting weight along the sagittal plane.
- **Side to Side weight transfer:** Shifting weight along the coronal plane
- **General weight transfer:** Shifting weight throughout the dance routine, in all directions.

Transitions

- **Directional transition:** Diadochokinesis.
- **Speed transition:** Rapidly changing pace or tempo.
- **Quality of movement transition**: Rapidly changing movement quality, for example from smooth to jarring.

Spine

- **Posture-Tall:** Example, Ballet posture
- **Posture – Relaxed:** Example, Latin dance posture
- **Posture – Slumped:** Slouching, kyphosis.
- **Spinal movement** –The ability to move the spine at full range of motion and transition between postures.

Alignment

- **Knee/Toe alignment (ankle)**
- **Hip/Knee/Toe alignment (knee)**
- **Back/Knee/Hip alignment (hip)**
- **Whole lower limb alignment**
- **Upper body alignment**
- **Rotation of leg:** the ability to rotate the lower limb while maintaining perfect alignment, without joint strain.

Quality of movement

- **Arms, extension/retraction:** Bartenieff fundamentals, patterning of upper limb [10]
- **Legs, extension/retraction:** Bartenieff fundamentals, patterning of lower limb [10]
- **General flow:** Laban concept of continuous movement, without un-choreographed starts and stops [10].

Jumping

- **Preparation, 2 leg movement of elevation**: Effectively gathering force for release into the jump from a position with both feet on the floor.
- **Preparation, 1 leg movement of elevation**: Effectively gathering force for release into the jump from a position with only one foot on the floor.
- **Landing, 2 leg movement of elevation:** Even distribution of force and correct alignment during landing with both feet landing on the ground simultaneously.
- **Landing, 1 leg movement of elevation**: Even distribution of force and correct alignment during landing on one foot only.
- **Release and absorption of force in movement of elevation (quality of movement)**: Even distribution of force during both takeoff and landing (soft versus hard landing), with jumps that look fluid and seamless from start to finish.

Fig. 22.2 DFMS: dance fundamental movement skills

breakdown of the dance skills into basic elements. As noted earlier, these movement skills are informed by Laban Movement Analysis and Bartenieff Fundamentals, but they are comparable to traditional sports movement concepts in simplicity and interpretation. In developing the DFMS, we merged the abstract and complex dance theories with the simple and objective athletic skill sets, and created a set of "dance fundamental movement skills" that is meant to be accessible, simple, and applicable in many educational environments. We sought to bring specialized dance knowledge into the realm of broader practical applications across a spectrum of dance practice, providing an accessible tool for nonspecialists and specialists alike.

We noticed that the specific activities in sports fundamentals could be further broken down into yet more basic components of movement. For example, "running" can encompass balance skills, transitional skills, weight transfer, and whole-body alignment. If any one of these components is missing, the efficient and safe execution of the movement may suffer. For example, observing extra noise produced while running such as slamming feet or "heavy feet" indicates a suboptimal biomechanical state. Noisy running feet indicate a lack of muscle control and improper weight distribution through the feet [2]. The slamming sound tells the observer that too much force is being sent through the feet and tibiae to the knees in a shock pattern instead of being distributed more diffusely through the soft tissues. From a dance aesthetic perspective, students are expected to be able to float noiselessly across the floor; however, their inability to do so could have more serious biomechanical implications. If not addressed, this habit can translate into excessive strain on the joints leading to potential injury, including the possibility of stress fractures [2, 33]. We therefore deduced that "running" should be further broken down into more basic elements—in this case the skill at issue is the proper weight transition and distribution through the feet. In our classes, after teaching students to experiment with rolling weight through their feet and practicing various silent movement and transition activities for several weeks, the audible slamming reduced significantly.

Another example of the need to subdivide traditional sports movement fundamentals into smaller skill sets is demonstrated by a youth in a Footprints summer program. This student struggled to jump due to poor knee/toe alignment (varus knees), which made it both difficult and uncomfortable to attempt that motion. While "jumping" is a sports fundamental skill (and one of Théleur's basic movements for ballet), we again argue that this is too advanced, as it cannot be accomplished well without more basic skills, such as good body alignment. In this case, the physical challenge resulted in behavioral issues as the student tended to stop participating in dance activities whenever jumping was a featured component. The dance instructional team, being aware of the anatomical reason behind the struggle, modified the routines to allow successful and comfortable participation. For example, the expansive and explosive aesthetic of a leap can be accomplished using only the upper body. Combining both types of different jumping movements with some students using the upper body and some students using the lower body in a piece of choreography can visually enhance the piece. Choreography was altered so this student could avoid jumping while still contributing aesthetically to the piece and participating with the whole group. Consequently, the student's willingness and happiness to participate in the program increased and behavioral issues lessened.

In a subsequent case, the team went further to help the student address the underlying cause of the knee condition (collapsing foot arches), including helping the student pick out insoles and providing strengthening and stretching techniques particular to their condition. The team readily acknowledge that these latter interventions required specialized knowledge and may not be appropriate in all situations, but all that was required for the youth to happily participate was an awareness of the challenges and willingness to modify and personalize instruction. This situation illustrates one of the major goals of the FMT: to increase awareness for students and instructors, while providing simple activities that can help, if not correct, the underlying issues. It also raised the issue of the high level of corporeal expectation required of dancers. Neither of the participants with varus knees had been assessed as having a medical anomaly. According to the medical doctors who assessed both of these individuals, both were capable of participating fully in athletic pursuits, and no medical interventions were prescribed. From a dance perspective, despite this history, both faced clear barriers to fully participating in dance. This reinforces an essential consideration for practitioners: When a high level of performance is expected, the body and fundamental skills must be operating at that same high level, which may be beyond what is considered normal in everyday activities [36].

Method

Development Phase

Dance Fundamental Movement Skills were first explored by FDP in 2015 with four after-school classes in two locations in Calgary with a total of 34 children with no severe physical disabilities. There were two age-group classes in each location: a younger age group 5–7 years and older age class 8–13 years. These after-school classes spanned the academic year and formed the participant base from whom the DFMS was developed. The same dance skills were then taught and refined with an older-age group during a summer camp program in 2016 with 33 students, aged 8–16 years. Thus, the development phase occurred over a full year's time. Both males and females participate in FDP; however, the majority of participants are female. FDP does not collect additional demographic information. During the weekly, hour-long classes, in addition to learning choreography and a variety of dance styles, children explored physical movement skills using a mix of exercises and activities. The same instructors taught throughout the year, and thus each class had a consistent format with warm-up and cool-down included. The styles and routines taught varied throughout the year, as one of the missions of FDP includes a wide exposure to various genres. This was incidentally helpful to the investigators, as they could observe a variety of movement patterns and determine fundamental skills covering a broad range of dance genres, as opposed to what may have been missed in a single genre. For example, spinal mobility in African Dance is very different from Ballet; however, after observing both (and more) investigators could see the importance of not only the mobility of the spine required to dance, but also the awareness of how to move the spine appropriately in any given situation.

A year-long investigation and development process began in the fall of 2015, with a team comprised of two primary investigators working with five Footprints Dance Project instructors. One of the investigators was an anatomy consultant and the other, an artistic director. The Project instructors and investigators were all veteran dance teachers crossing a variety of genres, including Highland, Ballet, Contemporary, Hip Hop, and African dance. The project goal was not research-oriented. Funding was provided for program development and evaluation, not human-subjects research. At no point during development did such research occur.

While compiling background information for the FMT, the investigators noted the lack of existing data relevant to their observations. As such, to ensure the guide was both accurate and effective, they compiled their observations and expertise through a lengthy development process. The fall semester classes were observed to determine the specific skills to include in the guide, while the remainder of the school year was spent developing relevant exercises and fine-tuning which skills and activities to include in the guide. Segments of every dance class were video recorded by the instructors and sent to the investigative team for review. Instructors would film activities provided by the investigators, as well as their own choreographed routines in each class. In addition, observations from several in-person class audits throughout the year were considered in the analysis.

The investigators viewed the class videos independently and noted any observations. They then met in person each week and discussed their observations, drawing on their background knowledge as former dancers and informed by the work of authors such as Anne Gilbert and Shirley Murray [37, 38]. They focused on Laban Movement Analysis as well as the basic biomechanics of dance movement to determine strengths and weaknesses in the class and identify key areas of development. A key skill was defined as something essential for success in all, or most, dance activities regardless of genre. When missing, these skills significantly affected the dancer's ability to participate and succeed. These key skills became the Dance Fundamental Movement Skills (DFMS) referred to in the guide [2]. A total of 33 skills were identified for inclusion in the guide. Some broad categories were broken down into more specific skills. For instance, in the category of "balance," to reflect static versus dynamic balance and allow for differences between a single or double leg stance, four skills were identified: simple balance on one leg, simple balance on two legs, complex balance on one leg, and complex balance on two legs.

Another category identified was "transitions," as we observed the fundamental importance of being able to change direction, tempo, and the quality of movement. Agility for changing direction is valued in sports such as soccer, and our team remembered doing change of direction drills in school. In many of the routines, when it seemed like students struggled to follow along or keep up, through repeatedly watching the videos and different segments featuring directional changes it became clear that the biggest issue was in fact the students' physical ability to quickly and smoothly change direction. We also observed this during changes in tempo and quality of movement; such as transitioning from a robotic or jerky segment into something smooth and flowing. A similar issue was noticed with weight transfer through the body, as problems with the distribution of weight during movement caused additional effort requirements and poor biomechanics. This could be seen with the noisy running mentioned earlier and resulted in difficulty producing smooth movements.

Another important skill identified by the team members in the development phase of the project was motivation and confidence. Canada Sport for Life lists motivation and confidence as essential indicators of success [5, 15], and this concept is also reflected in the dance literature [39]. Dance teachers noted that children who were confident and motivated were eager to try new skills regardless of their initial level of competence. A child who was confident in themselves, motivated, and accustomed to being celebrated for their effort was more likely to try something repeatedly, whereas students missing any of those skills would either try once and quit after failing, or even refuse to try at all. Therefore, developing confidence and motivation were deemed equally important skills to physical movement skills.

During the video and in-class observations, the Footprints team noticed that students who were lacking or performed poorly in specific skills identified as fundamental, would subsequently struggle in movement sequences that relied on those skills. For example, with poor lower body alignment, any high impact or strength-based activity such as a *jeté*, would be compromised. Basic balance issues meant any pose, such as an arabesque, was more challenging. Difficulty with any transitional skill, such as moving from an extended or open position to a closed position, led to problems in managing tempo or directional changes. Teachers realized that the students were not “bad” at dance; rather, they were missing some essential skills that were necessary to perform the desired movements.

The Footprints Dance Project Movement Tool (FMT), A Free Open-Access iCourse

Once a skill was identified as fundamental, exercises and activities were developed by the dance anatomy consultant to combine dance activities with physiotherapy exercises and incorporate the targeted basic skill development into games and dance routines. This was an iterative process, as each class exposed something different to the investigative team, and while some skills were clearly fundamental from the onset, such as balance, some took longer to isolate, such as directional transitions. Recall that a fundamental skill is something without which a dancer struggles with even basic movements and cannot progress, not a specific movement, such as a plié. Specific movements become easier to master once fundamental skills have improved, which can be done with simple exercises and activities. Examples include such activities as one-legged freeze dance for static balance (called simple, single leg balance in the guide) or storytelling that incorporates slow knee bends to work on lower limb alignment.

Feedback from instructors, participants, and the investigative team determined if an activity was effective and well received. Feedback was collected via an ongoing discussion between team members both in person and through written notes and observations shared after each class. The instructors would provide their video and notes; the investigators would review them, ask for clarifications, and then meet to determine the next step. This next step would then be given to the instructors in time for them to plan the next class. Participants communicated both directly with their instructors during and after each class, and with one of the primary investigators after in-class observations and after the program conclusion.

Once team members agreed upon the efficacy of the dance exercises that were created to target all 33 fundamental skills, all of these dance activities were compiled into a teaching guide called the *Footprints Dance Project - Movement Tool (FMT)*. The guide was made available through an open-access iCourse to provide a teaching resource for those working with children in dance. The guide explains the concept of fundamental movement skills and is organized into categories. Each category is described with simple games and dance exercises for developing specific dance movement skills. The guide can be used as part of a dance program, either in studios or in schools, and can also be easily incorporated within a warm-up or cooldown for sports teams [2].

Many of the key concepts in the Dance Fundamental Movement Skills (DFMS) are standard movement properties with associated technical terms. We simplified some of these terms in the Footprints guide to make it accessible to many users. For example, *diadochokinesis* is described in the transition category as "directional transitions" and is explained as the ability to change direction, either up/down, front/back, or side/side. This renaming was a decision taken by the investigative team to make the guide less intimidating for a wider audience.

Preliminary Observations of the FMT Program Outcomes

After the FMT skill-specific exercises were implemented in the Footprints school-year classes, dance instructors and investigation team observers independently noted varying degrees of improvements in DFMS in all participants. Dance teachers reflected on their personal observations and written notes through the year, while the investigation team used the video footage to establish pre- and post-comparisons. Weight transfer, posture and spinal awareness, and transition skills were most notably improved for all 34 participants, with individual differences across categories. Overall, improvements in the younger age group (5–7 years) were most clearly discerned; their skill progress surpassed that of the older dancers by the end of the year. This observation was noted for further study, as it may reflect dance-specific developmental windows, such as the sport-specific windows seen in Lloyd and Oliver and Canadian Sport for Life [16, 40]. A qualitative report was compiled for funding oversight; however, the investigators realized a quantitative assessment would be best able to document program effectiveness and explore skill development in the future.

Quantitative Assessment Tool (DFMS-A)

The current methods of physical skill assessment are generally time consuming and often require specialized equipment, such as a pressure sensing mat for determining weight distribution. At the time of the DFMS development, no comprehensive skill assessments were available that fit the needs of the program. Thus, the Dance Fundamental Movement Skills Assessment (DFMS-A) was created using only equipment already in use: two cameras and a projector that connected to a laptop computer. DFMS-A was devised to provide a framework to analyze the relevant movement skills. The purpose of the DFMS-A is to provide a method of assessment that can assess an entire class in an hour, is diverse enough to analyze each of the 33 identified skills including confidence and fitness, can accommodate a large variation of ages and skill levels, and is still fun enough to engage the various age groups. It also needed to be standardized to reduce bias and variability. We decided that a dance routine would be the best way to observe all the skills in use, and that using video recordings both to administer and evaluate would allow for standardization and efficiency.

Versatility One of the criteria that we deemed necessary in the creation of the DFMS-A was that it needed to be versatile in application. The goal was to create one standard type of evaluation for all participants, effectively targeting each of the skill categories while accommodating both the lowest and highest level of performer. Therefore, we selected movements that allowed for individuals to adjust the level of difficulty. For example, within a side kick, a participant could raise or lower the leg, to increase or decrease the difficulty level, respectively. Or, in an "airplane" balance where the participant stands on 1 foot leaning forward with one leg raised in the air behind them and arms stretched to the sides like an airplane (Dekasana yoga pose), a participant could adjust the degree of leaning to match their skill level. In the complex balance poses, which include a side plank, a participant could keep things simple with both feet and hands on the ground or could elevate the pose to 1 foot and arm in the air.

Standardized delivery The setup for the DFMS-A involves a projector for teaching the movements, and a filming area with 2–3 cameras set up for assessment. The DFMS-A is a pre-recorded follow-along style video. This enables the entire class to learn the routine at the same time when the instructor plays the video. Participants watch a segment, try out the movement, and move on to the next segment. Pauses are built into the video. After learning each segment, the video then puts the whole routine together and participants can practice once through with music before the final assessment.

The final assessment segment of the video has the participants follow along doing the routine they just learned while being filmed. With one participant, two cameras are used, one anterior and one lateral view. With two participants, three cameras are used so each participant has a recorded lateral view. Including time for explanations, organization, and practice, the initial teaching takes less than 20 min, with the filming area using <5 min blocks accommodating two students each. Thus, a minimum of 16 students can comfortably be assessed in a 1 h class. With adequate space and staging, we believe the assessment can be run with up to three students at a time, increasing the 1 h capacity to 24.

Evaluation The recordings are analyzed outside of class time by a trained evaluator. Currently, there is only one evaluator; however, FDP would like to expand this in the future. Using a descriptive rubric, scores are assigned for each of the skills (Table 22.1). Scores are associated to three categories: "Fully Competent,"

Table 22.1 DFMS-A: dance fundamental movement skills sssessment

DFMS Assessment chart		Participant #:__________	Date:__________
Skill	**Developing**	**Intermediate**	**Full competence**
Confidence	1. 2. 3.	4. 5. 6.	7. 8. 9.
Motivation	1. 2. 3.	4. 5. 6.	7. 8. 9.
Comprehension	1. 2. 3.	4. 5. 6.	7. 8. 9.
Awareness	1. 2. 3.	4. 5. 6.	7. 8. 9.
Simple balance (static) 1 foot	1. 2. 3.	4. 5. 6.	7. 8. 9.
Simple balance (dynamic) 2 feet	1. 2. 3.	4. 5. 6.	7. 8. 9.
Complex balance (static) combination	1. 2. 3.	4. 5. 6.	7. 8. 9.
Complex balance, dynamic	1. 2. 3.	4. 5. 6.	7. 8. 9.
Front/Back weight transfer	1. 2. 3.	4. 5. 6.	7. 8. 9.
Side-to-side weight transfer	1. 2. 3.	4. 5. 6.	7. 8. 9.
General weight transfer	1. 2. 3.	4. 5. 6.	7. 8. 9.
Directional transition	1. 2. 3.	4. 5. 6.	7. 8. 9.
Speed transition	1. 2. 3.	4. 5. 6.	7. 8. 9.
Quality of movement transition	1. 2. 3.	4. 5. 6.	7. 8. 9.
Posture – tall	1. 2. 3.	4. 5. 6.	7. 8. 9.
Posture – relaxed	1. 2. 3.	4. 5. 6.	7. 8. 9.
Posture – slumped	1. 2. 3.	4. 5. 6.	7. 8. 9.
Spinal movement	1. 2. 3.	4. 5. 6.	7. 8. 9.
Knee/toe alignment (ankle)	1. 2. 3.	4. 5. 6.	7. 8. 9.
Hip/knee/toe alignment (knee)	1. 2. 3.	4. 5. 6.	7. 8. 9.
Back/hip/knee alignment (hip)	1. 2. 3.	4. 5. 6.	7. 8. 9.
Whole lower limb alignment	1. 2. 3.	4. 5. 6.	7. 8. 9.
Upper body alignment	1. 2. 3.	4. 5. 6.	7. 8. 9.
Arms extension/retraction	1. 2. 3.	4. 5. 6.	7. 8. 9.
Legs extension/retraction	1. 2. 3.	4. 5. 6.	7. 8. 9.

(continued)

Table 22.1 (continued)

Preparation 2 leg movement of elevation	1.	2.	3.	4.	5.	6.	7.	8.	9.
Preparation 1 leg movement of elevation	1.	2.	3.	4.	5.	6.	7.	8.	9.
Landing 2 leg movement of elevation	1.	2.	3.	4.	5.	6.	7.	8.	9.
Landing 1 leg movement of elevation	1.	2.	3.	4.	5.	6.	7.	8.	9.
Release & absorption of force in movement of elevation	1.	2.	3.	4.	5.	6.	7.	8.	9.
Rotation of leg	1.	2.	3.	4.	5.	6.	7.	8.	9.
General flow	1.	2.	3.	4.	5.	6.	7.	8.	9.
Fitness	2			5			8		
Accuracy of test	2			5			8		
Total									
				Scored by ____________________					

DFMS scoring key
DFSM assessment rubric
Developing competence
1. Never present/correct
2. Occasionally present/correct, 15% of the time
3. Occasionally present/correct, 25% of the time
Intermediate competence
4. Occasionally present/correct, 35% of the time
5. Present/correct half of the time 50%
6. Present/correct more than half of the time 60%
Fully competent
7. Present/correct more than half of the time 75%
8. Present/correct more than half of the time 90%
9. Present/correct all of the time 100%

"Intermediate Competence," or "Developing Competence." Scores in the range of "Developing Competence" should be the first areas of focus for instructors; however, in higher levels of performance where a score of 9 is optimal, even scores within the range of "Fully Competent" may need to be improved. Note that a score of 9 will be very rare, as it represents absolute perfection in that skill area. For example, the moment in the Chinese Acrobatic Ballet when the ballerina performs an arabesque on pointe, on 1 foot, on the head of her partner would represent a 9 in balance [41]. We expect the majority of participants to score in the "Intermediate Competence" range.

The scoring system is primarily related to the rate of consistency in a participant's performance during which they produce the correct movement. For instance, in the "Developing Competence" area, a score of 1 means that the skill is never present/correct, a score of 2 means that the skill is occasionally present/correct, approximately 15% of the time, and a score of 3 means that it is occasionally present/correct approximately 25% of the time. We hypothesize that an average healthy individual would score a 5, meaning the movement skill was both present and correct half of the time. Some readers may find this score low; however, the movements chosen for DFMS-A are designed to expose areas of weakness. Additionally, as in the acrobatic example above, the gold standard is extremely high. Most people can stand on one leg, but how many can fluidly adopt a single leg stance without any hesitation or wobbles while maintaining perfect alignment?

Considerations The participants are not made aware of the purpose of the video. They are told only that the purpose of the filming is to look at "how their bodies move." They are also instructed to "do their best and have fun." They are not told specifics about the movements (such as "keep your feet parallel"), only what the movements are, with a demonstration. For instance, the video will instruct them to do a knee bend but will not tell them to keep their knees over their toes. The purpose of providing practice time to do the movement sequence is not to help them succeed with individual movements, but to alleviate the negative impact of not understanding what they are supposed to do. The entire approach of the video has the unique benefit of negating the "white coat effect," whereby participants focus on the specific task because they know they are being assessed, thus skewing the authenticity of the results.

Another consideration to ensure that performance is reflective of daily practice and capabilities is the appropriate selection of filming groups. We recommend filming be performed with groups of 2–3, and it is the responsibility of the instructor to select the pairings with regard to group dynamics. Some children will feel too self-conscious alone in front of the cameras but will be more at ease with a friend. A more disruptive child could escalate negative behaviors or adopt a positive focus, depending upon the choice of partners. These are important considerations to assure reliability and validity of scoring. Children may score artificially lower on the skills due to these environmental factors. To account for this factor, the DFMS assessment has a final category based on the discretion of the examiner and instructor: Is this an accurate representation of the child's abilities?

The DFMS-A is not designed to be a medical assessment and is not a pass/fail metric. Its purpose is only to reflect areas of growth and development, and help the instructor monitor progress and design more effective classes. The DFMS-A is currently undergoing several stages of validation, and the results of the preliminary IRB-approved study have been submitted for publication in a peer-reviewed journal. The preliminary study compared the DFMS-A with three standard physical assessments of balance: Y balance test, Single Leg Stance (SLS) test, and Functional reach test. Pearson Correlations demonstrated significant correlations between the DFMS-A and Y balance and SLS tests, respectively ($r = 0.745$–0.974; $p < 0.008$), with minimal correlation found with the Functional Reach test. Intra-rater reliability was tested 1.5 years after the original assessment was completed, and demonstrated high reliability (>85%) [42, 43]. This result suggests the DFMS-A balance test could be applied in the medical field as a comprehensive balance assessment despite its original development as only a teaching aid and program evaluation tool.

Discussion

General Context

Studies show that there is positive correlation between established fundamental skill development in sports and success in athletics [13, 15]. In the dance realm, proficiency in basic movement concepts, such as effective weight transfer, reduces injury and permits dancers to excel in increasingly challenging movement patterns [33]. However, the importance of these skills extends well beyond physical performance. Fundamental movement skills and motor skills in general are linked to positive social and behavioral development [13, 44], improved cognitive development [45–47], and increased academic success [47–49]. Physical activity is essential for mental health and cognitive development in children, yet the majority of Children in North America fail to reach basic physical milestones and consistently lag in fundamental movement skills development. The gap between expected and actual ability has been increasing through the years, demonstrating the gradual worsening of skill development in children [50]. This issue is expected to negatively affect children's future ability to participate in athletic endeavors and ultimately result in poor physical and mental health outcomes overall.

Thus, the repercussions of systemic failure to teach these skills at an early age can result in serious consequences. Practitioners should be aware of these potential outcomes when working with young populations, and understand how participation in physical activities impacts much more than physical health. For examples of how dance can impact social and psychological well-being of youth, see "Beyond the Physical" inset, and Case Examples 2 and 3. These case examples, and numerous scientific studies, demonstrate how dance can be an effective therapeutic tool, even in dealing with significant social and personal trauma [50–53]. However, without established fundamental movement skills or teachers who can accommodate different abilities, this tool could be inaccessible to those who need it most.

Case Example 2

Being short in stature, 'Tory' was bullied from an early age. Ostracized in class by her peers, she found refuge in soccer where she physically excelled and was well accepted by her team mates. Her success in soccer increased her social isolation within the classroom. When Tory joined the community dance program she was connected with a group of like-minded individuals all from different ethnic backgrounds and all of different shapes and sizes. Most diverse, though, was the range of skills and aptitudes. Her new network was noncritical of her size, which afforded her the opportunity to consistently be placed front and central. She radiated enthusiasm and rallied the others to excel to the benefit of the ensemble. The noncompetitive nature of dance allows students to challenge one another without a winner or loser and without a right and wrong answer.

Social isolation and bullying is deeply ingrained within today's school culture. This is fueled by the competitive nature of most physical activities performed within schools. Many children have trouble finding a supportive environment where they can express themselves without criticism.

Andrea Pass, Artistic Director of Footprints Dance Project, Calgary, Canada.

Case Example 3
'Sue' experienced sexual abuse from her brother from a young age. When it started she confessed to not even knowing that it was wrong. As her awareness grew, she confided in her mother who rejected it as a baseless accusation. Isolated and distraught, she sought therapy to address the psychological consequences. After 2 years of intensive treatment she returned into the community through a youth dance program. Dance allowed her to establish a new relationship with her body through new pathways of emotional regulation. It allowed her to reconnect some of the shattered fragments of her experience and express them with movement. With her revitalized self-perception, she became an advocate for dance and the strength of dance to build back self-esteem.

Dance programs can provide opportunity for social contact to those who've encountered traumatic experiences. It can act as a cornerstone in an individual's recovery, allowing them to foster new relationships and master their emotions.

Andrea Pass, Artistic Director of Footprints Dance Project, Calgary, Canada.

Future Directions and Applications

In summation, what was originally a curriculum development project transitioned into a more in-depth exploration of DFMS and ultimately a novel assessment and validation study. During the first year of the project, the six-member team identified 33 fundamental movement skills essential to dance, through systematic observations of an existing dance program, in Alberta, Canada. Exercises and activities were then designed to improve each skill. These exercises and activities were compiled in the teaching resource (the FMT), which was developed in the second year and can be easily incorporated into dance classes to improve fundamental movement skills in students. After publication of the FMT, the DFMS-A underwent a preliminary validation study at the University of South Florida, with further validation ongoing. Once fully validated, the DFMS-A can become a useable tool both for evaluating the FMT and to explore other areas of interest involving DFMS.

Observations during the development of the guide and the DFMS Assessment tool highlighted the lack of available data concerning the connections between fundamental movement skills and other health aspects. This includes physical health and development, mental health and development, and social health and development. While it is well established that exercise plays a role in all these items, there is a paucity of information on the effect that fundamental movement skills have on the motivation to participate in future physical activities. The prevailing attitude seems to be that those who do not participate in physical activities either face barriers to participation, such as financial restrictions, or they simply just do not want to exercise. We are interested in exploring the connection between fundamental movement skills and the latter category, hypothesizing that motivation to move is developed at an early age with confidence and competence as essential cofactors. Once validated, the DFMS-A may provide an easily administered test of movement skills that could prove useful to other researchers. It may also be useful to those examining physical health and movement skills, such as physiotherapists working in schools who are looking for simplified methods of assessment.

My colleagues and I are also interested in expanding the DFMS and DFMS-A to accommodate a wider range of abilities. For example, exploring how the balance component changes with a dancer in a wheelchair, or how extension and retraction can be modified for individuals with mobility impairments and differences. An additional area of interest is bridging the communication gap between dancers and medical professionals. Presenting dance concepts in a manner accepted by the majority of medical professionals and presenting medical information to artists in an equally appreciated manner is a challenge in itself. An additional layer of complexity is effectively communicating the value of fundamental movement skills to the general public, who is schooled in neither field. The *Footprints Movement Tool* is an initial attempt to bridge these divides and we look forward to developing it further. Once further validation of the DFMS-A has been completed, we hope that this assessment becomes widely available to practitioners looking to evaluate these skills in the various populations with whom they work.

Acknowledgments Funding for this project was provided by four grants:

- The Royal Bank of Canada 'Learn to Play' Grant for 2016 & 2017;
- The Canadian Tire 'Jumpstart' in 2016 & 2017;
- The Alberta Foundation for the Arts 2016 & 2017; and
- Alberta Culture and Tourism 2017.

The program was supported and developed through Footprints Dance Project in Calgary, Canada. Special thanks to the following people involved in the Move Tool development: Lori Goods (Dance Teacher), Dr. Gregory Gutierrez (Physio Consultant for assessment), Conor Hearn (Course Layout/Video Editor), Shelby Holt (Dance Teacher and Contributor), Louise Huneck (Editor), Nicole Pemberton (Dance Teacher), Andrea Pass (Artistic Producer/Project Lead), Assessment validation is ongoing at the University of South Florida with Juanita Patterson-Price and Dr. Gregory Gutierrez.

Appendix: Supplemental Material 1

Beyond the Physical

Andrea Pass, Artistic Director of Footprints Dance Project, Calgary, Canada.

As Nietzsche once quipped, "We should consider every day lost on which we have not danced at least once." Today's youth face myriad challenges brought on by our rapidly changing world: From challenging political, economic, and environmental change, to rapid technological evolution; from cyberbullying and Internet radicalization to increasing obesity rates, youth must adapt quickly or face issues unknown even a generation ago. With casualties mounting in the alarming proliferation of opioids and a lack of confidence in the world's political authority, the manifestation of youth behavioral issues is significantly impacted. The most vulnerable of these exist in the low-income sector of the population. Here, parents working multiple jobs are often absent, and a void exists for positive role models and supervision to help guide youth into adulthood.

Authoritarian responses to youth behavioral issues are ineffective at treating the root causes. Dance and physical literacy can provide a range of benefits faced by at-risk youth. While often considered frivolous, Dance is a fundamental form of art and expression. Dance allows expression using the body and can help to form the foundation of confidence, resilience, self-advocacy, and social connectedness.

As humans, we strive to increase our well-being through social interaction. In turn, these connections foster coping mechanisms to deal with the complexities of our changing world. Participation in Dance offers the opportunity for social interaction, independence and autonomy. It improves our self-perception and the mastery of our bodies. For youth, taking part in dance improves self-efficacy (the individual's belief in their ability to achieve goals). It influences and builds confidence and self-esteem. Dance provides many opportunities for socialization and allows socially isolated individuals the opportunity for increased social contact.

Given the many problems children face today in our modern world, we need solutions that aid in behavioral development and target root problems. While it's long been understood that physical activity aids physical and social development through a range of mechanisms, a well-structured dance program provides all the health benefits while adding many psychosocial benefits. Not everyone can be an accomplished athlete, but everyone can benefit for the fun and social environment fostered by Dance.

References

1. Footprints Dance Project. Footprints dance project. http://footprintsdance.com/. 2013. Accessed 2018 Oct 18.
2. Pass A, Patterson-Price J. Footprints dance project – movement tool. https://footprints.myicourse.com/. 2017. Accessed 2019 Apr 17.

3. Fortier MS, Hogg W, O'Sullivan TL, Blanchard C, Sigal RJ, Reid RD, et al. Impact of integrating a physical activity counsellor into the primary health care team: physical activity and health outcomes of the physical activity counselling randomized controlled trial. Appl Physiol Nutr Metab. 2011;36(4):503–15.
4. Prescription to Get Active. Welcome to prescription to get active. https://www.prescriptiontogetactive.com/. 2017. Accessed 2017 Dec 13.
5. Canadian Sport for Life. Sport for life. http://sportforlife.ca/. 2018. Accessed 2018 Oct 18.
6. Beaulac J. A promising community-based hip-hop dance intervention for the promotion of psychosocial and physical well-being among youth living in a disadvantaged neighbourhood: University of Ottawa; 2008.
7. Beaulac J, Bouchard D, K E. Physical activity for adolescents living in a disadvantaged neighbourhood: views of parents and adolescents on needs, barriers, facilitators, and programming. Leisure. 2009;33(2):537–61.
8. Lander NJ, Barnett LM, Brown H, Telford A. Physical education teacher training in fundamental movement skills makes a difference to instruction and assessment practices. J Teach Phys Educ. 2015;34(3):548–56.
9. Van Rossum T, Morley D. Designing a movement assessment tool: Exploring the dilemmas of primary school teachers and movement experts. International Physical Literacy Conference; Toronto. 2017.
10. Kamla JD, Freeman GG. Fundamental motor skills and movement concepts: cornerstone of physical education programs for ages 3 to 8. Global J Health Phys Educ Pedagogy. 2014;3(2):150–60.
11. SHAPE America. National pe standards. https://www.shapeamerica.org/standards/pe/. 2013. Accessed 2019 June 22.
12. Ev B, Barnett LM, Zask A, Dietrich UC, Brooks LO, article BJR. Can we skill and activate children through primary school physical education lessons? "Move it groove it"—a collaborative health promotion intervention. Prev Med. 2003;36(4):493–501.
13. O'Brien W, Belton S, Issartel J. Fundamental movement skill proficiency amongst adolescent youth. Phys Educ Sport Pedagogy. 2015;21(6):557–71.
14. Australian Fundamental movement skills guide. The victoria fundamental motor skills manual for teachers. 2009.
15. Physical Health and Education Canada. Fundamental movement skills. http://www.phecanada.ca/programs/physical-literacy/what-physical-literacy/fundamental-movement-skills. 2017. Accessed 2018 Nov 15.
16. Lloyd RS, Oliver JL. The youth physical development model: a new approach to long-term athletic development. Strength Cond J. 2012;34(3):61–72.
17. Chatzihidiroglou P, Chatzopoulos D, Lykesas G, Doganis G. Dancing effects on preschoolers' sensorimotor synchronization, balance, and movement reaction time. Percept Mot Skills. 2018;125(3):463–77.
18. Payne H, editor. Dance movement therapy: theory, research and practice. 2nd ed. New York: Routledge; 2006.
19. Mainwaring LM, Krasnow DH. Teaching the dance class: strategies to enhance skill acquisition, mastery and positive self-image. J Dance Educ. 2010;10(1):14–21.
20. Schroeder K, Ratcliffe SJ, Perez A, Earley D, Bowman C, Lipman TH. Dance for health: an intergenerational program to increase access to physical activity. J Pediatr Nurs. 2017;37:29–34.
21. Batcup DC. A discussion of the dance movement psychotherapy literature relative to prisons and medium secure units. Body Mov Dance Psychother. 2013;8(1):5–16.
22. Williams FC. The embodiment of social dynamics: a phenomenon of western pop dance within a filipino prison. Res Danc Educ. 2013;14(1):39–56.
23. Guzmán A, Robinson L, Rochester L, James I, Hughes J. A process evaluation of a psychomotor dance therapy intervention (dancin) for behavior change in dementia: attitudes and beliefs of participating residents and staff. Int Psychogeriatr. 2017;29(2):313–22.
24. MOMO Mixed Ability Dance Theatre. Momo mixed ability dance theatre. http://www.momodancetheatre.org/. 2017. Accessed 2017 Dec 12.

25. Brew M. Axis dance company. http://www.axisdance.org/?gclid=EAIaIQobChMI0c31_aWH-4wIVB9lkCh0AoQqQEAAYASAAEgKdaPD_BwE. Accessed 2019 Jan 17.
26. Morris ML, Baldeon M, Scheuneman D. Developing and sustaining an inclusive dance program: strategic tools and methods. J Dance Educ. 2015;15(3):122–9.
27. REVolutions Dance Inc. Revolutions dance. http://www.revdance.org/about. 2013. Accessed 2019 June 22.
28. ILL-Abilities™. Ill abilities international dance crew. https://www.illabilities.com/. 2017. Accessed 2019 June 13.
29. Kimmerle M, Cote-Laurence P. Teaching dance skills: a motor learning and development approach: Andover, NJ: J. Michael Ryan Pub; 2003.
30. Koff SR, Magill RA. Book review: teaching dance skills: a motor learning and development approach susan r. Koff & J Dance Med Sci. 2004;8(4):145–6.
31. Alberta Learning. Physical education program of studies https://education.alberta.ca/media/160191/phys2000.pdf. 2000. Accessed 2018 Nov 22.
32. Bartenieff I, Lewis D. Body movement: coping with the environment. New York: Routledge; 2002.
33. Hackney P. Making connections: total body integration through bartenieff fundamentals. 6th ed. New York: Routledge; 2002.
34. SOBHD. Highland dancing: the textbook of the scottish official board of highland dancing. 8th ed. Edinburgh: Lindsay Publications; 2015.
35. Théleur EA. Letters on dancing, reducing this elegant and healthful exercise to easy scientific principles. London: Sherwood & Co.; 1832. 104 p.
36. Gose RL. Extraordinary dancing requires extraordinary (motor) learning. J Dance Educ. 2019;19(1):34–40.
37. Gilbert AG. Creative dance for all ages. American Alliance for Health, Physical Education, Recreation, and Dance: Reston; 1992.
38. Murray SC. The magic of movement: aesthetic movement principles for sport & dance: Alligator Press; 2005. ISBN: 0973881003, 9780973881004.
39. Krasnow G, Wilmerding MV. Motor learning and control for dance: principles and practices for performers and teachers. Human Kinetics: USA; 2015.
40. Canadian Sport for Life. Developing physical literacy: a guide for parents of children ages 0–12: Canadian Sport Centres; 2016.
41. Hyuuga A. Incredible swan lake ballet. https://www.youtube.com/watch?v=xI_olzX7Ycw. 2009. Accessed 2019 June 13.
42. Patterson-Price J, Gutierrez G. Validating the dance fundamental movement skills assessment for balance. [article]. In press 2020.
43. Patterson-Price J, Gutierrez G, editors. Dance fundamentals movement skills assessment. Third USF-PAMA Southeast Regional Conference "Lifecycle of the Performing Artist". Tampa; 2018.
44. MacDonald M, Lord C, Ulrich D. The relationship of motor skills and social communicative skills in school-aged children with autism spectrum disorder. Adapt Phys Act Q. 2013;30:271–82.
45. Davis C, Yanasak N, Allison J, Tomporowski P, McDowell J, Austin B, et al. Exercise improves executive function and achievement and alters brain activation in overweight children: a randomized, controlled trial. Health Psychol. 2011;30(1):91–8.
46. Goldinga A, Boesb C, Nordin-Batesc SM. Investigating learning through developmental dance movement as a kinaesthetic tool in the early years foundation stage. Res Danc Educ. 2016;17(3):235–67.
47. Keuna LL, Hunt P. Creative dance: Singapore children's creative thinking and problem-solving responses. Res Danc Educ. 2006;7(1):35–65.
48. Beaulac J, Kristjansson E, Calhoun M. Bigger than hip-hop? Impact of a community-based physical activity program on youth living in a disadvantaged neighbourhood in Canada. J Youth Stud. 2011;14(8):961–74.
49. de Waal E. Fundamental movement skills and academic performance of 5- to 6-year-old preschoolers. Early Childhood Educ J. 2019;47(4):455–64.

50. Cohen SO, Walco GA. Dance/movement therapy for children and adolescents with cancer. Cancer Pract. 1999;7(1):34–42.
51. Bradt J, Goodill SW, Dileo C. Dance/movement therapy for improving psychological and physical outcomes in cancer patients (review). Cochrane Database Syst Rev. 2015;(10):Cd007103.
52. Harris DA. Dance/movement therapy approaches to fostering resilience and recovery among African adolescent torture survivors. Torture. 2007;17(2):134–55.
53. Jeong YJ, Hong SC, Lee MS, Park MC, Kim YK, Suh CM. Dance movement therapy improves emotional responses and modulates neurohormones in adolescents with mild depression. Int J Neurosci. 2005;115(12):1711–20.

Chapter 23
Promoting Resilience and Fostering Mental Health Wellness Among University Dance Students

Emily Wright and Miranda Layman

Introduction: Mental Health Wellness in Higher Education

Evidence shows that university students face increasing mental health challenges that pose risks to their success. A 2016 report from the Center for Collegiate Mental Health summarizing clinical data from 139 college and university counseling centers reveals that rates of students who exhibit "threat-to-self" characteristics (non-suicidal self-injury and suicidal ideation) rose for the sixth consecutive year [1]. This report also found a 50% increase in university student visits to mental health services even though there were no increases in rates of pre-existing mental health concerns. A 2017 survey of 621 counseling centers conducted by the Association for University and College Counseling Center Directors relates that university students most frequently identify *anxiety* (48.2%) as a mental health concern, followed by *stress* (39.1%), depression (34.5%), suicidal ideation (25.2%), specific relationship concerns (22.9%), family concerns (21.2%), interpersonal functioning problems (18.8%), sleep problems (15.8%), and loneliness/social isolation (15.5%) [2]. In a systematic review of literature addressing the emotional and mental health needs of university students, Storrie et al. identified several common impacts of the emotional distress related to mental health challenges. They include poor grades, greater frequency of academic probation, decreased emotional and behavioral skills, increased social isolation, increased conflicts, and inadequate finances [3].

In responding to the increasing mental health concerns among students, colleges, and universities face many challenges in their endeavor to improve student access to

E. Wright (✉)
Independent Scholar, Charlottesville, VA, USA
e-mail: emily@emilywrightdance.com

M. Layman
Belhaven University, Jackson, MS, USA
e-mail: mlayman@belhaven.edu

S.-H. Lee et al. (eds.), *Perspectives in Performing Arts Medicine Practice*,
https://doi.org/10.1007/978-3-030-37480-8_23

mental health services [4]. For example, institutions face shrinking and restricted budgets that inhibit their ability to allocate resources to mental health services. Further, research indicates that university faculty and staff often lack knowledge about specific mental health diagnoses and/or the skills to work with students in ways that balance accessibility with academic integrity [5]. A course instructor may wonder what kind of accommodations are appropriate for a student whose anxiety makes sleeping difficult and who may struggle to complete assignments or get to early morning classes on time [6]. Despite increased utilization of mental health services, university students often do not seek treatment for mental health problems. In a survey of 2785 students at a large, public university, Eisenberg et al. found that between 37% and 84% of students with positive screens for depression or anxiety, did not seek mental health services that offer free access to short-term psychotherapy as well as basic health services [7]. While further research is needed to examine the factors contributing to underutilization of mental health services, these findings suggest that "education and awareness campaigns may be especially effective in reducing unmet needs for mental health services" [7, p. 600].

Mental Health Wellness in University Dance Students

Addressing mental health issues in the general university population is complex; but university dance students present a unique set of mental health disorders that require special attention. The stressors of the academic environment are compounded by the pressures of pre-professional dance training and long hours of intensive physical activity. Furthermore, the emphasis on performance-orientation can encourage maladaptive dispositions and self-destructive behaviors [8]. Unfortunately, limited research has considered the role of mental health in postsecondary dance education. The National Association of Schools of Dance offers recommendations for "musculoskeletal health and injury prevention" but does not include mental health wellness in its standards and guidelines for university dance programs [8, p. 67]. We searched *the International Bibliography of Theater and Dance with Full Text, PsychARTICLES, SPORTDiscus with Full Text*, and *PubMed databases* using the keywords dance, students, university, education, and mental health within the parameters for scholarly, peer-reviewed publications. This search yielded 88 articles, only six of which addressed topics relevant to student dancers' mental health. The key concepts addressed in the literature were low self-esteem, poor body image, performance anxiety, training distress, and psychological distress due to physical injury [9–14]. Van Staden et al., in their phenomenological study of a small group of professional ballet dancers, found further that the professional training environment influences the development of role-identity rather than self-identity, maladaptive perfectionism, hyper-awareness of surveillance, internalized pressure to achieve at the expense of personal needs, neurotic defensiveness, a lack of social support and failure to trust, envy, competition, and difficulty with career transitions due to uncompromising attitudes toward the physical body [8, pp. 21–23]. Using these concepts as a framework, we developed an inquiry to explore what our dance student population knew about mental health wellness and identify what specific mental health challenges faced them.

Utilizing the inquiry data, we created a one-semester mental health wellness initiative program aimed at increasing dance students' awareness of campus and community mental health services and helping with practical strategies to promote mental health wellness. Parallel to the wellness initiative program, we prompted dance faculty and staff to modify department wellness screenings and technique class absence policies in ways that acknowledge mental health as a vital component of dance curricula.

Initial Inquiry

We designed the initial inquiry using approaches from sequential mixed methods research procedures [15]. We began with an exploratory survey of 84 dance students to determine their baseline knowledge of mental health wellness and to gauge their interest in specific topics related to mental health issues. Then, we conducted a 13-member focus group as a means to expand upon the findings of the survey data. While the topic of mental health challenges naturally arose over the course of our pilot and wellness initiative, we emphasized the promotion of mental health wellness in accordance with World Health Organization recommendations [15]. The pilot initiative utilized ethical research practices in the research design, data collection, analysis, interpretation, writing, and dissemination of the study, including careful consideration of the potential benefits to participants; voluntary participation and informed consent prior to data collection; confidentiality of survey participants; protected access to data collected; and transparency concerning intent to publish findings [16, pp. 87–92]. Our inquiry was approved by the Institutional Review Board of Belhaven University. Finally, it should be noted that our pilot inquiry was conducted at a small, liberal arts university whose mission is to integrate education and career preparation with Christian religious formation. While the impact of religion on mental health wellness is beyond the scope of this study, we acknowledge that the long history of antagonism between Christianity and the mental health community is an important factor in a study of attitudes toward and practical application of mental health wellness [17]. In the initial inquiry, we included a question about Christian perspectives on mental health in the survey, and we explored this topic in more depth with the focus group.

Initial Inquiry Procedure

Using Insel and Roth's Connect Core Concepts in Health, we developed an 18-item inquiry in order to evaluate student awareness of mental health wellness as well as highlight the key components of wellness promotion, including: awareness of psychological health and its impacts on general well-being, knowledge of resources and practices to cultivate mental health wellness, and an understanding of the influence of social, cultural, and/or religious attitudes toward mental health [15, 18–20]. Participants were asked to indicate their agreement/disagreement (strongly disagree, disagree, neither agree nor disagree, agree, strongly agree) with a series of statements about mental health wellness. Inquiry responses were anonymous, and participants could choose to skip any question. The inquiry also included demographic information and informed consent procedures. All undergraduate and graduate dance students in attendance at the weekly department meeting were invited to participate in the initial inquiry, which was administered via the online platform SurveyMonkey during a weekly dance department meeting.

Initial Inquiry Participants

Eighty-one undergraduate and 3 graduate dance students between the ages of 18 and 24 years opted to participate in the pilot study survey. One participant identified as American Indian/Alaskan Native, 3 as Asian/Pacific Islander, 3 as Black/African American, 1 as Hispanic, 75 identified as White or Caucasian, and 1 as Multiple Ethnicities. Seventy-nine participants identified as Female and 5 identified as Male.

Initial Inquiry Findings

In terms of understanding and awareness of mental health wellness, more than 95% of survey participants agreed or strongly agreed with the statement, "I understand what mental health wellness is and how it impacts my personal, social, and academic life"; while fewer than 5% neither agreed nor disagreed. Yet 24% of participants either disagreed or strongly disagreed that they know what to do to practice mental health wellness in their own lives. Fifteen percent also disagreed with the statement, "I know what resources are available to me on campus and in the community to support my mental health wellness." In terms of social support, 57% agreed or strongly agreed that they are comfortable discussing mental health wellness with friends, family members, and/or faculty; 31% were neutral; and 12% either disagreed or strongly disagreed. Sixty percent of participants agreed or strongly agreed that they know what to do if someone else shared a mental health challenge with them, 30% were neutral, and 10% disagreed or strongly disagreed. Finally, 62% of participants agreed or strongly agreed that they receive positive messages about mental health wellness from friends, family members, and/or faculty, 25% were neutral, and 13% disagreed or strongly disagreed. The inquiry did not ask participants to distinguish between friends, family, and faculty in terms of social support for mental health wellness. While it is perhaps encouraging that a majority of participants believed they understood what constitutes mental health wellness, as well as practices and resources available, significant minorities of

Table 23.1 Participant interest in mental health wellness topics

Campus resources for mental health	16
Community resources for mental health	27
Practices to cultivate personal mental health wellness	63
Challenges to mental health wellness	35
Christian perspectives on mental health wellness	52
Mental health wellness in dance-specific contexts	66

dance student participants did not. Further, the increase in percentages of participants who were neutral or disagreed with statements about social support concerning mental health wellness suggest that further research on the social factors of mental health wellness in university dance communities could be fruitful.

Participants were also asked to indicate one or more topics related to mental health wellness they wanted to learn more about. To this question, 16 wanted to learn more about campus resources, 27 community resources, 63 practices to cultivate personal mental health wellness, 35 challenges to mental health wellness, 52 Christian perspectives on mental health wellness, 66 mental health wellness in dance-specific contexts (such as dance training and performing) (see Table 23.1). A space was also provided for participants to list additional topics of interest, questions, or comments about the survey in general. Finally, participants were asked to indicate their interest in participating in a focus group on psychological well-being. Twenty-six survey participants also indicated their interest in participating in a focus group.

Focus Group Procedures

As a means to expand upon the initial survey, a 90 min focus group was conducted to afford the researchers with a deeper sense of students' understanding and concerns related to mental health wellness. Since an element of the pilot study was to explore new ways to promote general well-being among university dance students, the focus group also enabled us to facilitate collaborative, spontaneous dialogue around these topics and generate the possibility for new, creative solutions to arise [21]. The focus group was moderated by one of the researchers in a semi-structured format in which the moderator used the survey questions as a framework for discussion, while also asking open-ended questions, such as "What do you do to cultivate mental health wellness in your life?" and "How can we develop resilience in the midst of life's challenges?" The open-ended questions allowed for the possibility of new questions and discussion topics to emerge. The session was audio-recorded for note-taking and transcription purposes. The moderator reviewed informed consent and confidentiality procedures with focus group participants, then initiated the discussion with a preliminary review of the initial findings from the pilot survey.

Focus Group Participants

Of the 26 survey participants who indicated their interest, 13 ultimately participated in the focus group. All focus group participants were undergraduates (1 sophomore, 9 juniors, and 3 seniors). Twelve participants identified as White or Caucasian and 1 identified as Black or African American; 12 participants identified as Female and 1 identified as Male.

Focus Group Results

Over the course of the discussion, the following themes emerged:

Disconnection between theoretical understanding and lived experience of mental health. While reflecting on their understanding of psychological wellness and its impact on their lives, focus group participants identified a gap between their ability to understand mental health on an intellectual level and their capacity to practically address these issues in their lives. For instance, one participant observed that reading about the characteristics of a mental health condition was very different than witnessing a friend live with that condition in real life. As dancers, they seemed particularly interested in learning about mental health from kinesthetic and sensory perspectives that they thought would contribute to a deeper understanding of the lived experiences of mental health wellness. They also suggested that there is no singular model for mental health wellness for all. Instead, they expressed interest in learning a diverse range of practices that could contribute to wellness in different contexts or stages of life. In addition to understanding how systems of university dance training present challenges to wellness, focus group participants expressed a desire to learn greater self-awareness to enable them to adapt to these challenges. As one participant observed,

> [Coming to college] was a really big shock for me because I was raised in a smaller environment with people I'd known my entire life. And coming into a place with a new pool of people where everyone is coming from different walks of life… Everyone is trying to navigate those relationships, trying to understand whose issues are whose and not really even knowing who you are. I struggled with that a lot my freshman year. I've started to learn a little bit more about emotional boundaries between people and choosing how and when to engage with someone who's struggling.

Learning practical tools to develop greater self-awareness could improve university dance students' transitions to college and contribute to the potential for more successful interpersonal interactions as well.

Inseparability of mental health wellness from everyday life challenges. Although the focus of the pilot initiative was mental well-being, focus group participants quickly shifted the conversation to the difficulty in separating wellness from everyday life challenges. Another focus group participant observed:

> I was thinking about the idea that mental health is just the absence of anxiety [or other disorders]. But, in reality, we're going to deal with a lot of those things. How can you be mentally well, but still approach issues like anxiety? Because it's not this thing you can just get rid of. How do you work with it? Not just to survive, but to thrive. That's an idea that's hard to get out of people's minds—it's not just the absence of something that makes you healthy.

Of course, there is a difference between dealing with occasional feelings of anxiety and a medical diagnosis of clinical anxiety. Yet, this participant identified that everyone at some point in life will deal with mental health challenges. For her, a key component of well-being is the normalization of challenges and the cultivation of strategies that foster resilience.

Mental Health and Interpersonal Interactions. Pre-professional dancers spend a significant amount of time and energy learning to attune their awareness to their bodily and emotional states as a means to project particular qualities in performance. For example, in dance courses, students typically wear clothing (such as leotards, tights, or fitted t-shirts) designed to allow instructors to see their anatomical alignment while dancing. However, student participants observed that these attire requirements are sometimes a source of self-consciousness and can lead to comparison and competitiveness. Further, studies show that the use of mirrors as an aid to learning and refining also contribute to decreased body image satisfaction [22]. Thus, these professional tools are not always compatible with practices that contribute to healthy interpersonal relationships. While discussing the role of social context for psychological health, focus participants seemed to recognize the unique challenges for dancers as a result of the close physical proximity and extended time periods that they often spend together. One respondent reflected:

> Something I've noticed more recently is how much other people's feelings and how they're expressing themselves affects me. Whenever I'm surrounded by a lot of negativity, I become more negative... So [I'm learning to] evaluate the situation and ask, "Is this a realistic reaction to this situation?" And if someone else is freaking out about it, "How can this not affect me? How can I maybe help them through it and not just join them in their response?

Student/Teacher Power Dynamics. Finally, focus group participants recognized that the dance classroom environment, in which faculty assess students on the basis of technical and creative performance, often complicates the transparency needed to address mental health wellness head-on. As one student put it, "I'm afraid that if I tell my professor I'm struggling with anxiety and panic attacks, they might give me less feedback in class or not cast me in their next work." While the university has a trained mental health counselor who can provide safe and confidential counseling, students report that the demands of their schedules often conflict with the limited hours available for appointments. Thus, staff members who do not assess students, such as the dance athletic trainer, become the preferred confidants for students with mental health challenges, further complicating trust relationships between students, faculty, and staff.

Focus group participants' insights clarified and expanded our understanding of the survey data results. They also point to several areas for further research, including the development of kinesthetic and sensory approaches to mental health education, the effects of specific professional dance practices on perceived well-being, the role of interpersonal dynamics in university dance environments, and the effects of power dynamics and disclosure of evaluation of mental health status in the university environment. The results of our focus group data were key to the design of the second component of our project, a mental health education initiative.

Mental Health Education Initiative

We designed our educational initiative to be as responsive as possible to the initial findings that emerged from the pilot data. The focus group themes revealed that students needed a better lived understanding of mental health wellness, tools and resources to address it, methods for navigating the influences of their social environment, and reassurance that disclosure would be supported by instructors and not result in negative consequences. Thus, we aimed to address these themes within our three-part educational initiative comprised of a collaborative faculty/student presentation at a dance department-wide meeting, a community guest lecture hosted by the Institute for International Care and Council, and a department-wide mental health wellness day. We devised the initiative based on standards for health promotion in higher education established by the American College Health Association (ACHA), which include:

- Alignment of health promotion with the mission(s) of the institution
- Utilization of a socio-ecological[1] approach, which addresses health promotion at multiple levels—especially at the level of campus and community
- Collaboration with interdisciplinary partners
- Development of approaches that acknowledge diversity and foster inclusive communities [23]

Collaborative Faculty/Student Presentation During a one-hour department-wide meeting, a dance faculty member partner and a Junior dance major co-delivered a 15 min presentation on mental health and well-being. We presented content based on areas of interest indicated in our survey responses, and the collaborative student/faculty nature of the presentation emphasized a socio-ecological approach to wellness promotion. The presentation included a definition of mental health wellness as "state of well-being in which every individual realizes his or her own potential, can cope with the normal stresses of life, can work productively and fruitfully, and is able to make a contribution to her or his community" [24] and descriptions of the ways in which psychological health impacts thoughts, bodily sensations, behaviors, and emotions. This presentation also promoted organiza-

[1] The term "socio-ecological model" refers to an ecological model for health promotion, which highlights the many intersections of individual and social factors that contribute to overall well-being on university campuses, including interpersonal, organization, community, and systemic structures [24].

tions and tools available to students to support well-being at different levels, including: student-led organizations, faculty and staff, and campus organizations, such as the Office for Career and Calling. We concluded with a dance faculty-led breakout session that gave students the opportunity to ask questions or share feedback in smaller groups. Involving faculty in this effort was both a means of heightening their awareness of student needs and a means of addressing the issue of power dynamics mentioned in the focus group. This effort, while small-scale, was significant in creating space for open dialogue between faculty and students around this topic.

Community Guest Lecture As part of their ongoing work on mental health in religious contexts, the Institute for International Care and Counsel hosted a campus-wide guest lecture. In keeping with ACHA guidelines, we included a community guest lecture in our initiative as a means to develop cross-campus, interdisciplinary partners. Approximately 20 dance students joined a general audience for a talk by Dr. Matthew Stanford, director of the Hope and Healing Institute in Houston, Texas, whose mission is to provide religious organizations with educational resources that bridge the gap between pastoral care and mental health service providers [25]. In keeping with the religious mission of the university, this talk centered on Christian approaches to mental health through the lens of biblical literature.

Mental Health Wellness Day The culmination of our pilot initiative was a Mental Health Wellness Day, including a keynote session with our campus counselor, followed by breakout sessions led by dance faculty [26]. The sessions were designed in response to student survey data as well as the responses of focus group participants. Our camp counselor, who has a personal background in dance and sees a number of dance students in individual sessions, conducted a 90 min session in which she addressed the concepts of cognitive distortions and positive stress as they relate to dance training. This session gave students the opportunity to learn cognitive behavioral strategies to address thought patterns that might contribute to mental health challenges in the classroom or studio. Students then had the option to participate in various faculty-led sessions, including the use of religious literature for positive thinking, mindful meditation, and taking time for fun and playfulness. We designed a range of serious and light- hearted options for each session so that students could choose according to their interest and energy level.

Preliminary Outcomes

In response to the preliminary findings of our pilot initiative, our department continues to prioritize faculty and staff education as a means to develop best practices for mental well-being in university education and implement them in a dance-specific context. The ACHA suggests that many students facing mental health challenges may feel more comfortable seeing a healthcare professional over a mental health professional, which is consistent with the dance athletic trainer's experience in our department [27]. We are continuing to explore ways to empower students to seek support from mental health professionals to ensure they are receiving care from qualified professionals. For example, our dance athletic trainer has revised the pre-participation health screening process to include evaluation of mental health. Further, our department has developed a mental health policy and procedures manual to address issues like class absences as a result of mental health challenges and procedures for mental health crises.

Pre-participation Health History Evaluations and Mental Health Screenings

Our original pre-participation health history evaluation (PPHHE) was a two-step process in which all dance majors and minors enrolled in dance courses were required to provide documentation of an annual physical conducted by their primary care physician and to participate in a yearly, dance-specific health screening conducted by the dance athletic trainer. While our original screening focused almost exclusively on physical health components, we have revised these guidelines to include a mental health evaluation in the general physical exam and during the dance-specific health screening. Mental health screening questions are modified from guidelines provided by the National Collegiate Athletic Association's Sports Science Institute, including:

- I often have trouble sleeping.
- I wish I had more energy most days of the week.
- I think about things over and over.
- I feel anxious and nervous much of the time.
- I feel stressed out much of the time.
- I feel stressed out during dance activities.
- I often feel sad and depressed.
- I often struggle to feel confident.
- I don't feel hopeful about the future.
- I have a hard time managing my emotions (anger, frustration, impatience).
- I have feelings of hurting myself or others [28].

Any "yes" response to these questions results in a follow-up discussion between the dance student and the dance athletic trainer to determine if the student should be referred to a licensed mental health professional for further evaluation. Data collected from these screenings can be used to assist in early identification of potential mental health concerns, for referral to mental health providers, and to support continuity of care for dance students with pre-existing diagnoses of mental health challenges.

Mental Health Policy and Procedures Manual

Our department has also implemented a Mental Health Policy and Procedures Manual, which provides dance faculty, staff, and students with a definition of mental health wellness, identifies specific members of the healthcare team who will oversee potential incidences, and outlines the necessary steps to manage an acute or chronic mental/behavioral health situation. These guidelines mirror procedures outlined for acute and chronic physical injury or illness. While we do not expect that these policies and procedures will resolve all difficulties, we anticipate that they will assist dance faculty in providing sufficient resources to care for those with mental health challenges. We also anticipate that these revisions will create additional opportunities for further conversation around mental health wellness and contribute to the further normalization of mental health conversations in our community. The manual encompasses the following items:

1. *Holistic Healthcare for Dance Students*: The university and the dance department prioritize the physical, mental, emotional, and spiritual wellness of each student.
2. *Definition of Mental Health Wellness*: Mental health wellness is defined as the emotional, psychological, and social well-being of a person [24]. For the purpose of these guidelines, mental health issues will be categorized as acute or chronic. Acute emergencies are defined as sudden changes in mental conditions (i.e., perceived suicide attempt or changes in mental status). These conditions may require referral to mental health professionals and/or hospitalization. Chronic conditions include, but are not limited to, depression, anxiety disorders, and/or other previously diagnosed mental conditions.
3. *Identification of Mental Health Wellness Personnel*: The dance athletic trainer is the primary point of contact for screening and referral to a qualified mental health provider for the diagnosis and/or treatment of acute or chronic mental health conditions. The dance athletic trainer will collaborate with faculty, the campus counselor, the Dean of students, and residence hall staff in the on-going assessment of dance activities that impact a mental health condition.
4. *Pre-Participation Health History Evaluation (PPHHE)*: The Dance Department takes a proactive approach to mental health concerns by including a mental health screening as part of new and returning dancer students' PPHHE. At-risk dance students identified through the PPHHE screening will have a follow-up conversation with the dance athletic trainer and may be provided an additional, more detailed questionnaire. The dance athletic trainer will determine if the

dance student needs a referral for further evaluation by a licensed mental health-care team.

5. *Treatment Protocols for Mental Health Conditions*: Dance students are not required to disclose a mental health diagnosis. However, if a condition necessitates accommodations, such as a reduced course load or extended test-taking time, they are encouraged to disclose this information to the Office of Student Care. The dance athletic trainer can assist in the monitoring of symptoms and connect dance students with campus and community mental health services to ensure consistency of treatment.
6. *First Aid for Mental Health Crises*: If a dance student reports a mental health emergency, such as inability to perform daily tasks, rapid mood swings, increased agitation, threats of harm to self or others, isolation, and/or paranoia, the dance athletic trainer or supervising staff/faculty will assess the immediacy of the situation and notify the appropriate mental health professional or call for emergency assistance. In the event of a mental health crisis, the dance athletic trainer will serve as the liaison between the student seeking treatment and faculty to ensure proper treatment and smooth transition to classes and rehearsals.
7. *Class Absences*: Dance students experiencing mental health challenges that affect class participation are encouraged to make an appointment with the campus counselor and to communicate with faculty in affected classes. Per university policy, students who miss more than 20% of classes will fail the course except in the case of extenuating circumstances to be considered in consultation with the Dance Chair, Dean of Students, and University Registrar. Students who receive class attendance accommodations for mental health challenges may be expected to demonstrate adherence to appropriate treatment protocols and report consistent follow-up care to Dance Department Chair.

Conclusion

In sum, our mental health wellness initiative encompassed an exploratory student survey, a focus group, and an educational intervention designed to address the information generated by the survey and focus group. The focus group themes revealed that students needed a better lived understanding of mental health wellness, the tools and resources to address it, methods for navigating the influences of their social environment, and reassurance that disclosure would be supported by their instructors and not result in negative consequences. Our educational initiative sought to attend to those key themes through a collaborative faculty–student presentation, a guest lecture, a mental health wellness day, and revision of our departmental policies and procedures. We have not collected formal data on the outcomes of these efforts thus far, but, informal feedback from faculty and staff has been positive. Given the complexity of mental health issues in university dance populations, limitations of our initiative include a lack of research studies that address the overlapping concerns of university students and pre-professional dance training and a need for more sophisticated methods of data collection. The preliminary results of this pilot initiative also point to avenues for future research, including the impact of the university dance environment on mental well-being and the role of the student/teacher relationship in reporting mental health conditions. In the future, our department plans to explore the integration of mental health wellness practices in specific dance course syllabi as well as the role of mentorship in destigmatizing and normalizing mental health challenges.

Based upon our experiences, we suggest that other educators consider implementing surveys and/or focus groups to glean a point of reference for what their students know, or want to know about mental health, and then consider several educational interventions during the semester to address key issues such as a mental health wellness day, co-led faculty/student presentations, and/or guest presentations by mental health professionals. We found that collaborating with our campus resources and creating partnerships was highly important as well as reflecting upon departmental policies and practices as a full faculty. Through sharing our initial data and program experiences, we hope to expand the conversation on mental health in university dance students to other performing arts departments as a means to share resources and best practices with other institutions.

References

1. Center for Collegiate Mental Health. 2016 annual report. 2017. https://sites.psu.edu/ccmh/files/2017/01/2016-Annual-Report-FINAL_2016_01_09-1gc2hj6.pdf. Accessed 23 Apr 2019.
2. LeViness P, Bershad C, Gorman K. The Association for University and College Counseling Center Directors annual survey. 2017. https://www.aucccd.org/assets/documents/Governance/2017%20aucccd%20survey-public-apr26.pdf. Accessed 23 Apr 2019.
3. Storrie K, Ahern K, Tuckett A. A systematic review: students with mental health problems—a growing problem. Int J Nurs Pract. 2010;16:1–6.
4. Collins ME, Mowbray CT. Students with psychiatric disabilities on campus: examining predictors of enrollment with disability support services. J Postsecond Educ Disabil. 2008;21:91–104.
5. American College Health Association. National college health assessment executive summary. 2017. https://www.acha.org/documents/ncha/NCHA-II_FALL_2017_REFERENCE_GROUP_EXECUTIVE_SUMMARY_UNDERGRADS_ONLY.pdf. Accessed 24 Apr 2019.
6. Gooblar D. How to help a student in a mental-health crisis. Chronicle of Higher Education 2018. https://www.chronicle.com/article/How-to-Help-a-Student-in-a/245305. Accessed 24 Apr 2019.
7. Eisenberg D, Golberstein E, Gollust S. Help-seeking and access to mental health care in a university student population. Med Care. 2007;45:594–601.
8. Van Staden A, Myburgh CPH, Poggenpoel MA. Psycho-educational model to enhance self-development and mental health of classical dancers. J Dance Med Sci. 2009;13:20–8.
9. National Association of Schools of Dance. National association of schools of dance handbook 2018–19. Reston: National Association of Schools of Dance; 2018.
10. Grove J, Main L, Sharp L. Stressors, recovery processes, and manifestations of training distress in dance. J Dance Med Sci. 2013;17:70–8.

11. Quested E, Duda J. Perceived autonomy support, motivation regulations and the self-evaluation tendencies of student dancers. J Dance Med Sci. 2011;15:3–14.
12. Alimena S, Air ME, Gribbin C, Manejias S. Utilization of routine primary care services among dancers. J Dance Med Sci. 2016;20:95–102.
13. Air ME. Psychological distress among dancers seeking outpatient treatment for musculoskeletal injury. J Dance Med Sci. 2013;17:115–25.
14. Scoffier-Mériaux S, Falzon C, Lewton-Brain P, Filaire E, d'Arripe-Longueville F. Big five personality traits and eating attitudes in intensively training dancers: the mediating role of internalized thinness norms. J Sports Sci. 2014;14:627–33.
15. World Health Organization. Prevention and promotion in mental health. Geneva, Switzerland; 2002.
16. Research Design CJW. Qualitative, quantitative, and mixed methods approaches. 3rd ed. Los Angeles: Sage; 2009.
17. Sullivan S, Payne JM, Cheney AM, Hunt J, Haynes TF, Sullivan G. The pew versus the couch: relationship between mental health and faith communities and lessons learned from a VA/clergy partnership project. J Relig Health. 2014;53(4):1267–82.
18. Stanford M. Where is mental health in the Bible? Institute for International Care and Council: Jackson; 2018.
19. Here to Help. Wellness modules 2015. http://www.heretohelp.bc.ca/wellness-modules. Accessed 4 Jan 2018.
20. Insel PM, Roth WT. Connect core concepts in health. 12th ed. New York: McGraw-Hill Education; 2012.
21. Merriam SB. Qualitative research: a guide to design and implementation. San Francisco: Jossey-Bass; 2009.
22. McParland JL, Flowers P. Nine lessons and recommendations from the conduct of focus group research in chronic pain samples. Br J Health Psychol. 2012;17:492–504.
23. Radell SA, Keneman ML, Mandradjieff M, Adame DD, Cole SP. Comparison study of body image satisfaction between beginning and advanced-level female ballet students. J Dance Med Sci. 2017;21:135–43.
24. American College Health Association. Standards of practice for health promotion in higher education, 3rd edition. 2012. https://www.acha.org/documents/resources/guidelines/ACHA_Standards_of_Practice_for_Health_Promotion_in_Higher_Education_May2012.pdf. Accessed 3 Jan 2018.
25. World Health Organization. Mental health: a state of being. http://www.who.int/features/factfiles/mental_health/en/. Accessed 20 Nov 2017.
26. Hope ad Healing Center & Institute. About the HHCI. https://hopeandhealingcenter.org/about-us/. Accessed 1 Feb 2018.
27. American College Health Association. Considerations for integration of counseling and health services on college and university campuses. Linthicum: American College Health Association; 2010.
28. National Collegiate Athletic Association Sports Science Institute. Inter-association consensus document: best practices for understanding and supporting student-athlete mental wellness. https://www.ncaa.org/sites/default/files/HS_Mental-Health-Best-Practices_20160317.pdf. Accessed 5 Jan 2018.

Chapter 24
Development of a Multidisciplinary Approach to Wellness and Injury Management at an Intensive Youth Orchestra Summer Festival

Regina Campbell

Introduction

The life cycle of a musician may begin as early as age three and rigorous training often begins before the age of eight. Like elite athletes, classical musicians often feel driven to practice for hours at a time so they can perform at a high level [1–4]. Playing-related musculoskeletal problems (PRMPs) are common in adult musicians [5–8] and can result in the inability to play for a period of time. Injuries sustained are thought to relate to physical demands reflecting the particular instrument [5, 7, 8] (see Chap. 13, *Musculoskeletal and Associated Conditions in the Instrumental Musician*). Studies also suggest PRMPs are common in children and that risk factors may be similar [9–11].

Along with physical injury risk exposure, musicians, like sport athletes, are under intense psychological pressure from performing in public. Unlike the athlete community, however, the musical community can be a challenge for implementing best practice models of healthcare due to negative cultural perceptions of injury [12]. Competition and shame due to negative connotations of inferior technical competency as a causative factor for injury among musicians can lead to reluctance to admit pain and seek care [13, 14]. A complex relationship develops between performance-related pain and a range of psychosocial factors [15].

Promoting wellness and early intervention with injury treatment may avoid lost time for musicians performing across the life cycle [16, 17]. A team of specialists who understand healthy practice strategies and implement injury prevention measures tailored to musicians may reduce the incidence of playing-related musculoskeletal disorders in musicians [18]. In this chapter, I describe the evolution and beginning implementation of a Health and Wellness Series program designed to

R. Campbell (✉)
Performing Arts Physical Therapy, PC, Winchester, MA, USA

S.-H. Lee et al. (eds.), *Perspectives in Performing Arts Medicine Practice*,
https://doi.org/10.1007/978-3-030-37480-8_24

prevent and treat playing-related musculoskeletal disorders and psychosocial issues amongst student musicians at the BUTI, a summer music program in western Massachusetts.

Boston University Tanglewood Institute (BUTI)

The Boston University Tanglewood Institute [19] is a summer music program for students ages 14–20 years. It is comprised of a summer orchestral program, a wind ensemble, piano program, and instructions in voice, composition, and harp. Each year, BUTI hosts approximately140 students and employs specialist teachers in all areas of instruments, composition, voice, and conducting. Duration of the program varies: for example, for harp, 4 weeks, wind ensemble, 4 weeks, piano, three or 6 weeks, and the orchestral program 8 weeks. Orchestral students are required to play daily 3 h orchestra rehearsals and 1–2 h chamber music rehearsals. In addition, orchestral students have weekly lessons and practice on their own another 1–3 h per day.

History and Evolution of the Health and Wellness Series Program

In Summer 2015, the administration began to notice some time loss from playing and paid attention to injury reports from teachers and the nursing staff. Although no formal data were collected, an administrative member recollected many reports of incidences about injuries amongst the approximate100 orchestral students. For example, a cellist dropping out due to a Repetitive Strain Injury (RSI) and Carpal Tunnel Syndrome, three upper strings students requiring time off from rehearsals and concerts, and several teachers reporting student pain and injury complaints. In the midway of the summer program, a physical therapist (the author of this article) was invited to conduct a 2 h injury prevention workshop by the administration. Over 100 students and 10 faculty attended the workshop.

The first hour of this workshop was a didactic presentation with Power Point slides. It contained information pertaining to the Performing Arts Medicine Association and National Association of Schools of Music four areas of Performing Arts Health (Musculoskeletal, Auditory, Voice, Psychological) with focus on prevention of musculoskeletal playing-related injuries. The presentation reviewed basic anatomy of the trunk and upper extremity muscles, bones, and joints. It described common injuries sustained by musicians and how to recognize them in their own bodies, including tendonitis in the wrists/hands, forearms and rotator cuff, back and neck strain, brachial plexus compression at the thoracic inlet, cubital tunnel, and carpal tunnel, and disorders of the TMJ and embouchure. The importance of early treatment, measures for self-treatment, and when to seek professional help were outlined. Ergonomics and posture for all instruments and vocalists were discussed. The presentation content also addressed efficient solo practice routine management, including the importance of score study and auditory learning pathways as ways to avoid overplaying. Participants were taught to take breaks every 20 min, and to do warm-up and cool-down exercises away from the instrument with light cardio, stretches, and sensory integration methods. General wellness considerations of getting enough sleep, hydration, nutritional support, cardio exercise, and stress management through meditation were reviewed.

The second hour of the 2015 workshop was experiential. First, the students were guided through demonstration and verbal instructions in the light cardio, stretching (trunk, neck and upper extremity muscles), and sensory integration routine discussed during the first hour of the presentation. The instructor then observed and analyzed several students' playing technique and ergonomic approach to their instruments. This was very well received as instrumentalists of each group enthusiastically volunteered to participate in the demonstration. Faculty who attended the workshop also engaged by giving recommendations for instrument setup, posture, and playing technique.

Following the workshop in 2015, the BUTI administrator and I discussed over a period of several months ways to implement health and wellness classes and physical therapy intervention in future summer programs. The primary goal was to reduce and prevent injury rates, allowing the students to remain as fully participatory as possible in the BUTI program. We also wanted to introduce the students to tools to develop lifelong learning of wellness habits in their preparation for musical careers.

In 2016, the BUTI administration continued to receive anecdotal reports of pain and injury, but again, no attempt was made to collect systematic data. The BUTI administrator associated with the development of the wellness program reported that out of the approximate 140 students at the festival, one clarinetist and three upper string players required time off from rehearsals and concerts. Teachers continued to report unofficial remarks to administrative staff about student injury complaints. There was no information available about what those students did to address the problems.

A wellness series of classes began in response to positive reception of the 2015 workshop. Weekly classes were held for 1 hour at 7 AM including the following disciplines: Body Mapping[1]—2 sessions; Feldenkrais[2] —2 sessions; Physical Therapy stretching and strengthening group exercise class—1 session; Alexander Technique[3]—1 session; and Trager—1 session. Physical Therapy referrals for

[1] Body Mapping is an offshoot of the Alexander Technique. Body Mapping guides musicians to recognize the movement foundation to music-making by developing an understanding of how the body is connected from head to toe along with its design for movement. It trains movement along with the musician's senses and attention.

[2] Feldenkrais Method uses gentle, mindful movement to facilitate body awareness.

[3] Alexander Technique is a system of body awareness designed to promote well-being by ensuring minimum effort in maintaining postures and carrying out movements.

injured students were made via the Institute's nurse to my private office. Two students were followed for PT evaluation and treatment sessions.

Average class size in the wellness series began at 14 but dropped to 5 by the end of the program. The drop in attendance raised concerns for the program organizers. The administration and clinicians speculated that possible reasons for decreased participation may have been the early morning class time, demand on students for extra rehearsals, student perceptions of needing to practice more toward the end of the program, or student burn out with demands on their time toward the end of the program. Despite the Institute's recognition of student injuries and the perceived merit of the wellness program, no one administered student or faculty surveys to formally assess the program. Fortunately, these issues were taken into account in the planning of the program for the following years.

Beginning of BUTI Health and Wellness Series Program 2017

The BUTI received a grant from the Whitney family whose daughter is a former student of the program for the support of a 5-year Wellness Series. This grant provided for physical therapy assessment and triage clinics, and classes in Body Mapping, Feldenkrais Method, Alexander Technique, Yoga, and mental skills training [17]. Signs on bulletin boards on campus and emails to faculty promoted participation in the physical therapy clinics as well as the wellness classes.

Physical Therapy Assessment and Triage sessions were made available twice a week for 2 h each. The drop-in sessions consisted of a brief PT screen of student reports on the injured area. The PT screens included provocation tests for repetitive strain injury and peripheral nerve compression, static and dynamic postural assessment with musical instruments, and targeted strength and range of motion testing. Patient history was obtained regarding practice habits and ensemble requirement details. Students were triaged to determine if time was needed for rest from ensemble rehearsals.

After completing the brief physical therapy screen, students were provided immediate instruction on independent pain management, warm-up routines away from the instruments prior to playing, and practice strategies. Recommendations for adaptation of musical instrument accessories (shoulder rests, chin rests, supportive equipment for woodwind and brass instruments) were given as well. Contact and discussion with the students' teachers in the program were facilitated for technique or instrumental issues and their interrelationship with the presenting injury. After the screening, some students were cross-referred to nursing and physical therapy and some signed up for the PT sessions directly. Nurses' clinical treatment included heat, ice, and medication. Data and treatment plan for students seen in the PT Assessment and Triage Clinics were recorded (Table 24.1).

When indicated, students were referred to my off-campus Performing Arts Physical Therapy office for follow-up pain management, manual therapy, exercise instruction, postural training, splints, spirometers, and instrument adaptations.

Table 24.1 Physical therapy injury screening: summer 2017 ($N = 12$)

Instrument	Injury	Follow-up plan
Bassoon	Forearm RSI	PAPT
Bass	RCT. Torn during spike ball game	PAPT. Referral to Ortho at MGH for surgical consult
Harp	Wrist joint pain	None necessary
Cello	Sought prevention info	None necessary
Violin	Cervical/thoracic strain	PAPT. No insurance. No treatment
Viola	Forearm RSI	PAPT
Voice	Parry Rhomberg	PAPT
Piano	Lumbrical RSI	None necessary
Piano	Cervical strain	PAPT.
Clarinet	Cervical strain	None necessary
Clarinet	Cervical strain	PAPT in Boston
Flute	TOS	PAPT
	Cubital tunnel syndrome	

Key terminology:
PAPT Performing Arts Physical Therapy
RSI repetitive strain injury
Parry Rhomberg rare connective tissue disease
TOS thoracic outlet syndrome
Cubital Tunnel Syndrome compression or stretching of the ulnar nerve at the cubital tunnel
RCT rotator cuff tear

Instructions on how to maximize private practicing were given in the PT session. These suggestions included utilizing score study, auditory learning, and taking breaks at least every 20 min for 5 min. Some students who presented with peripheral nerve compression involving motor weakness were told not to practice solo repertoire at all and to avoid practicing orchestral repertoire outside of rehearsals. Attending off-campus PT required parental permission for minor-aged children. Lengthy telephone conversations often ensued to discuss the injury, treatment during the duration of the program, and a follow-up plan in their home community after leaving the program. While the on-campus PT Assessment and Triage Clinics were covered by BUTI, the cost of the follow-up PT treatment sessions in the private practice during the duration of the program was not. Out- of-state insurance coverage issues were frequently problematic. These are challenges to be considered for any similar program implementation.

As a result of high dropout rate in class attendance toward the end of the program in 2016, the program organizers moved the classes to the evening TO allow for better attendance. The average wellness class size was 15 with the attendance ranging from 5 to 37. Two classes were more in demand: Body Mapping class was increased to three sessions and the Feldenkrais Method class became weekly.

Only one student out of approximately 140 dropped out in 2017. This was due to a sports-related injury, not a performance-related injury. Anecdotal reports were given for decreased time lost from rehearsals and performances due to injury.

Continuation of the Health and Wellness Series Program in 2018

The Health and Wellness Series grant continued into its second year in 2018. Weekly Physical Therapy assessment and triage clinics continued in the same fashion as in 2017. (Table 24.2). Again, students requiring follow-up PT intervention were seen

Table 24.2 Physical therapy injury screening: summer 2018 ($N = 21$)

Instrument	Injury	Follow-up plan
Double Bass	Cervical strain	Referral to PT in community
Double Bass	Low back pain	None necessary
Cello	Cubital tunnel syndrome	None necessary
Cello	B RCI Cervical/thoracic strain	PAPT
Cello	Left opponens strain	PAPT
Cello	Left lateral epicondylitis	None necessary
Viola	Left UT strain Low back strain	PAPT
Viola	Thoracic strain Chest/sternal pain	PAPT
Violin	Thoracic strain	None necessary
Violin	Cervical spasm, left TMJ pain	PAPT
Violin	Left forearm/wrist RSI	None necessary
Violin	Thoracic strain	PAPT
Violin	Thoracic strain	None necessary
Violin	Cervical/thoracic strain Left upper arm pain	PAPT
Violin	Cervical strain	None necessary
Bassoon	Opponens RSI Right cubital tunnel syndrome	PAPT
Oboe	Right DeQuarvains tenosynovitis Cervical strain	PAPT
Horn	Hypermobility joint syndrome Cervical strain	PAPT
Clarinet	Left TOS Right cubital tunnel syndrome h/o TFCC/EDC tear	PAPT
Trumpet	Cervical/thoracic strain	PAPT
Flute	Cervical/thoracic strain	None necessary

Key terminology:
B RCI rotator cuff injury
UT strain upper trapezius strain
RSI repetitive strain injury
TMJ temporomandibular joint
Left UE left upper extremity
h/o history of
TFCC triangular fibrocartilage complex
EDC tear extensor digitorum communis tear
TOS thoracic outlet syndrome

in my off-campus private office. Treatment for students who required follow-up physical therapy because of PRMP included pain management, manual therapy, exercise instruction, postural training, splints, spirometers, and instrument adaptations. Instructional approaches as similar to 2017 were provided.

Group classes also continued to be held as part of the Health and Wellness Series. No students out of the approximate 140 students in the program dropped out of the BUTI program in 2018. In 2018, evening wellness classes continued and were moved to a larger facility at BUTI to allow for greater numbers of student participation. The tools and information in the classes were intended to develop healthy habits that benefit the body and mind for life. In addition to the regular sessions in Body Mapping, Feldenkrais Method, Alexander Technique, a class in Yoga[4] and overcoming performance anxiety was added.

Conclusions

We observed that the attendance for all disciplines of the Health and Wellness Series in 2018 was clearly higher than the previous year. We notice, however, that attendance at the on-site Physical Therapy Assessment and Triage Sessions was not as high as one might expect considering injury rates described in the literature [9–11]. Reasons for this might be the limited time slots allotted for PT appointments, faculty and students not being aware of services offered, difficulty with direct access to care, and lack of free time to attend appointments. Psychosocial factors may also have contributed to low attendance. These issues, consistent with findings in prior studies [13, 14], may be attributed to feelings of competition with peers, shame due to negative connotations of inferior technical competency, and reluctance to admit pain.

During the years that on-site Physical Therapy was available at the BUTI, no students dropped out of the program due to playing-related injuries. In this chapter, we report that the 12 students who were seen in PT Assessment and Triage sessions in 2017 and the 21 seen in 2018 were able to continue playing in ensembles for the entire program.

On-site Physical Therapy services also allowed teachers in the program to communicate with the provider regarding instrument setup and playing technique and how these factors may have contributed to pain and injury. Recommendations for future programs similar to this model would be developing awareness of the resources, direct referral systems including via faculty, and seamless communication loop among the health care personnel. Particularly, early PT intervention for injury can help decrease time lost from rehearsals and performances [16].

During the BUTI Health and Wellness Series program, a strong community was forged among the healthcare staff, faculty, and parents surrounding the young

[4]Yoga is a Hindu spiritual and ascetic discipline, a part of which, including breath control, simple meditation, and the adoption of specific bodily postures, is widely practiced for health and relaxation.

musicians' life. This communication provided the student musicians, their families, local physical therapy providers, and teachers with the coordinated care for continued treatment upon finishing the program. The program has also provided students with tools for lifelong learning about wellness and injury prevention not only in music-making but also for healthy living through the mind-body awareness approaches of Alexander Technique, Body Mapping, Feldenkrais Method, Mental Skills training, and Yoga.

References

1. Watson A. What can studying musicians tell us about motor control of the hand? J Anat. 2006;208:527–42. https://doi.org/10.1111/j.1469-7580.2006.00545.x.
2. Hyde K, Lerch J, Norton A, Forgeard M, Winner E, Evans AC, Schlaug G. Musical training shapes structural brain development. J Neurosci. 2009;29:3019–25. https://doi.org/10.1523/JNEUROSCI.5118-08.2009.
3. Krause V, Scnitzler A, Pollok B. Functional network interactions during sensorimotor synchronization in musicians and non-musicians. NeuroImage. 2010;52:245–51. https://doi.org/10.1016/j.neuroimage.2010.03.081.
4. Hoenig K, Müller C, Herrnberger B, Sim EJ, Spitzer M, Ehret G, Kiefer M. Neuroplasticity of semantic representations for musical instruments in professional musicians. NeuroImage. 2011;56:1714–25. https://doi.org/10.1016/j.neuroimage.2011.02.065.
5. Ackermann BJ, Driscoll T, Kenny DT. Musculoskeletal pain and injury in professional orchestral musicians in Australia. Med Probl Perform Art. 2012;27(4):181–7.
6. Middlestadt S, Fishbein M. The prevalence of severe musculoskeletal problems among male and female symphony orchestra string players. Med Probl Perform Art. 1989;4:41–8.
7. Leaver RE, Harris EC, Palmer KT. Musculoskeletal pain in elite professional musicians from British symphony orchestras. Occup Med. 2011;61:549–55. https://doi.org/10.1093/occmed/kqr129.
8. Paarup HM, Baelum J, Holm JW, Manniche C, Wedderkopp N. Prevalence and consequences of musculoskeletal symptoms in symphony orchestra musicians vary by gender: a cross-sectional study. BMC Musculoskelet Disord. 2011;12:223. https://doi.org/10.1186/1471-2474-12-223.
9. Ranelli S. Hand and upper limb playing-related musculoskeletal problems in children learning instrumental music: the influence of gender, age and type of instrument. J Hand Ther. 2010;23(4):433.
10. Britsch L. Investigating performance-related problems of young musicians. Med Probl Perform Art. 2015;20(1):40–7.
11. McCready S, Reid D. The experience of occupational disruption among student musicians. Med Probl Perform Art. 2007;22:140–6.
12. Rickert DL, Barrett MS, Ackermann B. Injury and the orchestral environment: part I. Med Probl Perform Art. 2013;28:219–29.
13. Guptill CA. The lived experience of professional musicians with playing- related injuries: a phenomenological inquiry. Med Probl Perform Art. 2011;26:84–95.
14. Guptill CA. Injured professional musicians and the complex relationship between occupation and health. J Occup Sci. 2012;19:258–70. https://doi.org/10.1080/14427591.2012.670901.
15. Altenmüller E, Jabusch HC. Focal dystonia in musicians: phenomenology, pathophysiology and triggering factors. Eur J Neurol. 2010;17(Suppl. 1):31–6. https://doi.org/10.1111/j.1468-1331.2010.03048.x.

16. Chan C, Driscoll T, Ackermann B. The usefulness of on-site physical therapy-led triage services for professional orchestral musicians – a national cohort study. BMC Musculoskelet Disord. 2013;14:98–106.
17. Brown J. New initiative helps BU Tanglewood Institute students stay well to play well. In BU Today, July 26, 2019. http://www.bu.edu/articles/2019/new-initiative-helps-bu-tanglewood-institute-students-stay-well-to-play-well/. Accessed Aug 2019.
18. Zaza C. Prevention of musicians' playing-related health problems: rationale and recommendations for action. Med Probl Perform Art. 1993;8:117–21.
19. Boston University Tanglewood Institute. http://www.bu.edu/cfa/tanglewood/. Accessed Aug 2019.

Chapter 25
Clinical Care of Performing Arts Students in the University Setting: A Successful Model with Wide Potential

Jeffrey A. Russell

Introduction: The Case for University Performing Arts Healthcare

University performing artists are just as deserving and needful of clinical healthcare as any other performing artists. While their relative youth may provide extra durability and resistance to certain demands of their artistic endeavors, they nonetheless experience a substantial number of injuries, although available data on performing arts injury in this age group are focused primarily on dance [1–8]. University performing arts programs—by nature of their mission to educate, explore, and push boundaries—typically offer a progressive repertoire, regardless of the art form. This may be one reason for the injury rates seen in university-affiliated performers, and it is well established that performing artists overall, in universities and other venues, exhibit a high injury rate [1, 2, 6, 9–14]. In this chapter, "university" refers not just to institutions that technically or nominally are universities, but also to colleges, junior colleges, community colleges, conservatories, and other academic settings where performing artists typically are between the ages of 18 and 26. Moreover, this chapter is written with a broad view of what constitutes an "artist." Herein, any of the talented individuals associated with the wide variety of crafts required to produce a performance are categorized as performing artists, not just the stage performers themselves. This includes designers, stagehands, choreographers, stage managers, costume shop workers, and others.

J. A. Russell (✉)
Clinic for Science and Health in Artistic Performance, Division of Athletic Training,
School of Applied Health Sciences and Wellness, College of Health Sciences and Professions,
Ohio University, Athens, OH, USA
e-mail: jeff.russell@ohio.edu

S.-H. Lee et al. (eds.), *Perspectives in Performing Arts Medicine Practice*,
https://doi.org/10.1007/978-3-030-37480-8_25

Whereas students represent a vulnerable population being guided under the authority of (and, in some ways, essentially subservient to) professors, administrators, and others at their institutions, it is incumbent upon a university to ensure that any health conditions that present themselves are adequately managed. Indeed, university arts accreditation bodies that fall under the Council of Arts Accrediting Associations—specifically the performing arts ones: the National Association of Schools of Dance, National Association of Schools of Music, and National Association of Schools of Theater—require attention to the health and welfare of performing arts students as outlined in their accrediting documentation [15–17], though much laterality is given for how to accomplish this. Text from the handbook of the National Association of Schools of Dance [15] offers conceptual guidance in its standards that is common to all three of these accrediting bodies:

> Students enrolled in dance unit programs and faculty and staff with employment status in the dance unit must be provided basic information about the maintenance of health and safety within the contexts of studio practice, rehearsal, and performance.
>
> For dance majors and dance faculty and staff, general topics include, but are not limited to, basic information regarding the maintenance of musculoskeletal health and injury prevention. They also include instruction on facilities and equipment hygiene, and the use, proper handling, and operation of potentially dangerous materials, equipment, and technology as applicable to specific program offerings or experiences…
>
> Dance program policies, protocols, and operations must reflect attention to maintenance of health and injury prevention and to the relationships among: the health and safety of dancers; suitable choices of equipment and technology for various specific purposes; appropriate and safe operation of equipment and technology; and other conditions associated with health and safety in practice, rehearsal, and performance facilities.
>
> Specific methods of providing information and addressing injury prevention, technology, and facilities are the prerogative and responsibility of the institution. (pp. 67–68)

Within the framework that university performing arts students are deserving of specialized healthcare, the purpose of this chapter is to focus on outlining several mechanisms by which such care can be delivered while also considering some of the intricacies of doing so.

This chapter will:

1. Outline the facets of performing arts healthcare that should be addressed in a university setting.
2. Explain the challenges inherent in providing performing arts healthcare to university students.
3. Identify the roles of various professionals in providing care and which professionals should be considered as potential contributors to a comprehensive healthcare team.
4. Describe appropriate methods for providing performing arts medicine care to university performing artists.

Foundations of Providing Healthcare to University Performing Artists

Artists often are idiosyncratic in their approach to life. This must be respected if a healthcare professional expects to provide care effectively. Unfortunately, performing artists report many distasteful experiences with the healthcare profession [1, 18–20]. This may drive some artists away from traditional practitioners, but it surely frustrates all of them. This is not surprising; every individual deserves to be treated with respect and to be given the opportunity to explain their injury or disease to a qualified professional.

Factors in Healthcare Delivery

In its attempt to reconstitute the way healthcare is delivered in the United States, the Institute of Medicine [21], an organization formed under the congressional charter of the National Academy of Sciences, adopted six aims that originally were proposed by Gerteis et al. [22] in their book *Through the Patient's Eyes: Understanding and Promoting Patient-Centered Care*. These aims should be incorporated into any patient care and certainly are appropriate for inclusion in a performing arts medicine clinical venue, including one at a university. Most, if not all, of these seem as though they should be intuitive in any healthcare delivery, but, as stated above, clearly there is a disconnect between many healthcare practitioners and performing artists.

1. *Patients' values, preferences, and expressed needs should be understood and respected.* This is the fundamental characteristic that should be exhibited by any healthcare professional. In one study, 70% of surveyed dancers cited not being understood as their most common reason for having a poor experience with a practitioner [1]. Neglecting this facet is particularly egregious in the arts because of the presence of a broad range of views, tastes, lifestyle choices, gender identities, and, even, appearance choices such as clothing, hair style and color, makeup, and tattoos. Most university environments provide a haven for these modes of individualism. Artists whom some might view as far out of the societal mainstream gravitate toward the arts because they feel safer there from judgment and ridicule than they do in more traditional fields. Thus, it is necessary for those in healthcare to establish a rapport with artistic patients that is built on human value and respect, if not agreement. This then forms the foundation for the artist to receive healthcare advice and intervention.
2. *Patients' care should be coordinated and integrated.* Artists (and every other type of medical patient) become frustrated when caregivers appear to not be communicating with one another. Certainly there is room for individual differences in care approaches, second and third opinions, and other normal

alternatives. However, when continuity of care is disrupted because practitioners do not review prior records, or when they simply do not work together as a team in delivering care, patients are the ones who are adversely affected and a clash develops between a patient's needs and a provider's service.

3. *Clinicians should provide information, communication, and education to patients*. The days of clinicians "protecting" patients from their medical records are long over. While artists often do not have a scientific background, they nonetheless are capable of understanding medical terms and concepts when they receive proper explanations. Many clinicians would be surprised to find how astute artists are about matters of their medical care. Details matter in artistic performance, so the vast majority of performing artists have little trouble also comprehending the details of their injuries or conditions. Moreover, they have a legal right to this information as established by the Health Insurance Portability and Accountability Act (HIPAA) [23, 24].
4. *Clinicians should ensure physical comfort of the patient*. Pain as a physical construct spills over heavily to the emotions and affects activities of daily living along with the physical function of artistic endeavors. Artists' relationship to pain is substantially different than that of non-artists, and the "dance through it," "play through it," "get through it" mentality is widespread among artists [9, 25–30]. Interestingly enough, therefore, practitioners may never have the opportunity to address the physical comfort aspect of care—or the opportunity will be delayed until a patient's condition increases in severity—because many artists simply will ignore their symptoms and not seek healthcare.
5. *Clinicians should provide emotional support to the patient*. Performing artists often are naturally emotive in their responses, and this may impact their interaction with healthcare providers. In addition, the emotional dimension of wellness [31] may be the one dimension of wellness that is most tightly tied to each of the others. Thus, the importance of appreciating the emotions when caring for university performing artists cannot be overstated.
6. *Clinicians should involve family and friends in the patient's care*. Social support is a crucial aspect of patient care. Obviously this depends wholly on the patient's willingness to allow family and friends to be part of the process. Clinicians customarily are bound by confidentiality guidelines such as those of HIPAA. However, within this type of necessary constraint, performing arts students' parents, friends, classmates, and professors all can provide assistance with ensuring patient compliance, adherence, progress, and well-being.

Tzelepis et al. [32] suggest that patient-reported measures are the best way to identify the extent to which patients' needs are met and, thus, whether healthcare is truly "patient-centered." There is a wide variety of measures of quality musculoskeletal care [33], a presentation of which is beyond the scope of this chapter. However, it is important in any performing arts medicine system that the artists' view of their care is both considered and measured, rather than it being neglected by clinicians operating on the assumption that the artist-patients' needs are being met.

Artists generally are well attuned to signals sent by their bodies. Since many subscribe to somatic practices, they are trained to "listen" to what their bodies "speak." Additionally, performing artists have a keen sense of body awareness simply because their bodies are integral to their performances; that is, they have to pay close attention in order to accomplish their performing. This body sense can be both an advantage and disadvantage. It is advantageous when an artist can clearly explain symptoms that assist a provider in making a diagnosis. On the other hand, it may be a disadvantage when these "tuned in" sensations receive focus that is too heavy and, consequently, magnified to the extent that relatively minor issues are portrayed as major ones [34]. This may be a particularly acute problem if an artist feels that their performing career is threatened [25].

Factors in Artist Wellness

University performing artists are in an important training period of their careers. The academic environment lays the foundation—for better or worse—from which they launch into professional performance, education, administration, or other roles related to performing arts. In this formative stage, they also are able to establish—or eschew—healthy practices in physical fitness, nutrition, rest, alcohol consumption, tobacco and drug use, and other areas. Those decisions to establish or eschew may depend on the quality and frequency of positive messages and reinforcement offered by their professors, directors, healthcare providers, and other influencers in their university lives.

Also germane to a discussion of how individual differences affect performing arts healthcare in university students are the six dimensions of wellness defined by Hettler [31]. These apply to all individuals, but require special attention in students because of the concentrated, stressful nature of an academic environment. In practice, none of the six stands alone; they are intertwined and interdependent, and can be confounding if not sufficiently regarded by a healthcare practitioner. The six dimensions are:

1. Physical—pertains to one's tangible, anatomical, and physiological body
2. Emotional—pertains to one's feelings and reactions to circumstances
3. Intellectual—pertains to one's thought processes, learning, and decisions
4. Social—pertains to the communities of people of which one is a member, for example, family, friends, classmates, artistic collaborators
5. Occupational—pertains to the vocational work or career of a person (in students, this usually is considered to be their academic work)
6. Spiritual—pertains to one's connection to a personal, transcendent purpose that extends beyond oneself and the immediate environment

In order to understand how these six dimensions relate to the delivery of healthcare to artists, consider a dancer with a sprained ankle, a pianist suffering from DeQuervain's syndrome in the wrist, or a theater technician who sustained a concussion. In each case there is a physical injury, and that is what most healthcare practitioners focus on because, after all, that is what is obvious and urgent. However, in all three of these cases it is likely that the performers will require healing time away from their art form. This creates one of the most difficult challenges for any healthcare professional working with artists, whether at the university level or elsewhere: artists are reticent to take time away for injury management and recuperation.

In requiring any of the artists in the three examples above to take time off, the physical dimension immediately, significantly, and negatively impacts the emotional dimension—possibly eliciting anger, frustration, or depression; the occupational dimension—artistic classes, rehearsals, and performances will be missed, possibly lowering a student's course grades; the social dimension—removal from a community in which the artist has established camaraderie; and the intellectual dimension—the negativity of the circumstances, and sometimes desperation to return to artistic activity. The ultimate result of this may be poor decision-making in other areas of life. Moreover, if the injury is severe enough and time loss is extensive, the situation may influence the performer's spiritual sense of adding value to others and their connection to their life's purpose. It is easily seen, then, how what may seem to be a relatively straightforward physical injury can proliferate adversity across most, if not all, dimensions of an artist's wellness. In summary, it is incumbent on performing arts medicine practitioners to assess and attend to the breadth of their patients' beings when delivering care. With six dimensions comprising true whole person care, neglecting one or more of these will yield a *hole* in the patient's *whole*.

Factors Related to the Nature of Performing Arts

Finally, healthcare practitioners must understand certain differences between sports and performing arts, as even a sports medicine model—the best model on which to base performing arts medicine care—must be adapted and adjusted if it is to serve artists well. Table 25.1 provides a comparison between some aspects of a sports performance environment and their parallels in performing arts. (It is noted that the aquatic sports are an entirely different type of activity with their own peculiarities.) Healthcare workers showing performing artists that they recognize the distinctions and are willing to accommodate their care plans accordingly is part of patient-centered care in performing arts medicine and will make the care delivery much more effective and enjoyable for both parties.

Certainly traditional athletes strive for excellence and perfection; however, the pursuit of perfection can become the bane of the performing artist. What is considered a successful performance in sports may have many allowable failures. In baseball, for instance, errors are publicly posted on the scoreboard. Ice hockey players who commit an infraction are placed on display in the penalty box for all to see. In basketball, hitting only 50 shots out of 100 yields a very decent shooting percentage of 50%. On the other hand, imagine posting a dancer's choreographic misstep on an electronic display

Table 25.1 A comparison of features between university sports and performing arts

	Sports	Performing arts
Attire	Uniforms, activity appropriate sportswear	Wardrobes, costumes
Footwear	Cleats, sneakers, skates, ski boots/skis	Character shoes, pointe shoes, ballet slippers, jazz shoes, pedestrian shoes, no shoes (e.g., modern dance)
Performing facilities	Stadium, arena, gymnasium, track, outdoor course, ice rink, ski slope	Studio, stage, theatrical set, movie set, backstage, prop shop, costume shop
Ground or floor surface	Grass, artificial turf, wood court, clay court, track, ice, snow	Wood floor, sprung wood floor, concrete, vinyl ("marley"), grass, artificial turf, roadway (e.g., marching band)
Practice/ rehearsal time	Relatively short practice times (usually, and when compared to performing arts)	Extensive practice and rehearsal times (often 6–10 h per day, sometimes more)
Seasons	Pre-season, in-season, off-season	Rarely a true off-season

above the stage or sending an actor who forgot a piece of his lines to sit for 2 min in the "penalty chair" at downstage right (or for 5 min if he forgot several lines!). How would we view a symphony musician, concert pianist, or opera singer who hits only 50 notes correctly out of every 100? The lunacy of such suggestions confirms the pressure artists are under to perform perfectly. This drive must be accounted for and thoughtfully managed by healthcare providers who care for the artists.

Specific caveats are present in many types of care. For example, the nature of performing arts costuming may prevent some types of taping or bracing that practitioners would be accustomed to applying in traditional sports. On the other hand, certain types of costuming may allow the application of musculoskeletal appliances crafted to facilitate participation while reducing the risk of further injury because the costume can hide the protective device. In dancers especially, necessary range of motion of the foot and ankle necessitates significant adaptation of standard sports taping techniques.

Footwear also can be a complicating factor in caring for artists. A pointe shoe has very little space for tape or padding applications, while a ballet slipper provides little support compared to a sports sneaker. A narrow, elevated heel on a character shoe may predispose a performer to ankle sprains. In modern or contemporary dancers who rarely wear any sort of shoes while dancing, choices for taping, padding, and orthotics are extremely limited, especially if they would compromise a dancer's crucial interface between the foot and the floor.

The likelihood of overuse and lack of rest is high in university performing artists, especially when the demands of a performing arts degree program are coupled with the already frequent tendency for students to work late at night and into early mornings. The typical lack of a true off-season—either self-imposed by students anxious to build their "chops" by gaining as much experience as possible or simply as a matter of the typical university calendar combined with students' elective summer intensives schedule—compounds this problem.

University Performing Arts Components Requiring Care

The primary performing arts disciplines found in university environments are dance, music, theater, and marching band. Activities such as gymnastics, rhythmic gymnastics, and synchronized swimming clearly have artistic components, but are classified as sports. In between pure performing arts and performance sports lie cheerleading and dance team (or entertainment dance). Artistic purists would exclude these two from performing arts, and some universities view them as sports teams, especially since their role is to support teams in competition by heightening the fan experience at athletic contests. However, often these groups' members fall into a gap where they do not receive medical attention from their university's intercollegiate athletic department, nor do they qualify as performing artists if their university provides a performing arts medicine clinic.

Two other considerations inform the categorization of performing arts in the university environment. First, theater may best be subdivided into performance (i.e., actors) and production (e.g., designers, stage managers, technicians, and so on), because these two divisions usually are under different types of demands. Second, while marching band is certainly music (and may be housed in the music department in most universities), a band's members may be drawn largely from students in non-music majors. For example, at Ohio University only about 15% of the 240 marching musicians are housed within the music school. The rest are spread through diverse areas of study across campus.

Theater initiates a fascinating discussion in performing arts medicine. Of the performing arts mentioned above, it may be the one that receives the least amount of attention from physicians, athletic trainers, physical therapists, and other healthcare professionals in a university setting. While stage combat may be one obvious theater subdiscipline in which potential injury can be surmised, less apparent is the physicality required of actors in many theater performances. Furthermore, the danger inherent in on-stage sets and props is not obvious because watching talented actors can lull an audience member into thinking that performing carries minimal risk. Even less conspicuous are the backstage spaces that actors must pass through during performances and where technicians work to produce the show.

Of course, virtually all performing art forms make use of stagehands, electricians, carpenters, lighting technicians, and similar individuals who support theatrical or entertainment performances. The opportunities for injury in these individuals are essentially limitless [35–38], with occupational health and safety serving as a crucial medical specialty in such venues.

Circus arts may be pooled with theater for the purpose of performing arts medicine care delivery. There is a small, but gradually increasing, body of literature pertaining to this art form [6, 39–45]. Intense, audience-thrilling, and danger-ridden Cirque du Soleil-style performances are the pinnacle of achievement in this genre; thus, the need for injury prevention and care is intuitive. Similarly, high-energy theatrical productions such as *Spiderman* have an added measure of injury risk, and, indeed, serious injuries do occur [46]. Finally, stunt performers are a population of performers whose likelihood of sustaining an injury seems predetermined, at least to the casual onlooker [47, 48]. While minimal medical literature exists on this topic [49, 50], and most universities do not administer training programs in stunt work, the inclusion of its artists in a performing arts healthcare program certainly is warranted whenever feasible.

Film, media, and visual arts represent artistic practices that may not be considered purely performing arts in a university context. However, film students may fall under the theater-related area of entertainment mentioned above, depending on the nature of their department and course of study. Although Ohio University's performing arts medicine clinic's remit does not officially extend to these majors, from time-to-time these students report with injuries because of the clinic's reputation for specialized, artistic-minded care. Clearly, individuals in these art forms are prone to physical afflictions and, therefore, deserving of healthcare; but, their care is not within the purview of this chapter.

Special Concerns Related to University Students and the Academic Environment

There are characteristics of a university environment and of university students that require recognition and accounting for when providing performing arts medicine care. These create stress on students beyond the obvious pressure of managing an academic workload and maintaining satisfactory grades. With a view toward the whole-person care described previously, possible detriments to several of the six dimensions described by Hettler [31] are relatively easy to deduce.

Being away from home, potentially for the first time or across a long distance, may manifest itself in a couple of different ways. One is the expected loneliness and missing parents, siblings, and hometown friends, especially until a university peer group is established. However, the stress of being away in a new place also may interact with the concurrent freedom from parent-imposed structure and ready availability of destructive social influences such as environments where alcohol and drugs are abused. Additionally, many students' angst stems from interpersonal problems with others, such as a boyfriend, girlfriend, or parent, or from constant worry about finances, which includes the increasingly common practice of incurring an overwhelming debt load to complete a university education [51, 52].

On top of stress exuding from the academic environment, additional stressors on university students exist in performing arts themselves. All performers must wrestle with negative feedback and not being called back during an audition process. Additionally, the countless hours dancers, musicians, theater performers, and other theater personnel spend honing their work and the fear that sustaining an injury or illness will remove them from performances or, worse, cause them to lose their place to another artist, are constantly present. As noted earlier, artists strive for excellence by the very nature of performing. However, taken to an extreme, perfectionism, overachieving, and overscheduling also seem to be common challenges throughout performing arts.

In dance, there is a tendency toward perfectionism and fitting oneself into a preconceived, yet often unrealistic, physical appearance mold. These two issues are especially prevalent in classical ballet. Most dancers practice with the ubiquitous mirrors; research suggests that in ballet mirrors may negatively impact dancers' perceptions of themselves [53], particularly high level dancers compared to low level [54]. Some evidence also suggests that mirrors reduce, rather than improve, the effectiveness of ballet teaching [55].

Medical literature about artistic performance anxiety is weighted heavily toward music [56–58], though dance is represented, as well [59]. Overall, any time one is required to perform in front of an audience the potential for performance anxiety—which can be absolutely debilitating in some artists—is present.

In theater, common sources of stress to which students may be subjected include learning and remembering one's lines, timing of stage entries and exits, and cues for lights, curtains, and the like. Unfortunately, errors in any of these are readily apparent on stage, which is the basic reason why they are stressful. Contending with performance anxiety also is a very real battle in theater. Other stressors may evolve from tension between a principal actor and their understudy and the extremely long and late-night hours university students often spend in their theater spaces. Furthermore, this latter time factor may directly conflict with the time students need to engage with their non-theater studies.

Healthcare Providers Who Work with University Performing Artists

Types of Healthcare Professionals

There is a wide variety of healthcare specialists who bring important expertise to performing arts medicine. As a general rule, performing artists benefit when healthcare providers work together as a team, and when artistic staff such as professors and directors are included. The Institute of Medicine's [21] admonition that patient care be coordinated and integrated is a key to ensuring the team approach is successful. Table 25.2 lists the healthcare professionals who commonly attend to performing artists. The involvement of any of these obviously depends on the framework with which a university's performing arts medicine program is created, the medical environment of a given campus and its surrounding community, and the resources available for enlisting these providers.

It is critically important within the context of performing arts that a firm distinction be made between healthcare professionals who are licensed to practice by their state or national professional association and non-licensed professionals who commonly interface with performing artists and may be presented with an artist's injury or illness. The latter category includes individuals like professors; teachers; artistic

Table 25.2 Types of healthcare professionals commonly working in performing arts medicine

Physicians
Doctor of Medicine
Doctor of Osteopathy
Specialties:
Orthopedic Surgery
Sports Medicine
Non-surgical Orthopedics (e.g., Sports Medicine Trained Primary Care Physician)
Physical Medicine and Rehabilitation (Physiatry)
Occupational Medicine
Osteopathic Manipulative Medicine
Otolaryngology/Laryngology
Neurology
Psychiatry
Primary Care (e.g., Family Practice, Internal Medicine, Gynecology, Pediatrics, Geriatrics)
Other specialists as needed
Doctor of Dental Surgery or **Doctor of Medicine in Dentistry** (Dentist)
Doctor of Podiatric Medicine (Podiatrist)
Doctor of Chiropractic (Chiropractor)
Allied Health Professionals
Athletic Trainer
Physical Therapist
Occupational Therapist
Certified Hand Therapist
Audiologist
Vocologist
Speech-Language Pathologist
Dietitian
Massage Therapist
Acupuncturist
Psychologist/Clinical Psychologist/Sports Psychologist
Licensed Professional Counselor
Complementary/Alternative Practitioners

directors; stage managers; Pilates, Yoga, Gyrotonics, Alexander, and similar somatic practice instructors; personal trainers; and kinesiologists. None of these people, as well-meaning as they may be, should undertake the evaluation and treatment of an injury or illness. However, their expertise—especially of the teachers and directors who are around the students virtually constantly and know the students best—should be viewed as extremely valuable to any healthcare professional providing performing arts care. A relationship established between a practitioner and the artistic and ancillary staff can be a key asset in patient compliance.

As an example, in dance it has been reported that the most common individual to whom dancers report their injuries is their dance teacher [1, 60]; as many as 80% of survey respondents indicated this was their practice [1]. While certainly logical that this occurs, dance teachers are not, in most cases, licensed as healthcare practitioners and should, therefore, avoid acting as such. Wang and Russell [1] recommend strong adherence to this principle, though they also encourage healthcare professionals to include teachers and other artistic personnel in communication linkages, so long as a patient gives permission for this to occur. This type of communication helps reduce anxiety in the artist and the performance production staff, while promoting the likelihood that follow-up care guidelines are understood and followed.

A word about complementary and alternative care providers is warranted here, as well. These are somewhat difficult to classify, and some of the professionals in Table 25.2 practice complementary (in addition to traditional methods) or alternative (in place of traditional methods) healthcare. Though many complementary and alternative practitioners' methods are not researched well, performing artists frequently gravitate toward this type of caregiver, presumably because, at least in part, they are dissatisfied with traditional allopathic practitioners. In one study of dancers, 6% of surveyed respondents indicated they visited a naturopath and 1% reported visiting a reflexologist [1]. In another study, 9% of dancers surveyed saw an Eastern medicine practitioner for their injuries [60]. However, it is suspected that the actual numbers of performing artists who consult complementary or alternative healthcare providers is considerably higher than that. The reader is referred to the National Center for Complementary and Integrative Health of the National Institutes of Health for further information about these techniques and research surrounding them [61].

Practical Guidelines for Performing Artist Patients and Clinicians

As previously mentioned, performing artists may be less than enthusiastic about healthcare practitioners, and most can recount unfavorable incidents they have experienced. Much of this can be avoided if both the artist-patient and the clinician approach the consultation correctly. Both parties have their own contributions to make to ensure success.

The artist should compile a list of specific symptoms associated with their clinical complaint and another list of questions that pertain to understanding the condition or injury and its treatment, and then take the lists to the healthcare appointment. The lists should be concise and focused, as they will form the framework for an intelligent conversation with one's healthcare practitioner.

An artist must respect the healthcare provider's time. While research has shown that many university dancers do not feel that their clinicians spent enough time with them [1], every practitioner is extremely busy and under great pressure to move through their clinic schedule. As a patient, the artist should not expect that all of their aches and pains can be evaluated in one visit ("Since I'm here, can you also look at…?"), or that they are owed unlimited amounts of conversation with the provider. Artists must be considerate, respectful, and try to view the visit from a healthcare delivery perspective as well as one's own.

Healthcare practitioners generally respond well to patients who are gracious and grateful. The artist should thank the practitioner for serving with their talents and skills, even if not 100% satisfied that every need was addressed or every question was answered. Clinicians are experts, but are neither omniscient nor magicians. The artist-patient will often be quite astounded by what can be accomplished and how well the patient–practitioner relationship develops when a gracious attitude is presented.

In caring for performers, healthcare practitioners can do much to ensure a successful visit and a content patient. Understanding the rigors of the artists' art forms and appreciating the physical and other sacrifices they make to participate in the arts are paramount. One way to do this is by attending arts performances, something that dancers have reported to be the most important indicator of their healthcare provider's interest in them [19].

During the appointment, the clinician should take sufficient time to learn how the artist's injury occurred and appreciate both the mechanism and the artist's valuable perspective about it. Furthermore, the practitioner must acknowledge how devastating the injury is to the artist's life and provide reassurance about both the diagnosis and the treatment. All in all, the elements of patient-centered care previously cited will serve as the underpinnings to support these efforts.

Practical Implementation of Care for University Performing Artists

Injuries to performing artists, including to university performers, are predominantly musculoskeletal in nature. Thus, any university performing arts medicine service should be well equipped to manage these. However, non-musculoskeletal injuries, conditions, and diseases are frequently encountered, with cardiovascular, internal/abdominal, infectious disease, gynecological, laryngological, and dental being the ones usually seen. Mental health conditions also frequently must be confronted, including eating disorders, substance use disorder, bipolar disorder, borderline personality disorder, anxiety disorder, depression, and others. In 2017, the percentage of Americans ages 18–25 years who suffered from a mental illness was 25.8%; females are substantially more likely than males to suffer mental illness in this age category (31.9–19.8%) [62]. The treatment of mental illness in performers should not be confused with the use of artistic methods and media as a psychological intervention. The latter includes the professions of music therapy, dance movement therapy, and drama therapy, to name a few. These comprise effective techniques for ameliorating a variety of mental illnesses; however, they are not germane to this chapter's topic.

Table 25.3 lists several types of services that will benefit university performing artists if the services are provided. While a university performing arts medicine clinic may not offer all of them, it will serve artist-patients well if mechanisms for referral to specialists in the appropriate fields are arranged prior to them needing to be implemented.

Table 25.3 Types of services ideally offered in university performing arts clinics

Injury evaluation
Injury treatment
Injury rehabilitation
Injury prevention
Taping, bracing, padding, consultation about musculoskeletal appliances, and adaptation of appliances and wardrobes for performances
On-site event care
Facility safety consultations
Emergency care
Fitness prescription
Nutritional counseling
Mental health counseling
Specialist care referrals
Surgical care referrals

Several different applications of performing arts medicine programs are available at universities around the United States, though such care is infinitely short of universal. Despite poor data availability that cannot identify an exact number, it is anecdotally accepted by clinicians who operate these programs that they are not commonplace, even though the number of university arts programs nationwide is considerable. Among United States universities, colleges, junior colleges, and community colleges, approximately 1203 have some type of dance program [63] (83 dance programs are accredited by the National Association of Schools of Dance [64]); 1579 have some sort of musical ensemble program [65]; 1182 report offering concert band [66]; 433 sponsor marching band programs [67] (643 music programs are accredited by the National Association of Schools of Music [68]); and 1905 have some type of theater or drama program [69] (184 theater programs are accredited by the National Association of Schools of Theatre [70]). While the data include overlap of programs within universities, the point of these tabulations is to demonstrate that there are numerous performing arts programs—and, therefore, very large numbers of potential artist-patients—embedded in American universities.

Implementing Healthcare for University Performers

There are several possible scenarios by which a university can deliver healthcare to its performing arts students and faculty. Funding is routinely the keystone issue that prevents more universities from proceeding with plans to implement a performing arts medicine program. The common denominator, however, is an alliance between the arts and the health sciences, and this must be established at the outset in order to set a foundation on which funding and all other components can successfully be built.

Common adjectives usually used in universities to describe this type of partnership are multidisciplinary (two or more disciplines working on a project, with each remaining essentially autonomous in its contribution), interdisciplinary (collaboration of two or more disciplines, with the knowledge of each being integrated for the project), and transdisciplinary (collaboration of two or more disciplines that is so close that the typical lines between them are blurred and, as a result, novel approaches to the project are created). While some may consider distinctions among these to be esoteric minutiae, there are points about the three paths to collaborating that should be contemplated by those spearheading a university-based performing arts medicine program.

At its core, performing arts medicine provided within a university certainly combines at least two disciplines, making it multidisciplinary. However, by its very name and how it operates, it also bridges divides between artistic (performing arts) and scientific (medicine) fields, thus making it interdisciplinary, as well. As summarized by Toomey et al. [71] interdisciplinary effort is "an integrated approach to answering a question that recognizes the limitations inherent in the compartmentalized system of academic research" (p. 1).

In practice, though, performing arts medicine encompasses qualities that are not just multidisciplinary or interdisciplinary, but also transdisciplinary, with the latter being the ultimate, altruistic hallmark of any university's healthcare plan for performing artists. Toomey et al. [71] frame the context for this: "Trans-disciplinary work moves beyond the bridging of divides within academia to engaging directly with the production and use of knowledge outside of the academy" (p. 1).

To practically apply this in performing arts medicine, then, a well-planned, well-executed program should strive to meet the more expansive, far-reaching definition of transdisciplinary by exerting positive, beyond-the-campus influence on the community in which the university is located, on the field of performing arts medicine, and on the health and wellness practices of professional artistic companies. For example, when properly trained, a university's performing arts students will become conveyers of this transdisciplinary effort as they bring their knowledge of proper wellness, self-care, and healthcare to the field upon graduating and seeking employment as artists.

Incorporating the above schema as a basis, I have developed performing arts medicine programs at three different universities and discussed with many colleagues how to construct their own versions at their universities. I also have been privileged to work with some of the most dedicated, hardworking people I know: the artistic colleagues—professors, directors, choreographers, performers, technicians, etc.—I have partnered with over the years. These experiences yield insights that hopefully will help the reader initiate a similar arrangement.

Invariably, there will be roadblocks to developing a university performing arts medicine program; as noted above, funding will be chief among these. At its core, no program will succeed without some permutation of an energetic, symbiotic partnership between the performing arts and the health sciences. Most of the time the process will be spearheaded by passionate arts faculty who recognize the need for such an offering and who pursue mechanisms for bringing the idea to fruition by contacting potential healthcare partners. Regardless of the methods incorporated or the challenges encountered, several characteristics within a partnership will increase the likelihood of success. Four principal pillars are described below.

Mutual respect The partnership will not—indeed cannot—subsist without respect between the artists and the healthcare providers. Backpedaling and apologizing are poor balms for the wounds of disrespect, and trust may never be restored if it is broken. It is very possible that, unless a healthcare practitioner comes from an artistic background (certainly a wonderful ally for any artist trying to establish a partnership for performing arts medicine), those from the arts and those from healthcare will have very different views about life, about the university environment and about how to solve problems. Rather than being wedges that divide, these differences should be celebrated, enjoyed, and explored for how they can add value to the partnership. In the end, everyone must remember and focus on the mission: to set up a mechanism by which performing arts students can receive healthcare. If one does not respect another as a person, he or she will never respect another as an artist or a healthcare practitioner.

Creativity First and foremost, artists are creative people. Healthcare workers typically are, as well, but in a different context. Thus, bringing creative partners together yields the kind of brainstorming and idea generation required to develop a plan and continue to retool it to accommodate to the university environment and overcome the adversity that is virtually guaranteed to arise. In other words, creative minds have the capacity to think "out-of-the-box" that is necessary to keep moving forward by assessing the current landscape and finding alternate routes.

There are many ways that performing arts faculty and their students can build mutually beneficial relationships with those in the health science departments, intercollegiate athletics, the student health center, or elsewhere. Two examples are inviting these colleagues to performances, potentially including an offer of complimentary tickets (remembering that one of the chief desires performing artists have for their healthcare providers is that the providers attend performances [19]) and bringing small, mobile performing ensembles to the buildings where healthcare colleagues work and non-arts students attend classes. Celebrating the creativity of the arts around non-artists has great potential for fostering collegiality.

Tenacity Closely allied with creativity, and certainly a logical corollary, is tenacity. Tenacity simply is a refusal to give up. It is one's creativity that continues to enable one's success; tenacity is the fuel that drives this forward and focuses one's effort to persevere when challenges and obstacles arise. Sadly, many artists are too acquainted with adversity; yet, as a result they have developed the ability to be tenacious. Whether struggling for jobs that make ends meet financially, finding funding for arts programs, or determining some way to manage an injury, artists continue to press forward in the face of difficulty and long odds. Although, to repeat, such circumstances are unfortunate, respecting the quality of tenacity and channeling its positive potential is a key aspect of bringing performing arts healthcare to a university environment.

A Healthcare Champion Ultimately, healthcare cannot be delivered unless properly qualified and licensed healthcare workers are accessible. Many arts faculty dream of—and even plan—programs to provide performing arts medicine care, yet are left unfulfilled because they cannot find a healthcare champion. That champion is the one who not only is passionate to partner with the arts faculty to establish a clinical environment that serves the performing artists in their university, but has the "chops" necessary to deliver the care or coordinate others to provide it.

Types of Facilities for University Performing Arts Medicine

To follow are four main methods by which university performing artists can receive healthcare. This is not an exhaustive list as there are many permutations that can be customized to a given university's environment. Nonetheless, these basic types offer some structure and ideas for a university that desires to initiate a program to care for its performers. Major advantages and disadvantages of each are provided in Table 25.4.

Performing Arts Medicine Clinic

This option is a bespoke facility dedicated exclusively to caring for performing artists at the university. In such a scenario, the university will have made a significant commitment to the specialized care delivery required by performers. In the majority of instances, the clinic will be staffed primarily by athletic trainers as these healthcare professionals are most familiar with working in university environments secondary to their traditional employment in intercollegiate sports. The care delivered to the artists will be essentially the same as that provided to the university's student-athletes. In some cases, the staff will be graduate assistant athletic trainers who concurrently study for a graduate degree in the university's athletic training curriculum. A full-time staff athletic trainer (or other type of practitioner) or a licensed healthcare professional faculty member in athletic training, physical therapy, or a similar field often is the clinical director or supervisor; but, in all cases the providers must be licensed by their state for the type of work in which they engage in caring for the performing artists.

Advantages Dedicated facility offering specialized care; provides greatest control over the clinical environment; if set up to operate like a traditional athletic training facility, patients may be seen with no out-of-pocket fees.

Table 25.4 Advantages and disadvantages of implementation methods for performing arts medicine programs

	Performing Arts Medicine Clinic	Athletic Department's Athletic Training Facility	Student Health Center	Community-based Practitioners
Advantages	Dedicated facility offering specialized care Provides greatest control over the clinical environment If set up to operate like a traditional athletic training facility, patients may be seen with no out-of-pocket fees	Fully operational and skilled clinical environment already familiar with caring for high ability patients No new facility setup (and associated expenses) required Good access to consulting healthcare professionals who already work with the athletic department	Location usually is on-campus or nearby Cost of program probably will not fall on the performing arts departments or require new funding	Requires virtually no outlay of resources by the university Artists have virtually complete control over which healthcare providers they visit
Disadvantages	Requires the greatest initial financial outlay and a recurring budget Must find a new clinic space or reconfigure space currently utilized for a different purpose Recruiting practitioners may be challenging because of the need for healthcare providers with a background in caring for performing artists	Traditional athletic trainers may not embrace caring for performing artists Geographic location may not be close to performing arts portion of campus Busy clinic schedule may preclude timely care for artist-patients Typical athletic environment may be foreign or intimidating to performing artists	Practitioners typically are skilled in primary care, but facility may not include specialists in performing arts healthcare Performing arts faculty who need injury attention likely are not welcome as clientele at facility intended for students	May not be geographically feasible for students to access care Specialization in performing arts medicine may not be available Waiting time to obtain an appointment can be lengthy Rapport with practitioners may be challenging Likely to be the most expensive option for artist-patients

Disadvantages Requires the greatest initial financial outlay and a recurring budget; must find a new clinic space or reconfigure space currently utilized for a different purpose; recruiting practitioners may be challenging because of the need for healthcare providers with a background in caring for performing artists.

Athletic Department's Athletic Training Facility

This is a logical place where many performing arts faculty start their search for healthcare providers empathetic to artists' injuries. In some institutions, arts professors are downtrodden by the disparity between the athletic "haves" and the artistic "have nots." The intercollegiate athletic department, therefore, is a place where they hope to obtain at least a sampling of the specialized sports medicine care afforded to the athletes. Certainly, in most schools, this is a well-functioning unit that delivers excellent and efficacious care. Unfortunately, the typical athletic training staff is heavily burdened with caring for the student-athletes, so they may not be amenable to overtures that request care for the institution's performing artists. Furthermore, unless the athletic trainers are highly motivated to provide healthcare to performing artists, there may be, as previously discussed, a gap between the care that the performers expect and the care that actually is delivered in the athletic training clinic. Even when a university's athletic trainers agree in theory that assisting the performers is a worthwhile endeavor, budgetary and other practical constraints may disallow them establishing a relationship between athletics and the arts.

Advantages Fully operational and skilled clinical environment already familiar with caring for high ability patients; no new facility setup (and associated expenses) required; good access to consulting healthcare professionals who already work with the athletic department.

Disadvantages Traditional athletic trainers may not embrace caring for performing artists; geographic location may not be close to performing arts portion of campus; busy clinic schedule may preclude timely care for artist-patients; typical athletic environment may be foreign or intimidating to performing artists.

Student Health Center

In this scenario, student performers obtain healthcare for their performing arts injuries in the same facility that provides primary healthcare to the student body at large. This is a relatively convenient method of receiving care and typically is included for all students via some sort of healthcare fee that is administered by the university. This type of facility usually is not staffed with performing arts medicine specialists; however, there are universities who intentionally build their healthcare program for performing artists into the existing framework of the student health center. Apart from such intentionality to hire specialists, the nurses, nurse practitioners, physician assistants, and physicians who form the main team of providers will have little to no background in the specialized care required by artist-patients. Nonetheless, this is a readily available and affordable method of administering healthcare. Particularly if the healthcare champion described previously can be located here, the arts faculty may be able to benefit their students by forming a very viable partnership with the student health center.

Advantages Location usually is on-campus or nearby; cost of program probably will not fall on the performing arts departments or require new funding.

Disadvantages Practitioners typically are skilled in primary care, but facility may not include specialists in performing arts healthcare; performing arts faculty who need injury attention likely are not welcome as clientele at facility intended for students.

Community-Based Practitioners

In the situation where a university does not commit resources to its own performing arts medicine program using one of the three arrangements outlined above, artists turn to healthcare providers in the local community around the campus. Of course, a possible, but the least desirable, method for doing so is to let the performers fend for themselves by finding their own providers and arranging payment either through health insurance or privately. Artists tend to use word-of-mouth to find those practitioners with whom they are happy [1], so it is not unreasonable to expect them to seek care in this fashion. However, it is preferable when the performing arts faculty can vet the caregivers in order to establish their credentials, quality of care, reputation, and willingness to see performing artists. Depending on the university's locale—metropolitan, suburban, or rural—access to the necessary specialties may be limited and the distances to their offices may vary substantially.

Advantages Requires virtually no outlay of resources by the university; artists have virtually complete control over which healthcare providers they visit.

Disadvantages May not be geographically feasible for students to access care; specialization in performing arts medicine may not be available; waiting time to obtain an appointment can be lengthy; rapport with practitioners may be challenging; likely to be the most expensive option for artist-patients.

Conclusion

The delivery of healthcare to performing artists in a university environment is a complex, but important, undertaking. This chapter has offered concrete concepts and methodologies for establishing this type of healthcare enterprise. Many considerations intersect to create the overall milieu of care. These include types of practitioners, specialties of care offered, quality of care, patient-centeredness, funding, and more. Fundamentally, a performing arts medicine offering at a university requires partnership, compassion, a fervent performing arts faculty, and a healthcare champion who is qualified and properly licensed to deliver care. Successful ventures of this sort at US institutions demonstrate that the programs are rewarding to implement and integral to the health and well-being of performing artists.

References

1. Wang TJ, Russell JA. A tenuous pas de deux: examining university dancers' access to and satisfaction with healthcare delivery. Med Probl Perform Art. 2018;33:111–7. https://doi.org/10.21091/mppa.2018.2018.
2. Weigert BJ. Does prior training affect risk of injury in university dance programs? Med Probl Perform Art. 2005;20:115–8.
3. van Merkensteijn GG, Quin E. Assessment of compensated turnout characteristics and their relationship to injuries in university level modern dancers. J Dance Med Sci. 2015;19:57–62. https://doi.org/10.12678/1089-313X.19.2.57.
4. Cahalan R, Kearney P, Ni Bhriain O, Redding E, Quin E, McLaughlin LC, et al. Dance exposure, wellbeing and injury in collegiate Irish and contemporary dancers: a prospective study. Phys Ther Sport. 2018;34:77–83. https://doi.org/10.1016/j.ptsp.2018.09.006.
5. DiPasquale S, Becker N, Green S, Sauers K. Self-reported injury and management in a liberal arts college dance department. Med Probl Perform Art. 2015;30:224–30. https://doi.org/10.21091/mppa.2015.4041.
6. Stubbe JH, Richardson A, van Rijn RM. Prospective cohort study on injuries and health problems among circus arts students. BMJ Open Sport Exerc Med. 2018;4:e000327. https://doi.org/10.1136/bmjsem-2017-000327.
7. White HM, Hoch JM, Hoch MC. Health-related quality of life in university dance students. Med Probl Perform Art. 2018;33:14–9. https://doi.org/10.21091/mppa.2018.1004.
8. Wanke EM, Kunath EK, Koch F, Davenport J, Weisser B, Groneberg DA, et al. Survey of health problems in musical theater students: a pilot study. Med Probl Perform Art. 2012;27:205–11.
9. Stanek JL, Komes KD, Murdock FA. A cross-sectional study of pain among u.s. college music students and faculty. Med Probl Perform Art. 2017;32:20–6. https://doi.org/10.21091/mppa.2017.1005.
10. Wristen BW, Fountain SE. Relationships between depression, anxiety, and pain in a group of university music students. Med Probl Perform Art. 2013;28:152–8.
11. Ramkumar PN, Farber J, Arnouk J, Varner KE, Mcculloch PC. Injuries in a professional ballet dance company: a 10-year retrospective study. J Dance Med Sci. 2016;20:30–7. https://doi.org/10.12678/1089-313X.20.1.30.
12. Allen N, Nevill AM, Brooks JHM, Koutedakis Y, Wyon MA. The effect of a comprehensive injury audit program on injury incidence in ballet: a 3-year prospective study. Clin J Sport Med. 2013;23:373–8. https://doi.org/10.1097/JSM.0b013e3182887f32.
13. Ackermann B, Driscoll T, Kenny DT. Musculoskeletal pain and injury in professional orchestral musicians in Australia. Med Probl Perform Art. 2012;27:181–7.
14. Liederbach M, Dilgen FE, Rose DJ. Incidence of anterior cruciate ligament injuries among elite ballet and modern dancers: a 5-year prospective study. Am J Sports Med. 2008;36:1779–88. https://doi.org/10.1177/0363546508323644.
15. National Association of Schools of Dance. National Association of schools of dance handbook 2018-19. Reston: National Association of Schools of Dance; 2018.
16. National Association of Schools of Music. National association of schools of music handbook 2018–19. Reston: National Association of Schools of Music; 2019.
17. National Association of Schools of Theatre. National association of schools of theatre handbook 2018–19. Reston: National Association of Schools of Theatre; 2019.
18. Thomas H, Tarr J. Dancers' perceptions of pain and injury: positive and negative effects. J Dance Med Sci. 2009;13:51–9.

19. Lai RYJ, Krasnow D, Thomas M. Communication between medical practitioners and dancers. J Dance Med Sci. 2008;12:47–53.
20. Air M. Health care seeking behavior and perceptions of the medical profession among pre- and post-retirement age Dutch dancers. J Dance Med Sci. 2009;13:42–50.
21. Institute of Medicine (US) Committee on Quality of Health Care in America. Crossing the quality chasm: a new health system for the 21st century. Washington (DC): National Academies Press (US); 2001.
22. Gerteis M, Edgman-Levitan S, Daley J, Delbanco TL, editors. Through the patient's eyes: understanding and promoting patient-centered care. San Francisco: Jossey-Bass Publishers; 1993.
23. Office for Civil Rights. Your Rights Under HIPAA. HHSGov 2008. https://www.hhs.gov/hipaa/for-individuals/guidance-materials-for-consumers/index.html. Accessed 27 Jan 2019.
24. Office of the National Coordinator for Health IT. Video 1–Your Health Information, Your Rights 2016. https://www.youtube.com/watch?v=3WsRzlutBQk&feature=youtu.be. Accessed 27 Jan 2019.
25. Anderson R, Hanrahan SJ. Dancing in pain: pain appraisal and coping in dancers. J Dance Med Sci. 2008;12:9–16.
26. Encarnacion MLG, Meyers MC, Ryan ND, Pease DG. Pain coping styles of ballet performers. J Sport Behav. 2000;23:20–32.
27. Tajet-Foxell B, Rose FD. Pain and pain tolerance in professional ballet dancers. Br J Sports Med. 1995;29:31–4.
28. Lampe J, Groneberg DA, Ohlendorf D, Wanke EM. Pain in female dancers and dance teachers: perception, assessment and related behaviour. Scand J Med Sci Sports. 2019;29:623. https://doi.org/10.1111/sms.13387.
29. Lampe J, Borgetto B, Groneberg DA, Wanke EM. Prevalence, localization, perception and management of pain in dance: an overview. Scand J Pain. 2018;18:567–74. https://doi.org/10.1515/sjpain-2018-0105.
30. Akehurst S, Oliver EJ. Obsessive passion: a dependency associated with injury-related risky behaviour in dancers. J Sports Sci. 2014;32:259–67. https://doi.org/10.1080/02640414.2013.823223.
31. Hettler W. The six dimensions of wellness – National Wellness Institute 1976. https://cdn.ymaws.com/www.nationalwellness.org/resource/resmgr/pdfs/sixdimensionsfactsheet.pdf. Accessed 30 Jan 2019.
32. Tzelepis F, Sanson-Fisher RW, Zucca AC, Fradgley EA. Measuring the quality of patient-centered care: why patient-reported measures are critical to reliable assessment. Patient Prefer Adherence. 2015;9:831–5. https://doi.org/10.2147/PPA.S81975.
33. Abrams GD, Greenberg DR, Dragoo JL, Safran MR, Kamal RN. Quality measures in orthopaedic sports medicine: a systematic review. Arthroscopy. 2017;33:1896–910. https://doi.org/10.1016/j.arthro.2017.04.014.
34. Meyers MC, Bourgeois AE, Stewart S, LeUnes A. Predicting pain response in athletes: development and assessment of the sports inventory for pain. J Sport Exerc Psychol. 1992;14:249–61.
35. Rossol M, Hinkamp D. Hazards in the theater. Occup Med. 2001;16:595–608.
36. Hinkamp DL, McCann M, Babin A. Occupational health and the arts. J Occup Environ Med. 2017;59:835–42. https://doi.org/10.1097/JOM.0000000000001027.
37. Rossol M. The health and safety guide for film, TV, and theater. New York: Allworth Press; 2011.
38. Morton J. Musical theatre: the hazards of the performer's workplace. Med Probl Perform Art. 2015;30:1–7.
39. Hamilton GM, Meeuwisse WH, Emery CA, Shrier I. Examining the effect of the injury definition on risk factor analysis in circus artists. Scand J Med Sci Sports. 2012;22:330–4. https://doi.org/10.1111/j.1600-0838.2010.01245.x.
40. Munro D. Injury patterns and rates amongst students at the National Institute of Circus Arts: an observational study. Med Probl Perform Art. 2014;29:235–40.

41. Shrier I, Halle M. Psychological predictors of injuries in circus artists: an exploratory study. Br J Sports Med. 2011;45:433–6. https://doi.org/10.1136/bjsm.2009.067751.
42. Shrier I, Meeuwisse WH, Matheson GO, Wingfield K, Steele RJ, Prince F, et al. Injury patterns and injury rates in the circus arts: an analysis of 5 years of data from Cirque du Soleil. Am J Sports Med. 2009;37:1143–9. https://doi.org/10.1177/0363546508331138.
43. Wanke EM, McCormack M, Koch F, Wanke A, Groneberg DA. Acute injuries in student circus artists with regard to gender specific differences. Asian J Sports Med. 2012;3:153–60.
44. Wolfenden HE, Angioi M. Musculoskeletal injury profile of circus artists: a systematic review of the literature. Med Probl Perform Art. 2017;32:51–9. https://doi.org/10.21091/mppa.2017.1008.
45. Long AS, Ambegaonkar JP, Fahringer PM. Injury reporting rates and injury concealment patterns differ between high-school cirque performers and basketball players. Med Probl Perform Art. 2011;26:200–5.
46. Holloway D. Espresso shots: attack of the "Spider-Man" back stage. 2010;51:7.
47. Robb D. OSHA fines 'MacGyver' producers for accident that left stuntman badly injured | deadline. Deadline 2019. https://deadline.com/2019/02/macgyver-stuntman-accident-osha-fines-producers-1202560583/. Accessed 20 Feb 2019.
48. Ramos D-R, Patten D. Disney, paramount & more hit with concussion suit from Stuntman Estate. Deadline 2019. https://deadline.com/2019/02/disney-paramount-columbia-darryl-hammond-lawsuit-the-longest-yard-invincible-1202560729/. Accessed 20 Feb 2019.
49. Watanabe-Suzuki K, Suzuki O, Nozawa H, Ishii A. An autopsy case of a stunt man who jumped into seawater riding a motorcycle: a case report. Med Sci Law. 2002;42:355–7. https://doi.org/10.1177/002580240204200413.
50. Horwitz J, Furman G, Nussbaum M, Shenker IR. Letter: dangers of stunt riding. N Engl J Med. 1974;291:1194–5.
51. Britt SL, Ammerman DA, Barrett SF, Jones S. Student loans, financial stress, and college student retention. J Stud Financ Aid. 2017;47:25–37.
52. Heckman S, Lim H, Montalto C. Factors related to financial stress among college students. J Financ Ther. 2014;5:19–39. https://doi.org/10.4148/1944-9771.1063.
53. Radell SA, Adame DD, Cole SP. Effect of teaching with mirrors on body image and locus of control in women college ballet dancers. Percept Mot Skills. 2002;95:1239–47. https://doi.org/10.2466/pms.2002.95.3f.1239.
54. Radell SA, Adame DD, Cole SP, Blumenkehl NJ. The impact of mirrors on body image and performance in high and low performing female ballet students. J Dance Med Sci. 2011;15:108–15.
55. Radell SA, Adame DD, Cole SP. Effect of teaching with mirrors on ballet dance performance. Percept Mot Skills. 2003;97:960–4. https://doi.org/10.2466/pms.2003.97.3.960.
56. Spahn C. Treatment and prevention of music performance anxiety. Prog Brain Res. 2015;217:129–40. https://doi.org/10.1016/bs.pbr.2014.11.024.
57. Brugués AO. Music performance anxiety--part 1. A review of its epidemiology. Med Probl Perform Art. 2011;26:102–5.
58. Matei R, Ginsborg J. Music performance anxiety in classical musicians – what we know about what works. B J Psych Int. 2017;14:33–5.
59. Walker IJ, Nordin-Bates SM. Performance anxiety experiences of professional ballet dancers: the importance of control. J Dance Med Sci. 2010;14:133–45.
60. Air ME, Grierson MJ, Davenport KL, Krabak BJ. Dissecting the doctor-dancer relationship: health care decision making among american collegiate dancers. PM&R. 2014;6:241–9. https://doi.org/10.1016/j.pmrj.2013.09.001.
61. National Center for Complementary and Integrative Health. National Center for Complementary and Integrative Health | NCCIH n.d. https://nccih.nih.gov/. Accessed 31 Jan 2019.
62. Substance Abuse and Mental Health Services Administration. National survey on drug use and health, 2017 annual report 2017. https://www.samhsa.gov/data/data-we-collect/nsduh-national-survey-drug-use-and-health. Accessed 21 Feb 2019.

63. Collegestate.com. College State: search for colleges based on dance activities. n.d. http://www.collegestate.com/activities/dance. Accessed 7 Feb 2019.
64. National Association of Schools of Dance. Home: national association of schools of dance. n.d. https://nasd.arts-accredit.org/. Accessed 7 Feb 2019.
65. Collegestate.com. College State: search for colleges based on music ensembles activities. n.d. http://www.collegestate.com/activities/music_ensembles. Accessed 7 Feb 2019.
66. Collegestate.com. College State: search for colleges based on concert band activities. n.d. http://www.collegestate.com/activities/concert_band. Accessed 18 Feb 2019.
67. Collegestate.com. College State: search for colleges based on marching band activities. n.d. http://www.collegestate.com/activities/marching_band. Accessed 7 February 2019.
68. National Association of Schools of Music. Home: national association of schools of music. n.d. https://nasm.arts-accredit.org/. Accessed 7 Feb 2019.
69. Collegestate.com. College State: search for colleges based on drama activities. n.d. http://www.collegestate.com/activities/drama. Accessed 7 Feb 2019.
70. National Association of Schools of Theatre. Home: national association of schools of theatre. n.d. https://nast.arts-accredit.org/. Accessed 7 Feb 2019.
71. Toomey AH, Markusson N, Adams E, Brockett B. United Nations Global Sustainable Development Report, Chapter 7 – Science Issues for the Attention of Policy Makers: Inter- and trans-disciplinary research: a critical perspective 2015. https://sustainabledevelopment.un.org/content/documents/612558-Inter-%20and%20Trans-disciplinary%20Research%20-%20A%20Critical%20Perspective.pdf. Accessed 5 Feb 2019.

Correction to: When Prevention Makes Good Music

Carina Joly

Correction to: Chapter 20 in: S.-H. Lee et al. (eds.), Perspectives in Performing Arts Medicine Practice, https://doi.org/10.1007/978-3-030-37480-8_20

The original version of this chapter was inadvertently published with an error in the figure citation, Fig. 20.3b. This has now been corrected as shown below:

In a standing position, the pelvis also plays an important role as it directly affects the upper body alignment. While standing up, through the practice of a sequence of alternating anterior and posterior pelvic tilts, participants are able to identify their pelvic postural habit. Due to long hours of activities in seated position, the iliopsoas muscle group may be shortened in certain individuals who have the tendency to stand throwing the weight toward the front (Fig. 20.3a). In these cases, iliopsoas stretches are highly recommended in order to enrich the amplitude of the pelvic movements and to bring more comfort when these individuals seek the neutral pelvic position.

The updated online version of the original chapter can be found at
https://doi.org/10.1007/978-3-030-37480-8_20

S.-H. Lee et al. (eds.), *Perspectives in Performing Arts Medicine Practice*,
https://doi.org/10.1007/978-3-030-37480-8_26

Editorial Review Board

Ruth Huntley Bahr, PhD is Associate Dean for the Office of Graduate Studies and Professor of Communication Sciences and Disorders at the University of South Florida. As a Fellow of the American Speech-Language-Hearing Association (ASHA), her areas of specialization include voice production, patient perceptions, dialectal variations, and prosody. Recent research focuses on voice treatment issues with seniors and spasmodic dysphonia. In her spare time, she does forensic consulting for the courts on speaker identification.

Candace M. Burns, PhD, ANP-APRN, FAAOHN is Professor at the University of South Florida (USF); Director of the Occupational Health /Adult-Gerontology Primary Care Nurse Practitioner Program, College of Nursing; and Deputy Director, USF Sunshine Education and Research Center. Her scholarship focuses on improving the health and safety of workers, especially nurses and veterans through the development of best practices. Her current research focuses on the health effects of occupational stress and coping strategies. She has authored over 70 peer-reviewed publications and 116 presentations at the international and national levels.

Stephanie L. Carey, PhD is a Research Professor at the University of South Florida, Department of Mechanical Engineering and Department of Medical Engineering. She is the research coordinator for USF's Center for Assistive, Rehabilitation and Robotics Technologies (CARRT). She has worked at the Tampa VA, University of Miami's Center of Excellence, The Miami Project to Cure Paralysis and for Peak Performance Technologies, now Vicon Motion Systems.

Dustin Hardwick, PT, DPT, PhD is an Assistant Professor at the Morsani College of Medicine, School of Physical Therapy and Rehabilitation Sciences at the University of South Florida. Hardwick has a Doctorate in Physical Therapy and PhD in Movement Sciences from Washington University in St. Louis. He completed his postdoctoral fellowship at the Cleveland Louis Stokes VA Medical Center. Hardwick's research interests focus on rehabilitation of the upper extremity in neurological disorders.

S.-H. Lee et al. (eds.), *Perspectives in Performing Arts Medicine Practice*,
https://doi.org/10.1007/978-3-030-37480-8

"The Editor"

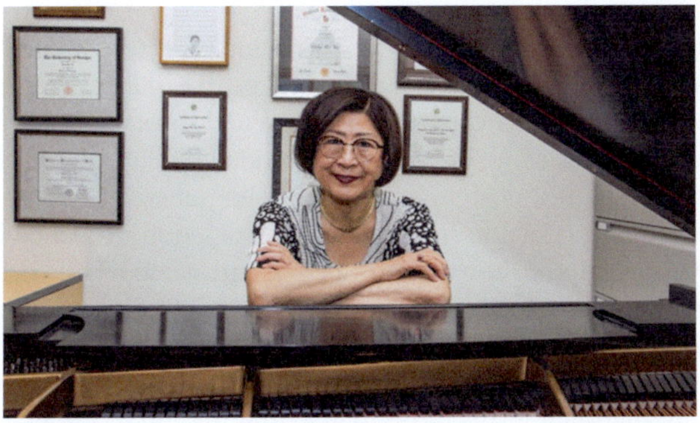

Sang-Hie Lee, PhD, EdD, MM is Professor of Music at the University of South Florida**.** She is the author of 65 scholarly publications and is featured in four Compact Discs by Ravello, Centaur, Capstone, and Alabany labels. Lee is the author of Scholarly Research for Musicians (Routledge) and the founding editor of the Cultural Expressions in Music Monographs Series (College Music Society).

S.-H. Lee et al. (eds.), *Perspectives in Performing Arts Medicine Practice*,
https://doi.org/10.1007/978-3-030-37480-8

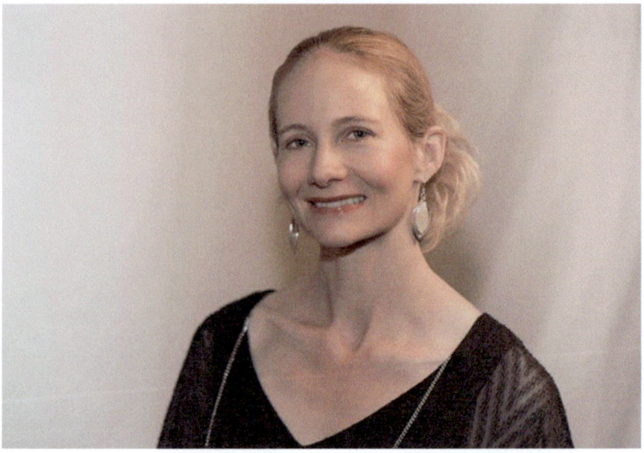

Merry Lynn Morris, MFA, PhD is Assistant Director for the University of South Florida Dance Program and has served on the dance faculty since 1998. Morris applies her movement expertise in novel and diverse ways, pursuing interdisciplinary endeavors that yield innovative products. Her interdisciplinary work includes disability studies, design, architecture, engineering, and health sciences. She is an active member of the International Association of Dance Medicine and Science (IADMS) and she has enjoyed being part of the USF-Performing Arts Medicine Collaborative since its inception, working closely with colleagues Sang-Hie Lee (founder) and Santo Nicosia on multiple initiatives.

Morris is active in the dance and disability community at local, regional, national, and international levels through teaching, research, leadership, and activism. She collaborates frequently with Arts4All Florida, a statewide arts and disability organization; works closely with REVolutions Dance, an integrated dance company and program based in Florida; and serves in Dance/USA's Dance and Disability Affinity Group.

Morris' artistic and scholarly research often explores the interface between human bodies and objects—the tension through which agency and power is negotiated in these relationships and the way identity is deconstructed/reconstructed. This interest coalesced with her work in disability, leading her to reconceptualize the design of assistive technology from a dance perspective. She has worked collaboratively across the domains of dance and engineering to invent new mobility devices for use in and outside of dance. The project has received national and international recognition and several patented chair prototypes have been developed. Morris has been featured/interviewed by MSNBC, PBS, CNN, NPR's *Science Friday*, the *Reader's Digest*, and the *Inventor's Digest* (cover story). Her invention has been featured at the *Smithsonian Institution* in Washington, DC, where she has also been a guest speaker and a profiled inventor (2018–2019). Her research scholarship appears in the *Journal of Technology and Innovation*, *Medical Problems of Performing Artists, Journal of Humanities in Rehabilitation, Research in Dance Education, Medical Science Educator,* and the *Journal of Dance Education.*

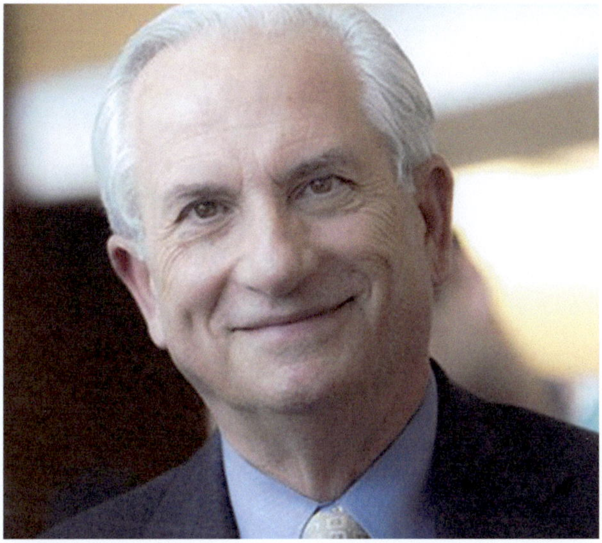

Santo V. Nicosia, MD is Distinguished University of South Florida Professor and Professor Emeritus in the Department of Pathology and Cell Biology at the University's Morsani College of Medicine. His academic career has spanned the fields of diagnostic gynecological pathology and cytopathology, ovarian cancer research, teaching, and administration, and has resulted in 176 manuscripts and 19 book chapters. Besides interests in medical history and cultural-health aspects of the Mediterranean diet, Nicosia has represented the College of Medicine in the Performing Arts Medicine Collaborative as Program Co-Chair for the past 10 years.

Index

S.-H. Lee et al. (eds.), *Perspectives in Performing Arts Medicine Practice*,
https://doi.org/10.1007/978-3-030-37480-8

MIX
Papier aus verantwortungsvollen Quellen
Paper from responsible sources
FSC® C105338

If you have any concerns about our products,
you can contact us on
ProductSafety@springernature.com

In case Publisher is established outside the EU,
the EU authorized representative is:
Springer Nature Customer Service Center GmbH
Europaplatz 3, 69115 Heidelberg, Germany

Printed by Libri Plureos GmbH
in Hamburg, Germany